Ziegler, Ernst

Pathological Anatomy and Pathogenesis

Inktank publishing

Ziegler, Ernst

Pathological Anatomy and Pathogenesis

Inktank publishing, 2018

www.inktank-publishing.com

ISBN/EAN: 9783747711552

A TEXT-BOOK

OF

PATHOLOGICAL ANATOMY

AND

PATHOGENESIS

BY

ERNST ZIEGLER
PROFESSOR OF PATHOLOGICAL ANATOMY IN THE
UNIVERSITY OF TÜBINGEN

TRANSLATED AND EDITED FOR ENGLISH STUDENTS

BY

DONALD MACALISTER M.A. M.D.
MEMBER OF THE ROYAL COLLEGE OF PHYSICIANS; FELLOW AND MEDICAL LECTURER
OF ST JOHN'S COLLEGE, AND PHYSICIAN TO ADDENBROOKE'S
HOSPITAL, CAMBRIDGE.

PART I—GENERAL PATHOLOGICAL ANATOMY

SECOND EDITION

London:
MACMILLAN AND CO.
1885

MAGISTRO SUO

CAROLO LUDWIG

EX PIETATE

DONALD MAC ALISTER

PREFACE

I HAVE first of all, at Professor Ziegler's request, to say something with regard to the German original of the text-book now offered to English students. His first design was to bring out a new and revised edition of Foerster's well-known manual of Pathological Anatomy. But as the revision went on, it became clear that the present state of our knowledge of Pathology could not be fitly represented without recasting and almost rewriting the whole work. It was therefore thought better that he should undertake an entirely new text-book, in which the subject should throughout be treated from a modern point of view. The great success of the first edition in Germany would seem to show that such a book was needed, and that the author's manner of treating the subject was approved by teachers of Pathology.

Professor Ziegler explains that a great part of his text is based upon observations made or verified by himself. Where he has drawn upon other sources he has carefully cited the needful authorities. "I am not blind to the fact," he adds, "that my statements and criticisms may bear too strongly the mark of my own personal views, and that these views may not be readily accepted by all pathologists. But I have nevertheless held it wiser not to introduce much matter of controversy into the text of a treatise intended mainly for students. Experience leads me to believe that the learner gains a readier and surer grasp of his subject when it is first presented to him as a uniform and coherent system of doctrine, even though the teacher's statement of it should border on the dogmatic. Once this grasp is gained it is easy for the more advanced student to master and to appreciate other theories and doctrines. I have given in smaller print full references to the literature of each subject discussed, and I have added such indications of its bearing as may prove useful to those who are engaged in pathological research."

The present English version was begun a year ago, on the basis of the first German edition. At that time there seemed to be no near prospect of a second German edition. In the first I found a considerable number of details which needed amendment or amplification in order to fit the book for the use of English students. The author very generously admitted my criticisms, and gave me full leave to make such changes as I might think useful. The work was well advanced, when a new edition of the first part was called for in Germany, and presently appeared. It embodied most of the improvements we had agreed upon, together with valuable additions. These I have now made full use of, so that this volume corresponds throughout to the second German edition. The matter in small print has had my special care, and I have verified a very large number of the references. The original contains few allusions to English or French memoirs; I have therefore made it my duty to add full notices of such as throw light on the subjects treated in the text, choosing both original contributions and papers serving as a clue to previous work. This feature, and the careful revision of the main text, will I trust help to make the text-book useful to English workers in Pathology, even though they may be familiar with German.

The first part—on General Pathological Anatomy and Pathogenesis—is now published. It is practically complete in itself, and on some subjects such as Malformations, Inflammation, Aetiology of tumours, and Bacteria, it gives a fuller account of modern teachings and discoveries than has yet appeared in any English manual. The second part—on Special Pathological Anatomy—is in course of publication in Germany. It is hoped that the English version of this part may be ready soon after the German edition is completed.

I owe more than I can well express to the kindness of Professor Klein; he has read through the proof-sheets of this volume, and has sent me many very useful suggestions and criticisms. Without his encouragement, and that of Professor Greenfield, I should not have ventured to undertake the work. I would also gratefully acknowledge the willing help I have received from my friends Professor Cossar Ewart, Dr J. F. Payne, and Dr S. H. Vines; and from one whose loss I shall never cease to feel—Frank Maitland Balfour.

The beautiful drawing of tubercle-bacilli, somewhat inadequately represented by Fig. 80, was kindly sent me by Dr Heneage Gibbes, of King's College, London.

In the multitude of references given I can hardly hope to have escaped all error. Any corrections or queries which may reach me shall therefore have my grateful attention.

DONALD MAC ALISTER

ST JOHN'S COLLEGE, CAMBRIDGE,
December 1882.

IN this second edition of the first part I have merely sought to correct the verbal inaccuracies which have come to my notice. I must postpone any more thorough revision until after the second part is completed.

November 1885.

CONTENTS

SECTION I.

MALFORMATIONS.

SECTION II.

ANOMALIES IN THE DISTRIBUTION OF THE BLOOD AND OF THE LYMPH.

SECTION III.

RETROGRESSIVE DISTURBANCES OF NUTRITION.

PAGE

SECTION IV.

PROGRESSIVE OR FORMATIVE DISTURBANCES OF NUTRITION.

SECTION V.

INFLAMMATION AND INFLAMMATORY GROWTHS.

SECTION VI.

TUMOURS.

SECTION VII.

PARASITES.

INDEX OF FIGURES

INTRODUCTION.

Life is known to us only in the concrete. It is indissolubly bound to a material substance. This substance, the basis of all the vital processes, is fashioned out of cells and their derivatives. All living organisms are made up of cells and cell-derivatives. The **cell** by itself appears originally as a microscopic mass of pale slimy finely-granular matter, the so-called **protoplasm**. It usually contains within it a **nucleus**, that is to say a structure like a tiny vesicle, whose form may be round, oval, rod-like, or irregular, and in whose interior we can make out by proper handling (1) small definite bodies, the **nucleus corpuscles** or nucleoli, (2) a net-like framework of **nucleus substance**, and (3) a clear fluid, the **nucleus juice**. The young cell is at first naked. Only in its maturer stages does it develope on its surface an optically distinct membrane or other structure according to the special tissue of which it forms a part.

The vital activity of the cell is of a threefold kind. It is directed in part toward its self-preservation, in part toward its propagation, and in part toward the ordering of its outward relations. VIRCHOW distinguishes these severally as the nutritive, formative, and functional activities. Many of the functions of the cell (including the chemical changes which always accompany them) cannot be directly observed and are only to be made out by their effects. Others again like motion, growth, and multiplication, can be observed in proper specimens under the microscope.

Every cell whether it be isolated or joined with others is influenced by the nature of its environment. This may work either to further or to hinder some or all of the functions of the cell. To a certain extent indeed the cell may exist unaffected by this influence in virtue of its own inherent properties, but the range of this independence is very limited. Let the external conditions deviate from the normal by more than a certain small amount and disturbances of the cell-functions at once show themselves. These disturbances may amount to the complete arrest of all signs of cell-life or even to the utter destruction of the cell as such.

M. I.

An *Amoeba* observed in a suitable liquid under the microscope manifests its vital activity by altering its form. It sends out fine prolongations from its pale finely-granular body-protoplasm. It fixes one or other of these to some object in its neighbourhood. Then its main mass flows towards them and blends with them again. If there be any fine particles suspended in the liquid and these happen to come within reach of the amoeba as it moves forward, the animal flows round about them as it were, and so takes them up into its substance.

Let us now change the external conditions by raising the temperature a few degrees. The result is that the movements, hitherto perhaps slow and languid, at once become more lively—the vital activity of the cell is increased. Raise the temperature higher still—the movements gradually cease. At a certain degree of warmth the cell becomes quite stiff and still, and only when the temperature is allowed to sink to its former level do the original movements gradually re-appear.

By cooling down the liquid we bring about a like result. The cell gradually ceases to move and becomes a mere inert globule. When the temperature is again raised it regains its power of movement.

Now add to the liquid a concentrated solution of common salt—the cell becomes turbid and shrivels up, its outline becoming irregular. Or pass a constant galvanic current through the liquid—the cell takes on a spherical form, becomes inflated, loses its fine granulation, becomes a mere vesicle with clear contents, and finally bursts.

These experiments show in clear and simple fashion how in consequence of changes in the external conditions the manifestations of life in the cell also change. The change may take the form of temporary increase, or of temporary diminution and arrest, or of permanent cessation. When the cell bursts we cannot pretend to doubt that it has ceased to exist as a cell: it is in fact dead. Even the shrunken salted cell, though its structure may be less affected, must still be regarded as dead, for in no way can we succeed in again obtaining from it any manifestation of life.

Permanent cessation of all the functions of the cell is what we mean when we speak of its **death**; even though at first sight the anatomical structure of the cell is not destroyed.

But in the first experiments the case is very different. When the temperature is raised or lowered in a moderate degree, only one of the cell-functions is suspended, the function of movement. The nutritive activity persists: hence it is that on readjustment of the temperature the motor activity is re-established. This cannot be spoken of as death. A condition in which there is not cessation of all the functions but only a partial suspension, diminution, increase, or alteration of any kind in some of them we distinguish as a morbid or diseased condition. The notion of **disease** is thus at the outset a physiological notion. We infer it primarily from the appearance of some abnormality among the accustomed manifestations of life. Disease is not an entity, capable of personification, of being placed in antithesis to health. The term **health** merely denotes that the vital functions are being performed in a manner which experience has taught us to regard as normal. So by disease we merely imply a phase of life whose manifestations deviate in some way from the normal type.

Restoration of the functions to the normal type is **recovery**: cessation of all function is **death**.

The causes of the diminution and extinction of a cell's vital activity may be internal as well as external. No cell is endowed with the power of living on indefinitely. Certain cells or rather unicellular organisms, it is true, have the power of producing a long line of descendants merely by continual subdivision of their own substance, and in this way their vital activity appears to persist for an indefinite time. But life protracted after this fashion has also its limits. In the first place, it is unlikely that all the cells derived by subdivision from the mother-cell should receive at their birth exactly the same share of vital energy. Granting then that in the process of derivation an unequal transmission of the vital properties of the mother-cell to the daughter-cells is possible, we must also admit that the less-favoured descendants must sooner or later fail in their power to overcome the normal agencies antagonistic to cell-life. But even if this be denied, the life of the cell becomes at once finite so soon as we pass from the simplest unicellular organisms to higher multicellular forms. When division of labour is set up within the organism, and the production of new individuals is no longer a function shared in by all the parts of it, then it follows of necessity that some of the parts, some of the constituent cells, must be destined to perish.

How long a cell can live cannot in general be exactly determined. It depends on the properties transmitted to it from the mother-cell. We may say broadly that a cell's life is shorter in proportion as it stands higher in the scale of development, and as its properties are more specialised. Thus for example the ganglion-cells and gland-cells of one of the higher animals are always short-lived, and often fail to produce any progeny at all. On the other hand the number of cell-descendants of a vertebrate ovum, or of an amoeba, is indefinitely large.

The death of a cell depending thus on internal causes is a physiological death. The gradual extinction of function which ushers it in does not fall within the category of disease: it is a phenomenon of age in the cell, a senile change, a senile retrogression.

Unlike this senile extinction of the vital processes a true disease is not a consequence of the indwelling and inherited properties of the cell. The efficient causes of a disease are always external.

In the observations we made on the amoeba it was heat or cold, an altered surrounding medium, or the galvanic current, which brought about disease and death. All these noxious influences are derived from without. And what we have here remarked in a single instance experience shows us to be universal. Autonomous as the cell may seem, it is yet unable without external impulsion to heighten its functions above the physiological standard, or on the other hand to check or to suppress them. We can therefore give a still more exact definition of the notion of disease. By the term **disease** we are to understand **a deviation of some of the vital manifestations from the normal, the deviation being conditioned by external influences.**

But in considering disease as thus defined we must not limit our attention to the case of a single individual, or we shall find our dictum contradicted by everyday experience. If we could observe under the microscope the successive generations of a unicellular organism, and follow with certainty the life-history of each, we should come upon individuals whose functions were abnormally performed, and that although it might be impossible to detect any injurious external influence at work. We should then have to confess that the abnormal behaviour was here, as in senile retrogression, conditioned by intrinsic properties. This would in fact be true, yet it would not contradict the above proposition—that disease can only arise through changes in the external conditions. If we had had before us a complete series of the cell's ancestors, and had noted all the phases of their lives, we should have found that the morbid phenomena of the last cell, though not immediately traceable to external influences, had yet already appeared in some of the foregoing generations. And there we should have found that external conditions existed which exercised a disturbing influence on the cell's life.

The morbid condition of the last cell then had not its origin in the cell's own lifetime. It was acquired from the mother-cell along with existence itself: the cell inherited it. We must thus distinguish **inherited** from **acquired** diseases.

What we have hitherto said of morbid life and death applies primarily to the individual cell. But the organism with which the physician and the surgeon have to deal is not unicellular. The human body is built up of millions of cells, and these cells differ one from the other in their morphological as well as in their physiological properties. Among unicellular organisms each single cell must exercise all the functions of life: but in many-celled organisms the principle of the division of labour is carried to a high degree of completeness. Different cell-groups have built up organs differing utterly in form and substance; even the component cells of the same organ are not all of the same nature. Notwithstanding this, we have no reason to suppose that what is true of the single cell is not also true of the various cell-groups.

The life of the entire organism as well as of the several organs is bound to the component cells: it is the activities of the latter which we perceive and accept as the manifestation of life. As disease of the unicellular organism is but abnormal action of the single cell, so human disease is but abnormal action of a multiplicity of cells.

Naturally the question becomes now much more complex. With the multiplication of the cellular elements, with their differentiation into diverse organs, arises the possibility of local disease. Nay it is all but inconceivable that, when the complex human organism is invaded by disease, each and every cell should thereupon simultaneously err from its normal function. As a fact experience shows that every disease has its local seat or seats: in other words it is not the entire organism which is diseased, but only some of its organs, or only individual cell-groups forming parts of organs. We have thus **organic** or **general** and **local** diseases. Which cell-groups become affected in any special case depends upon two factors: on the one side upon the external causes in operation, on the other upon the physiological nature of the tissue affected. A given injury does not affect every cell in the same degree. The vital properties of the cells of multicellular organisms are highly diverse, and so also is their power of resisting diverse influences. An injury that does not affect in the slightest the functions of one cell-group or organ may produce grave disturbances in those of another: a different injury may paralyse the tissues in one region, and in another stimulate them to increased activity. This difference in behaviour can depend only upon causes inherent in the cell and arising from its specific properties. It is the evidence of a specific **predisposition** of individual tissues to specific disorders.

On the other hand the influences which can injuriously affect the organism as such are innumerable, and the manner as well as the seat of their operation exceedingly various.

If then we duly regard the great variety of the causes of disease on the one hand, and on the other the equally great diversity of structure and therefore of predisposition among the tissues, we shall not be likely to under-estimate the difficulty that in most cases meets us when we try to determine the nature and the origin of a disease in man.

Here also it is true that the ultimate cause of disease is external; but the place and time and manner of its operation are far harder to determine than in the case of unicellular organisms. Sometimes it may be quite impossible to fix the ultimate determining factor, especially when an organ is attacked only in some of its elements and its functions are thus but slightly or imperceptibly affected.

There is still another fact to be considered—the **propagation** of disease from one organ to another. It often happens that an injurious agency which at first produces a morbid disturbance in one organ only, in its further progress invades another. This is brought about either by direct transition from one organ to its neighbour, or by actual transport of morbific matter through the blood-vessels and lymphatics to remoter regions. For example, a poison introduced into the intestine may be able to produce local disorder there; but if it be absorbed into the blood and so be carried to the various organs, it may further have the power of exciting grave functional disturbance in the brain; a different poison may leave the brain alone and influence the kidneys, and so on.

But this propagation of disturbance may take place in another way. Defective performance of its function by one organ is not always without influence upon other organs. A morbid condition of one very often involves the like in another. Thus disease of the liver and bile-ducts may throw back the secreted bile into the blood, and this impure blood will tend to inhibit the action of the heart. Again disease of certain ganglion-cells in the spinal cord is followed inevitably by the atrophy of certain muscles. Failing action of the kidneys may bring on the general affection called uraemia. Imperfect action of the lungs may bring on serious changes in the action of the heart.

Next to external influences **heredity** plays an important part in the genesis of disease. Unfortunately its influence is not easy to estimate; and it is often difficult, often impossible, to distinguish the inherited from the acquired.

The human organism takes its rise in the maternal propagation-cell, the egg; and its development dates from the instant when in the act of impregnation the egg receives a specific stimulus from the paternal spermatozoa. The impulse thereby communicated manifests itself by cell-division and multiplication. According to the laws of heredity, the properties of the paternal and maternal organisms are transmitted to the child that is to be; and it is hence probable *a priori* that morbid conditions of the parents may be likewise transmissible to the child. This as a matter of fact is the case. The transmission shows itself in two ways. In the first place there are actual diseases, such as syphilis, which are bequeathed by the parent to the child. They are such that even in the womb or shortly after birth, or later still in life, they make their appearance in like fashion with the parental disease and without the intercurrence of fresh injury from without. Such are inherited diseases in the narrower sense of the term. They originate in a diseased condition of the ovum or spermatozoon which is transmitted to their cell-progeny, or in a direct transference of some morbific agent from the tissues of the father or mother into those of the newly-generated organism. In the higher groups of animals the latter mode of transmission is the most likely one, and it has been actually demonstrated in certain special cases. They are not common.

More common than inheritance of a definite disease is inheritance of a morbid predisposition. By this is to be understood a certain debility of an organ or a tissue, not easy to define more exactly. This debility has arisen in the parents in consequence of some primary or inherited disease in them. In such cases an external cause is required to bring about the development of actual disease, and it is by no means necessary that the disease when it appears should be of exactly the parental type.

Inherited predisposition is oftenest observed in connexion with nervous disease, and just in this region is best exemplified the fact that the type of disorder need not be the same in the child as in the parent. It is probable that the external or determining causes have an influence in this modification of type.

Distinct from inherited disorders are those which the foetus acquires within the maternal organism after conception. It is true that the foetus is protected by the sheltering womb against manifold injuries to which in later life it becomes exposed. But it must not be forgotten that in this season of development, and especially in its earlier stages, its constitution is far frailer than in the mature condition. Nor must we leave out of account that its intimate relations with the maternal organism are in themselves a source of danger. Local changes in the uterus or in the foetal membranes, and disorders of the mother generally, must obviously have an influence on the development and life of the foetus. Experience proves indeed that the child *in utero* is subject to many and various diseases, and often enough perishes unborn. Certain diseases of the mother, such as small-pox, are directly transmissible to the foetus. Others inevitably involve its death.

As above said, local changes in the uterus and in the foetal membranes may also produce disturbances in the growing organism. To the investigator these do not show themselves primarily as disturbances of function: in the most favourable case he may perhaps be able to distinguish an abnormality in the movement of the heart or the action of a muscle. All that he finds on examination is the anatomical effect of the disturbance.

The foetus is an organism whose function is to grow. If any one part of the developing organism meet with an injury, or if by any means a local disorder anywhere arise, the consequence is a local disturbance of the process of growth. If in other respects the foetus developes normally and ultimately comes to be born, we shall find a corresponding abnormality in the conformation of the affected part. This may consist either in a defect, an overgrowth, an imperfect closure, or a misformation.

When the form or structure of a member deviates in this way from the normal, we describe it as a **congenital malformation.** It is the effect of a morbid process in the period of intra-uterine development, and may concern the whole or a part of the organism or of any one of its organs. Inasmuch as it is the effect of intra-uterine disturbance it is to be distinguished from acquired defect, mutilation, malformation, or overgrowth. The latter conditions arise in virtue of injuries sustained by the organism after it has become independent of the mother.

The question now arises, What are the special questions which fall to the lot of Pathological Anatomy in the investigation of morbid processes? Disease is nothing but a phase of life, in which one or more of the physiological processes is running an abnormal course. Is it then possible that the problems of life in disease can hopefully be attacked by anatomical methods? The observations that can be made during life upon diseased tissues such as the skin, the epithelia, the eye, show that these methods are practicable; and the experience gained at the post-mortem table, from the microscope, or through actual experiment, confirms after death the conclusions drawn from the living subject. All these show that anatomical tissue-changes lie at the bottom of the morbid phenomena observed during life: and that these tissue-changes are for the most part still recognisable after death. In other words they supply the justification for our previous postulate—that the diseases of man have always a local seat in some definite cell-group. Thus the primary and peculiar function of Pathological Anatomy is—to investigate with all possible exactness and detail the tissue-changes which are involved in the various forms of disease.

The information gathered in this field is already plenteous and important. Formerly diseases were of necessity classified symptomatologically; their names connoted certain groups of outward symptoms. Now, thanks to pathological anatomy, we are able to arrange them according to anatomical characteristics. We find this classification justified in practice by the constant recurrence of well-marked and specifically distinct anatomical changes in diseases whose whole course and character prove them to be in fact specifically distinct.

It cannot be gainsaid that as yet Pathological Anatomy has not succeeded in supplanting the clinical or symptomatic order of ideas. It is not yet possible in all cases to connect the morbid action of this or that organ with definite anatomical changes. We still must use the terms 'epilepsy,' 'diabetes,' to distinguish certain disorders; but that only implies that we are not yet able to replace the clinical conception by an anatomical one. It by no means implies that the several diseases are not dependent upon local changes in some special tissue or cell-group.

From the fact that we are sometimes unable to discover the seat of an affection we can only infer one of two things. Either the difficulties in the way of discovery are so great that we can only in certain favourable cases, not yet met with, succeed in overcoming them: *or*, that the tissue-change we are seeking eludes our optical appliances, inasmuch as it is not a change of gross structure, but one of chemical constitution and metabolism. This latter must at any rate be true of a vast number of trifling functional disturbances, whose transitory nature and slight intensity almost exclude the idea of a recognisable physical alteration of structure.

The various morbid tissue-changes which allow us in some measure to infer from the dead body the functional disorders experienced in life are either macroscopic or microscopic. A skilled eye can gather a great deal by mere inspection: and in this way a large number of diseases can be diagnosed on the post-mortem table. Still it very often happens that naked-eye inspection is insufficient: and it would in reality be much oftener so, if in previous similar cases the microscope had not already yielded us necessary information touching the minuter changes and the processes they involve.

Morbid changes have their seat in the cells, and in their derivatives the intercellular substances. It is therefore indispensable to a right understanding of these changes to call in the help of the microscope, and with it follow out the cellular and intercellular processes.

As a fact the microscope has in countless cases thrown an utterly unexpected light upon these processes, and the enormous advance of pathological anatomy in the last quarter of a century or so has been brought about simply by the exact attention bestowed upon them. VIRCHOW it was who inaugurated this new method and established it on a firm basis. Microscopic examination of cellular and intercellular changes, in connexion with naked-eye post-mortem examination, still remains the foundation on which our knowledge of disease and its nature must be based.

The amoeba, which under changed conditions of life becomes languid and finally dies, undergoes before the last event certain visible changes. These enable the observer to follow the process of dissolution if not completely at least through all its more important stages. It is plain that a simple experiment of this kind, made on a single cell, can exhibit but a fraction of the normal and pathological processes that take place among the cells, cell-colonies, and cell-derivatives of complex organisms. The cellular processes which underlie the various diseases are extremely manifold and extremely diverse. He who tries for the first time to penetrate deeper into their nature, and to educe the significance of the changes he observes, will hardly be able to accomplish at once his designs and desires. He must first become familiar with the essential facts of the subject, which have been gathered and sifted out by the fundamental investigations of VIRCHOW and the labours of FOERSTER, VON RECKLINGHAUSEN, KLEBS, COHNHEIM, EBERTH, RINDFLEISCH and many others.

The outcome of their labours is—that pathological processes fall into four great groups. If we follow the morbid processes in the order in which they attack the individual organism from its first beginning to its end, we naturally direct our attention first to those which affect its development.

The human being originates from a single cell by a process of continued cell-division. If for any reason a cell-group is not formed which naturally should be formed, the member or organ normally developed from this group will be lacking in the mature organism. A malformation is the consequence; and it is greater or less according to the number of cells undeveloped, and more or less obvious and striking according to the degree in which the symmetry and harmony of the whole is disturbed. When a structure is thus lacking or incomplete it is described as a **Hypoplasia** or **Aplasia**.

The second kind of morbid change ends also in defect of structure: not however through interference with growth, but through the destruction or degeneration of parts already formed. This may of course occur in the embryonic stage, and result in aplasia, or it may take place at a later stage as atrophy. These destructive or degenerative processes are not always alike: they may be rapid, or they may be slow and gradual; they may sometimes be extensive and obvious, sometimes strictly local and not at once perceptible. Changes of this kind are included under the term **Retrogression** or **Regression**.

In antithesis to these stand other processes distinguished as **Progression, Overgrowth,** or **Hyperplasia.** As the names indicate, the characteristic of these changes is an abnormally active growth, a too abundant cell-production. When they occur during embryonic life we have produced the so-called *Monstra per excessum;* in other words we have structures excessive in relative size or duplicated. When they occur at a later stage, in the growing, stationary, or declining periods of life, they result in overgrowth of the organism as a whole, or of single organs or their parts, or lastly in so-called tumours. We may describe such changes as **constructive** or **formative**. Constructive and retrogressive disturbances of nutrition are not to be regarded as wholly without correlation. On the contrary, progressive processes not infrequently succeed to retrogressive ones, the object here being, if we may speak teleologically, to replace parts which have been lost. In this case the process is described as **Regeneration**.

A fourth type of morbid tissue-change is that known as **Metaplasia**. Metaplastic processes are such as lead to the transformation of one species of tissue into another. Sometimes they are retrogressive in character, sometimes rather constructive. The most important and most striking instances of this form of tissue-change are afforded by the cells. But the intercellular substances may also, and not infrequently, undergo more or less complete metamorphoses. Thus although we chiefly turn our attention to the cellular processes as after all the most essential, we must not altogether leave out of account the behaviour of the intercellular substances. It is needful to note this, for the nature and condition of these substances have certainly some influence on the life of the cells themselves.

In each of these processes, retrogressive, constructive, and metaplastic, the condition of the circulatory system is of special importance. The regular and normal fulfilment of the function of circulation is essential to the maintenance of a tissue in its normal state. Disturbances of the circulation quickly bring about disturbances of function and changes in the tissues. Disturbances of the circulation play a distinct and highly important part in the process known as Inflammation. Unless we desire to limit this term to a single stage of the entire process, we may indeed say that the characteristic phenomena of Inflammation are those connected with the circulatory mechanism.

Pathological Anatomy has not fulfilled all its task when it has investigated the **morphology** of morbid change in cells and tissues. It must go on to determine the **genesis**, and the **causation** of morbid processes.

If we would obtain a satisfactory insight into the significance of the special changes that come before us, we must make it a first principle to compare these changes with each other, and with the known facts of physiology bearing on tissue-formation and degeneration. As our present ideas of the origin of specific forms of life only became possible after we had subjected animals to comparative examination and acquired an exact knowledge of their embryology, so also must we study disease comparatively and investigate with exactness the processes of histogenesis, if we are to attain a satisfactory understanding of morbid phenomena. The appropriate objects for investigation will in the first instance consist of the morbidly altered tissues taken from the human subject: but there will remain many questions for whose complete answer we must needs have recourse to experiments upon animals. The profound importance of these we may gather from the fact—that our knowledge of such diseases as can be artificially produced in animals is far more complete and thorough, than in the cases where the artificial methods have as yet failed us.

A knowledge of the **aetiology** of the several forms of disease is of the very highest import. It is beyond dispute that a perfect understanding of the causes of disease and their mode of action is the end and goal of all research in morbid anatomy; and it is the clear duty of pathologists to devote their energies to its attainment. If we could but define a disease, not according to its symptoms or its morbid anatomy, but strictly by referring it to its causes, we should gain far more than a clear comprehension of the affection; we should have done much to settle the therapeutic treatment.

It has long been known that certain diseases arise in consequence of the settlement of certain plants and animals in the human organism. Only of late years have we learned that the domain of these parasitic disorders, as they are called, is of wide and far-reaching extent. Formerly we were acquainted with such vegetable and animal parasites only as are relatively large in size and easy to detect: in the last twenty years our improved optical instruments have made us aware of a great number of minute and hitherto unperceived species of parasitic organisms. The Schizomycetes, or *Bacteria*, especially have been recognised in recent years as the causes of certain most grave diseases. The observations now before us make it probable that the 'bacterial' affections are very widely diffused. These investigations are of deep interest, and have vastly increased our store of facts concerning the diseases in question. It must not however be forgotten that the study of parasitic fungi can only make real and well-grounded additions to our knowledge of the associated diseases, can only in any measure yield us a true theory of them, can only lead us to a full understanding of the entire morbid process, when it has succeeded in making out the manner in which the fungi act, and the causal relation existing between fungus and disease.

Fungi have been detected in a large number of diseases, but only in a few cases have we gained an insight into their mode of affecting the organism. The mere presence of a fungus in the system cannot be described as disease. Disease only begins when, owing to the presence of the fungus, changes take place in the tissues of the organism which induce disturbance of their functions. Here then a wide field lies open to research. The detection of fungi in the diseased organism is but the first step towards discovery of the cause of the disease and its mode of operation. It is a long way from this first step to the full and complete explanation of the entire process. This hiatus in our knowledge must not be too little thought of. The smallest contribution to the filling up of the gap is at least as welcome as the discovery of a new fungus, —perhaps even more welcome. The pathologist must keep his attention well fixed in this direction. Even though it may lie beyond his present powers to follow the processes in which morphological change is no longer detectible, and molecular transformation recognisable only by the chemist takes its place, there nevertheless remains a vast region still accessible to his means of research. In dealing with fungi we have to do with formed elements, with cells in fact. The changes they produce are changes in cells and their derivatives: and in so much as relates to cellular processes and changes in formed protoplasm we have matter within the scope of anatomical investigation.

The path along which aetiological research has to proceed is twofold—examination of the altered human organ on the one hand, experiment on the other. The former in this case cannot lead us to much. Experiment is by far the more promising way. If a given fungus-disease can be produced in animals, it becomes at once possible to follow its spread and operation step by step: we are limited only by our instruments and modes of examination. It is thus in our power, in comparatively short time, to acquire information which not even centuries of post-mortem investigation would suffice to educe. This method of research is confessedly of somewhat limited reach. To say nothing of the technical difficulties which meet the investigator, the number of microparasitic diseases capable of transmission from man to the lower animals is small; or they run a course so different that their identity is not easily established. For such diseases therefore we are compelled to forgo this valuable aid. If we will not decline the task altogether we must adopt another method; we must endeavour to make out experimentally the biological properties of the several fungi, as they are found in the human body. If we are successful, we have made it at least possible to form an idea of their mode of working upon the system. Of recent years both methods have led to brilliant results.

But there are sources of disease other than parasitic—such as high temperature, cold, chemically active substances, etc. These must not be overlooked. Though they are for the most part not themselves amenable to anatomical methods, their effects upon the tissues are.

Knowledge of the morphology, the genesis, the aetiology of morbid changes is thus the aim and object of pathological anatomy. Its methods are post-mortem examination, direct or microscopic, on the one hand, experiment on the other.

On comparing the domain of the pathological anatomist with that of the clinical observer, it will not escape our notice that there is a gulf betwixt them. One has to do with death, the other with life: one with what has been, the other with what is and is to be. To bridge this gulf is the task of pathological physiology: hers it is to bind into one the scattered facts which pathological anatomy has gleaned; to discover and make sure the link that connects the morbid change with the disordered function. Standing with firm foot on the ground of anatomical research, and leaning on experiment as her staff, it is her part to explain to the physician the phenomena he has observed at the bedside of his patient. She analyses the complex of clinical phenomena into its elements, and from them reconstructs the natural types and species of disease. Through her mediation anatomical research joins hands again with practical medicine.

GENERAL

PATHOLOGICAL ANATOMY.

SECTION I.

MALFORMATIONS.

CHAPTER I.

GENERAL CONSIDERATIONS.

1. By **congenital malformation** we mean an anomaly in the form and make of the body as a whole, or of individual parts of it, referable to a disturbance of normal intra-uterine development. The degree of malformation may be very different in different cases. When the deviation from the normal is slight, affecting perhaps only a single part, we speak of it as a simple **anomaly**. The term malformation is not usually employed unless the misformed part or organ seriously disturbs the balance and harmony of the bodily form as a whole, seeming in fact to be ill-matched with the rest of the organisation. When the deviations from the normal are very considerable the affected individuals are spoken of as **monsters**.

Monsters fall into two great groups—the single and the double. In **single monsters** we have malformation occurring in a single individual. One or more parts of the organism may have been arrested in growth, and are therefore incomplete or wanting: thus we have monsters by defect (*monstra per defectum*). Or the structure and disposition of the parts may deviate from the normal, and thus we get monsters by perversion (*monstra per fabricam alienam*).

Double monsters are of several kinds. Two nearly similar individuals may have one or more parts in common; or a properly formed individual may have attached to it the ill-developed body of a second as an appendage; or lastly particular members may be doubled, or simply exaggerated in size (*monstra per excessum*).

The literature of malformation is rich both in comprehensive treatises and in accounts of individual cases. The following sketch is based on the works of FOERSTER (*Die Missbildungen des Menschen* Jena 1865); GURLT (Article *Monstrum* in the *Encyclopädisches Wörterbuch der medicinischen Wissenschaften*, vol. 24 and *Virch. Arch.* vol. 74); AHLFELD (*Die Missbildungen des Menschen* Leipzig 1880); and PERLS (*Lehrbuch der allgemeinen Pathologie* Part II 1879). FOERSTER, GURLT and AHLFELD give summaries of the ancient and modern literature of the subject. The student may also consult VROLIK's article on *Teratology* in *Todd's Cyclop. of Anatomy*, and LOWNE's *Catalogue of Teratological Specimens, Roy. Coll. Surg.* London 1872.

2—2

2. The human organism is developed from the ovum. This is a cell of definite and regular structure, which is set into activity by the impulse of impregnation. The rudiments of the several parts are produced by continued segmentation of the primordial cell. The morphological form of the embryo begins very early to appear, and depends ultimately on certain regular evolutionary processes which the several rudimentary organs undergo. These processes are histologically recognisable as lateral or central proliferations of the cell-complex, and the resulting outgrowths forthwith become differentiated into specific forms. The factors determining the special direction development is to take do not, in the first instance at least, lie in the external relations of the ovum, in its environment. They are rather to be sought in the inherent and inherited properties of the segmentation-cells. But at the same time the external relations are not without influence on the subsequent course of development. If these are abnormal, the process of embryonic growth may be thereby altered, arrested, or perverted.

Theoretically speaking the origin of a malformation may be of either of two kinds. On the one hand, the primary rudiment (in other words, the ovum) may have inherited a tendency to abnormal growth; on the other, a normal embryo may in the course of development be affected by disturbing influences from without which check its progress towards the perfectly developed form. Experience indicates that both events occur.

The recurrence of hereditary malformations in a family (such as excess of fingers or toes) can only be explained by the supposition that the abnormal tendency exists from the first in the embryo, having been transmitted to it from one or other parent. On the other hand the absence of one or more limbs, deficiency of the cranium, etc., observed only in isolated cases, are to be accounted for in a satisfactory way only by assuming that external causes of injury have affected the growing foetus.

Disturbing influences acting on the otherwise normal embryo play a far more important part than heredity in the genesis of malformations. This might be inferred from the fact that the term malformation has come to connote exclusively gross and obvious anatomical relations. These gross anatomical anomalies arise generally from external causes. The pathological peculiarities transmitted congenitally from parent to child manifest themselves less in anomalies of external form than in deficient or perverted function of the tissues, or in morbid predispositions. Such anomalies are to be detected only by minute anatomical examination, or they are incapable of anatomical demonstration at all.

3. **Monstrosities by defect**, as they occur in man, are of many kinds. Many of them affect most gravely the shape and fashion of the human form: others, of trifling character and affecting none but internal organs, can only be recognised by anatomical examination. The configuration of the body is most prejudicially affected

by defective closure, whether total or partial, of the larger body-cavities (pleural, peritoneal, or cerebrospinal); or, on the other hand, by defective development of the extremities.

The causes of malformation in any given case can only be approximatively determined, or referred to this or that hypothetical injury: nevertheless we can generally indicate the direction in which the cause of the defect is to be sought.

Monstrosities by defect are commonly malformations by arrest: they owe their existence to a local hindrance to the development of a normally constituted embryo. It is but seldom, and then chiefly in cases where the entire body is affected (as in dwarfs), that we can attribute the effect to heredity; even of such cases the hereditary ones form by no means the majority.

The influences which check and hinder growth are to be sought in alteration, injury, or disease of the uterus, or in disease of the foetus itself. To the first class belong defective development or disease of the membranes and placenta (uterine or foetal), adhesion of the amnion to the foetus, abnormally small quantity of *liquor amnii*, tumours of the uterus, concussions of the uterus with separation of the membranes, haemorrhages in the membranes or in their neighbourhood, etc. As concerns the foetus itself, its development may be disturbed by inflammatory affections which it acquires by transmission from the mother (Small-pox, Scarlatina, Endocarditis), or by inherited disease such as Syphilis. In the earlier stages of development abnormal twists or flexures of the embryo may be enough to cause very serious hindrances to growth.

The influences we have cited may act in various ways. Many arrest growth mechanically by simple pressure: others hinder the circulation so that the foetus or some of its parts receive too scanty a supply of blood, and thus the growth is retarded. Other affections, such as the inflammations, actually destroy parts already formed and so render their further growth impossible. Not infrequently several factors may act at the same time, or the malformation of one organ, like the heart, may involve detriment to the proper development of the others.

The point of time at which the disturbing influence makes itself felt may of course vary greatly, and so by consequence will vary the intensity of its effect. The earlier the injury the greater is usually its effect. The loss of a few cells in the earlier stages of growth may involve the absence of an entire organ or limb; while later on, after the general form is nearly complete, the same loss might not be noticeable at all. Malformations, in the narrower sense of the term, originate for the most part in the first three months of foetal life. By the end of that time the general form of the body and its members is well defined. Later disturbances give rise rather to changes that manifest themselves after birth as congenital disorders: they are therefore more fitly regarded as the anatomical basis of foetal diseases, than as true malformations.

GEOFFROY ST HILAIRE (*Histoire générale et particulière des anomalies de l'organisation chez l'homme et les animaux* Paris 1832—7) rejects altogether the doctrine of the primary perversion of the embryo (HALLER and WINSLOW) and refers the malformations by arrest entirely to mechanical influences. PANUM (*Untersuchungen über die Entstehung der Missbildungen* Berlin 1860) on the whole agrees with him, although he grants the possibility of a primary perversion. He produced malformations in embryo chicks by varying the temperature of the incubator, and by varnishing the egg-shells. DARESTE (*Recherches sur la production artificielle des monstruosités* Paris 1877) made like experiments, and produced malformations by arrest by placing the eggs vertically, varnishing the shells, raising the temperature above 45°C, and by warming the eggs in an irregular manner. He has lately (*Comp. Rend.* 1882) shown that abnormalities may be produced by prolonging the interval between the laying and the incubation of the egg.

On the significance of adhesions of the amnion to the foetus see JENSEN, *Virch. Arch.* vol. 42; FUERST, *Arch. für Gynäkologie* 1871; PERLS, *Allg. Pathol.*; DARESTE, *Comptes Rend.* 1882. If a malformation is to be produced, the original injury must of course not be too grave, otherwise the embryo would die outright. Above all things it is necessary that the apparatus of circulation should be maintained in working order. If the embryo dies, it is either expelled with its membranes from the uterus; or it is absorbed, in which case the membranes undergo further changes before they are finally expelled. A malformed foetus then can never sink below a certain minimum of development without perishing prematurely; unless indeed it manages to prolong its existence by attaching itself as a kind of parasite to a second simultaneously developing foetus. Compare Art. 13.

4. The malformations of single individuals, which we with FOERSTER have distinguished as *monstra per fabricam alienam* or **monstrosities by perversion**, consist exclusively of abnormalities in the viscera of the thorax and abdomen. To this class belongs the *Situs transversus* or right-and-left reversal of the position of the thoracic or abdominal viscera, or both. In this case we usually find, in addition to the change of position, other changes in the forms and relations of the misplaced organs. Here also we include the various malformations (mostly by defect) of the heart and great vessels. Lastly, we must mention the numerous malformations of the genital apparatus, especially those distinguished as true and false hermaphroditism.

The genesis of these malformations is in general to be referred to the factors cited in Art. 3. They are for the most part to be reckoned among the malformations by arrest.

For further details on this subject see the chapters relating to the several organs in the Special Pathological Anatomy.

5. **Double monstrosities**, *monstra duplicia*, have the entire body, or a part of it, duplicated. The duplicated parts are sometimes equally well developed, sometimes unequally. In the latter case one part is stunted, and appears as a parasitic appendage to a well-formed individual. We thus distinguish between **equal** and **unequal** double monstrosities.

Older theories had it that double monsters arose through the adhesion of two originally distinct ova (MECKEL, GURLT, G. ST HILAIRE). It was even assumed that the membranes of two separate ova might disappear at the point of contact, and then that the two foetuses might become fused together, so to speak. This view is no longer upheld.

All double monsters originate from a single ovum and are fashioned on a single blastodermic vesicle.

According to KOELLIKER, the first rudiment of the embryo appears as a round opaque white spot on the wall of the blastodermic vesicle. This is the embryonic area (*area embryonalis*), formerly misnamed the germinal area. The embryonic area originates in a thickening of the epiblast (ektoderm), produced by a multiplication of the cells of this outer layer of the bilaminar blastodermic vesicle. The embryonic area next becomes pear-shaped. At the same time there appears at its posterior extremity a rounded thickening, which is continued into a somewhat conical prolongation. This thickening is the earliest rudiment of the primitive streak, in other words it is the region of the epiblast or ektoderm from which the mesoblastic layer is to begin to grow. From the primitive streak the mesoblastic layer spreads between the epiblast and hypoblast till it extends over the whole of the embryonic area, and at length passes its boundaries. It thus forms a marginal zone, called the vascular area (*area vasculosa*), around the embryonic area. When the primitive streak has existed for some time, there appears in front of it the medullary groove. Thereupon the embryonic area becomes differentiated into a vertebral zone adjoining the medullary groove, and an outer lateral or parietal zone. The various parts and members of the embryo are produced by the progressive development of both zones.

The genesis of a double monster may be accounted for in various ways. In the first place it is conceivable that two embryonic areas may arise on the surface of a single blastodermic vesicle. These as they grow may come into contact, and fuse with each other to a greater or less extent. Another possibility is—that in the same embryonic area two primitive streaks may appear and subsequently two medullary grooves: these may remain distinct, or may in part become blended. Thirdly, we may suppose the primitive streak to be single, while the medullary groove is developed in duplicate either throughout or in some part of it. Finally, it may happen that in certain cases the duplication occurs at a still later stage, affecting either single parts of the vertebral or parietal zones, or the rudiments of the several organs as they develope from these zones.

Each of these hypotheses assumes—that at some time or other a duplication occurs in parts which normally are developed as single. In the first, the date at which duplication appears is that at which the embryonic area is first formed. In the others, the duplication takes place within the embryonic area itself. In the first three cases, the duplication occurs in structures which are axial: in the fourth, it may be limited to parts which are lateral.

We are compelled to accept the hypothesis that a duplication of some part or parts of the blastodermic vesicle or embryonic area can take place, if we are to account for the genesis of double monsters. The only question is—how far it is possible for a duplication which has already taken place to disappear again, owing to subsequent fusion. For example, it may be asked—whether from two originally distinct embryonic areas nothing but separate homologous twins can ever develope; or whether the twin rudiments can unite again at some later stage. This question cannot as yet be definitely answered, so far at least as concerns embryos of the age at which the blastodermic layers have become completely differentiated. On the other hand, it may readily be believed that two embryonic areas which are actually in process of formation may encroach on each other and so unite. Here we have to do not with a fusion of two formed and separate structures, but merely with a grouping or arrangement of cells (due to identical processes) taking place round two centres close to each other, instead of round a single one. It is perhaps best, in dealing with the genesis of the double malformations, to avoid assuming the occurrence of secondary fusion or reunion of primarily distinct rudiments; and to refer them all to incomplete cleavage or duplication. The ultimate causes of such cleavage are unknown to us: it is likely that they are partly internal and partly external.

The views of different authors on this subject (the genesis of double monstrosities) are very various. Some, like FOERSTER, VIRCHOW, OELLACHER, AHLFELD, and GERLACH, pronounce for the theory of cleavage. Others, such as SCHULTZE, PANUM, and MARCHAND, think that rudiments already more or less completely distinct may reunite. According to RAUBER, two or more primitive streaks may be formed on a single embryonic area; and these may meet at some point in their length and there fuse together. This is the 'Radial' theory. MARCHAND maintains that two rudimentary embryos are formed, and then unite. The duplication of the embryo is, he thinks, referable to causes anterior to the segmentation, inherent therefore in the ovum before impregnation, or involved in the process of impregnation itself. In support of this hypothesis he adduces some recent observations on invertebrates, which make it probable that the admission of two spermatozoa to the ovum may lead to the formation of two centres of segmentation. In other cases it is said that two blastodermic vesicles may be formed, and give rise to a double monstrosity. L. GERLACH lately attempted to produce double monsters experimentally. He varnished over a number of hen's eggs before incubation, leaving nothing uncovered but a Y-shaped space over the region of the primitive streak. Out of a number of trials he obtained on one occasion a *duplicitas anterior* (Art. 14), in addition to various other malformations. He infers that in chicks at least it is possible to produce double monstrosities by artificial means.

See FOERSTER, *Die Missbildungen des Menschen* Jena 1865; PANUM, *Untersuchungen über Entstehung der Missbildungen* Berlin 1860 and *Virch. Arch.* vol. 72; DÖNITZ, *Reichert's Archiv für Anat. u. Physiol.* 1866; DITTMER, *Reichert's Archiv* 1875; AHLFELD, *Archiv für Gynäkol.* vol. 9 and *Die Missbildungen des Menschen* Leipzig 1880; RAUBER, *Virch. Arch.* vol. 71; MARCHAND, *Realencyclopädie der gesammten Heilkunde*, Art. *Missbildungen*; L. GERLACH, *Sitzungsberichte d. phys. med. Soc. zu Erlangen* 1880; CLELAND, *Journ. of Anat.* 1874.

CHAPTER II.

MALFORMATIONS BY ARREST IN SINGLE INDIVIDUALS.

a. Arrested development of the embryo as a whole.

6. If the development of the embryo as a whole be interrupted, one of two results will follow. When the disturbance is grave the further development of the embryo is rendered impossible; it either ceases to live forthwith, or it dwindles away and ultimately perishes unborn. A slighter disturbance may not exclude a certain amount of development, and as a result there is born a foetus whose general form is normal, though in size it is small and puny. A dead foetus cannot remain for long unchanged; sooner or later it undergoes certain retrograde alterations. In most cases, foetus and membranes are expelled from the womb: and this constitutes abortion. In other cases, that is to say, in the earlier stages of its development, the embryo may be absorbed and so disappear, the membranes undergoing a different fate. Most commonly they are expelled at once; but at times they remain and pass through further changes. In this latter way is generally formed the so-called **fleshy mole** (*mola carnosa;* otherwise clot- or blood-mole). This is a flesh-like mass consisting of membranes and altered blood-clots. The clots form the greater part of the mass; they are the result of haemorrhages from the maternal placenta, and are not infrequently the efficient cause of the death of the foetus.

In other cases, the villi of the chorion undergo a peculiar degeneration, increase in size, and at length form a mass of club-shaped or spherical translucent cysts. These give the ovum at first sight the appearance of a bunch of grapes (whence the German name *Traubenmole,* or grape-mole). The manner in which cyst grows out of cyst, and the absence of stems uniting the pedicles, render this comparison somewhat inexact. In England this 'cystic degeneration' of the membranes is often described as a **hydatidiform mole**.

A still rarer product of completely arrested development is the so-called **lithopaedium**. The foetus dries up into a kind of mummy, while its superficial parts and the tissues enclosing it become calcified. This effect is oftenest found when the situation of the ovum is abnormal.

The second result of a general arrest of growth is **dwarfing** of the entire body (*Microsomia* or *Nanosomia*). Sometimes in dwarfs the proportion between the several parts is abnormal; for example, the head is often inordinately large.

b. *Arrested development of parts of the body.*

7. Malformations depending on imperfect closure of the cerebro-spinal cavity.

(1) **Acrania** (*Hemicephalus, Cranioschisis*) is a frequent malformation: it consists in an entire absence of the bones and integuments forming the vault of the skull. In most cases the brain is also lacking (*Anencephalia*), and the base of the skull is covered with a vascular mass of connective tissue, enclosing a variable number of cyst-like structures. More rarely there is found a pocket-like fold of dura mater, containing some brain-detritus. The forehead being imperfectly formed the eyes project strongly, and give these monsters a toadlike appearance. The parietal bones are entirely absent. The tabular portions of the occipitals, temporals, and frontals, may be wanting in whole or in part. If the supra-occipital be also wanting, while the upper cervical vertebrae remain unclosed, the monstrosity is spoken of as *Cranio-rachischisis*. In such cases the upper part of the spinal cord is also wanting or rudimentary.

The production of Acrania is referred by G. ST HILAIRE, FOERSTER, and PANUM to the collection of fluid in the cerebral vesicles prior to the fourth month of gestation (*Hydrocephalus*). DARESTE and PERLS dispute this view, on the ground that in Acrania the base of the skull is generally convex toward the brain, and cannot have been subjected to pressure tending outwards such as hydrocephalus would produce. They therefore regard the cause of Acrania to be some pressure exerted on the cranium from without. PERLS maintains that this external pressure may be exerted by the head-fold of the amnion: this may he thinks be stretched too tightly over the cranial flexure, and so arrest the proper development of the cranial vault.

Quite recently LEBEDEFF has offered a new explanation of Anencephalia and Acrania. He thinks these are due to the production of an abnormally sharp cranial flexure in the embryo. This occurs when the cephalic extremity grows at an unusual rate in the longitudinal direction, or when the head-fold of the amnion is retarded in its development. In consequence of the sharp flexure the closure of the medullary plate to form the medullary canal is prevented; or else the medullary canal already formed is obliterated. This explains very easily the subsequent absence of the brain, and of its membranous and bony coverings. The cystic structures found upon the base of the skull LEBEDEFF believes to originate from the folds of the medullary plate, which sink into the substance of the mesoblast, and are then constricted off from the main mass.

(2) **Hernia cerebri** and **Spina bifida** are terms used to describe minor deficiencies in the walls of the skull or of the vertebral column, through which the contents of their respective cavities protrude. In the case of the skull, a sacculation appears on the surface, which contains either fluid (*Meningocele*), or brain-substance (*Encephalocele*), or both (*Hydroencephalocele*). The fluid may lie either in the subarachnoid tissue, or in the dilated and sacculated ventricle; in the latter case it is enclosed on all sides by brain-substance (*Hydrocephalus externus* and *internus*).

Hernia cerebri is oftenest found in the occipital region, and at the root of the nose. The size of the sac, as also the size of the opening in the skull-wall, are very various.

The malformation known as *Spina bifida* is generally limited to the sacral and lumbar regions of the vertebral column. The herniated sac is covered by the integuments, and contains either fluid only (*Hydrorachis externa* or *Spinal meningocele*); or fluid with a thin layer of cord-substance (*Hydrorachis interna* or *Hydromyelocele*). In the latter case, the central canal is dilated by the fluid.

An interesting series of cases of Spina bifida will be found described in *Med. Times and Gaz.* 2, 1858.

(3) **Cyclopia** or **Synophthalmia** is a malformation in which the orbits form a single continuous cavity. This may be either very small, containing a mere rudiment of an eye or none at all, or larger in size and containing one eye or two lying close together. The nose is wanting, or represented by a snout-like projection just beneath the common orbit. When the brain is examined, we find instead of the cerebral hemispheres an undivided pointed vesicle running from behind forwards: the optic nerve is often either absent or single, and the olfactory nerve is likewise wanting. The other parts of the brain may also exhibit various malformations. The malformation as a whole depends on the defective development of the primary cerebral vesicle, in consequence of which the optic vesicles remain either unevolved or in close contact with each other (PERLS). DARESTE thinks the cause is arrested development of the head-fold of the amnion.

References: FOERSTER, *l.c.*; DARESTE, *l.c.*; PERLS, *Allgemeine Pathologie* II 1879; LEBEDEFF, *Virch. Arch.* vol. 86; MARCHAND, *l.c.*; ACKERMANN, *Die Schädeldifformität bei der Encephalocele congenita* Halle 1882.

8. Fissural malformations depending on imperfect union of the branchial arches.

(1) **Cleft palate** (*Cheilo-gnatho-palatoschisis*). In this deformity a fissure extends from the upper lip through the alveolar process of the superior maxilla, the superior maxilla itself, and the palate. The hard palate is cleft along its line of junction with the vomer; in the soft palate the fissure passes along the middle line; in the alveolar process it goes between the exterior incisor and the canine tooth. If the fissure is bilateral, there appears a yawning aperture above the mouth, which is wider and deeper according to the stage at which the development of the vomer, intermaxilla, and lip was arrested.

Very often the fissure affects only the upper lip (*Labium leporinum*, **hare-lip**); less often the palate alone, or the palate and superior maxilla. The slightest degree of fissure is probably represented by a slight notch or scar in the upper lip, or in another direction by a bifurcation of the uvula. Even slight fissures of this kind may however be bilateral.

These varieties of fissure depend on an imperfect union of the superior maxillary and palatal processes of the first branchial arch with the nasal process of the frontal, the intermaxilla, and the vomer. This union should normally take place in the third month. In some cases the cause of the cleft has been found to be a morbid adhesion of the amnion to the face. The malformation may be hereditary.

(2) **Schistoprosopia** and **Aprosopia**. If the development of the first branchial arch, and of the nasal process of the frontal, be still more seriously interfered with, we have instead of the middle of the face a mere gaping cavity. Cleft-palate has become cleft-face. In extreme cases, eyes and nose being also absent, there may be no face at all.

(3) **Agnathia**, or absence of the inferior maxilla, is due to arrested development of the inferior maxillary process of the first branchial arch. In consequence of this deficiency the lower half of the face seems cut away, and the ears come almost into contact with each other (*Synotia*). In special instances the superior maxillary process is also rudimentary, and the malformation is accompanied by Cyclopia, with imperfect cerebral development.

(4) In consequence of the partial persistence of a branchial cleft, we sometimes meet with fissure of the neck, the so-called **Fistula colli congenita**. This oftenest takes the form of an opening a little above and external to the sterno-clavicular joint: more rarely the opening is in the middle line, or higher up in the neck. Generally there is but one opening; sometimes however there are two symmetrically placed. The fistular canal is for the most part narrow and lined with mucous membrane; it passes

upwards and inwards and as a rule ends caecally: now and then it opens into the trachea or the pharynx.

Sometimes such fistulae have dilatations: or these may take the form of closed cysts filled with fluid (*Hydrocele colli congenita*), or of cavities containing epidermoid cells and cellular detritus (*Atheromata*). Fistulae and cysts of this kind are usually formed in the site of the third or fourth branchial cleft. Their hereditary character has been established in numerous instances.

On cervical fistula see HEUSINGER, *Virch. Arch.* vols. 29 and 33, *Deutsche Zeitschrift für Thiermed.* II (1875); REHN, *Virch. Arch.* vol. 62; NEUMANN and BAUMGARTEN, *Arch. für klin. Chirurgie* XX; VIRCHOW, *Virch. Arch.* vol. 35; SCHEDE, *Arch. für klin. Chirurgie* XIV.

9. Fissural malformations depending on imperfect closure of the pleuro-peritoneal cavity.

The ventral surface of the embryo, which is that directed towards the blastodermic vesicle, begins about the third or fourth week to close in by converging marginal growth. This at first takes place only from the anterior and posterior ends, but afterwards at the lateral borders also. At the end of this stage the only communication between the intestinal cavity and the vitelline or umbilical vesicle is by means of the omphalomeseraïc or vitelline duct. In the sixth week the duct becomes obliterated, but it happens not infrequently that the part next to the intestine persists as **Meckel's diverticulum**; this takes the form of a cylindrical or club-shaped sacculation of the ileum.

Clefts of the **abdominal wall**. The complete closure of the body-cavity occurs in the eighth week, but this is liable to several forms of interruption. The slightest degree of abnormality is that in which a peritoneal protrusion, containing a coil of intestine, persists at the site of the umbilicus. This forms a hemispherical bulging, from the apex of which the umbilical cord arises (*Hernia funis*). This malformation is common; the sac is usually small; it is less usual for the hiatus in the abdominal wall to be considerable. Cases however occur in which a fissure extends for nearly the entire length of the anterior belly-wall (*Gastroschisis* or *Fissura abdominalis*); this may even extend to the thorax (*Thoraco-gastroschisis*). In the latter case the development of the *laminae laterales* towards the umbilical vesicle must have been very early arrested. It is even possible for the funis to be absent altogether, and then the umbilical vessels pass direct to the placenta. Occasionally the fissure is altogether unclosed: in other instances a kind of hernial sac is formed by the peritoneum and the amnion stretched over it.

Now and then we find that the abdominal wall is duly closed in the neighbourhood of the umbilicus, while a fissure persists either above it or below it. If below it, the fissure is usually associated with imperfect closure of the allantois and so of the urinary bladder. The internal mucous surface of the bladder in this case appears externally, and is pressed forwards and everted by the intestines behind. The genital groove remains unclosed, and the external genitals are ill-developed. This is known as *Inversio*, *Ectopia*, or *Ecstrophia vesicae*.

Clefts of the **thoracic wall**. If the fissure is small and merely affects the sternum, it is described as *Fissura sterni*: if it is wider, so that the heart is covered only by membrane and integument, and protrudes, it is called *Ectopia cordis*.

The efficient causes of these imperfections of development are seldom demonstrable. It may be that they depend in part on morbid adhesions of the borders of the *laminae laterales* to the amnion. Very frequently they are found in individuals affected with malformations in other parts, such as the genitals or anus.

See BUHL, *Klinik der Geburtskunde von Hecker und Buhl* 1861; WEDL, *Wiener med. Jahrbuch* 1863; AHLFELD, *Arch. f. Gynäk.* V; PERLS, *Allg. Pathologie* II 1879. On intestinal diverticula see LOCKWOOD, *Brit. med. Journ.* I, 1882; ROTH, *Virch. Arch.* vol. 86.

10. Aplasia of the extremities and of the hip- and shoulder-girdles.

Defects in the development **of the limbs** are by no means rare. Different classes are distinguished according to the degree of malformation.

(1) *Amelus*. Limbs entirely wanting or replaced by wartlike stumps. Trunk generally well-formed.

(2) *Peromelus*. All the limbs stunted.

(3) *Phocomelus*. Limbs consisting merely of hands and feet, sessile upon the shoulders and pelvis.

(4) *Micromelus* (*Microbrachius*, *Micropus*). Limbs regular in form, but abnormally small.

(5) *Abrachius* and *Apus*. Absence of upper limbs, while lower are well-formed; and *vice versâ*.

(6) *Perobrachius* and *Peropus*. Arms and thighs normal; forearms and hands, legs and feet malformed.

(7) *Monobrachius* and *Monopus*. Absence of a single upper or lower limb.

(8) *Sympus*, or Siren-monster. Lower limbs coalescent, being first rotated backwards so that the external surfaces come into contact. The pelvis is usually malformed, as also the external genitals, bladder, urethra, and anus. Feet may be wholly absent or represented by single toes (*Sympus apus*): or there may be one (*S. monopus*) or both feet (*S. dipus*) at the end of the undivided extremity.

(9) *Achirus* and *Perochirus*. Absence or stunted growth of the entire hand or foot is seldom observed. More frequently we

find absence of single fingers or toes (*Perodactylus*); or coalescence of two or more (*Syndactylus* or 'webbing').

(10) Of the several bones those most commonly wanting are the radius, fibula, patella, clavicle, and scapula.

See FOERSTER, *l.c.*; GRUBER, *Ueber angeborne Defecte der Hand*, *Arch. f. Anat. u. Phys.* 1863; VOIGT, *Ueber congenitalen Radiusdefect*, *Arch. d. Heilk.* 1863; JULLIARD, *Sympodia*, *Gaz. méd. de Paris* 1869. Many cases of malformation of the limbs have been attributable to constriction and even amputation by folds or bands of the foetal membranes, or by loops of the umbilical cord. Compare ABELIN and BLIX, *Jahresber. der gesammt. Med.* 1863; BAMBEKE, *Annal. de la Société de Méd. de Gand* 1861; BAKER BROWN, *Obstet. Trans.* VIII (1867). DARESTE explains the formation of the siren-monster by supposing that the tail-fold of the amnion has pressed too tightly on the caudal end of the embryo.

c. *Malformations and Malpositions of the organs.*

11. We have seen that the form of the body as a whole is liable to manifold irregularities, resulting from disturbances in its development. The several organs may likewise, and from like causes, deviate in form and structure from the normal. Especially is this the case with the genital organs and with the heart, which very often exhibit anomalies depending on arrested development. But malformations affecting the alimentary canal, the kidneys, the lungs, or the brain, are by no means rare. These will more naturally fall to be discussed in connexion with the pathological anatomy of the respective organs.

Very frequently too we meet with **malposition** of the organs. This reaches its highest degree in the so-called *Situs transversus* (or *inversus*) *viscerum*; this is a right-and-left reversal of the viscera, the contents of the thorax and abdomen being transposed as if reflected in a mirror. It occurs in single as well as in double monsters.

But apart from the viscera, malpositions also occur in connexion with the extremities. Under this head must specially be mentioned congenital dislocations, or displacements of the articular ends of bones from their sockets: and also abnormal positions of the foot, the hands being less often misplaced.

According to the position of the foot we distinguish four types—

(1) **Pes varus** (commonly though less strictly called *Talipes varus*), or club-foot. The inner border of the foot is directed upwards, the outer downwards; the heels inwards; the astragalus projects strongly outwards; the scaphoid bone lies beneath the inner malleolus. The calf-muscles and tendo Achillis are shortened.

(2) **Pes valgus**, or flat-foot. The outer border of the foot is directed upwards, the inner downwards; the sole outwards. The peronei and extensor muscles are shortened.

(3) **Pes equinus**, or (as we might call it) tip-foot. The heel is drawn upwards; the tendo Achillis shortened.

(4) **Talipescal caneus**, or hook-foot. The toes are drawn up towards the front of the leg. The tibialis anticus, the peroneus longus and brevis, and the extensors, are shortened.

References on *Situs transversus*:—K. E. VON BAER, *Entwickelungsgeschichte* I p. 51; VALSUANI, *Annali univ. di med.* Feb. 1869; GRUBER, *Arch. f. Anat. u. Phys.* 1865; BUHL, *Mittheil. Münchner pathol. Inst.* 1878; HICKMAN, *Trans. Path. Soc.* 1869; VALLIENNE, *Étude sur les transpositions viscérales* Paris 1881.

Transposition of the abdominal viscera alone is much more uncommon than complete transposition of all the viscera.

References on Congenital Dislocation: HUETER, *Gelenkkrankheiten* 2nd edition; KÖNIG, *Lehrb. der Chirurgie* II; GRAWITZ, *Virch. Arch.* vol. 74; KRÖNLEIN, *Deutsche Chirurgie* Part 26, 1882.

The ordinary surgical text-books give details concerning the various congenital deformities of the hands and feet. On the genesis of club-foot see ADAMS's *Jacksonian Essay* London 1873.

CHAPTER III.

DOUBLE MONSTROSITIES AND MALFORMATIONS.

a. *Cleavage affecting the undifferentiated embryo.*

a. Complete cleavage of the axial structures.

12. Forms in which the development of the **segments** is **equal.**

(1) **Homologous twins**; these are produced when the development of the divided rudimental embryos goes on without check or hindrance. Homologous twins are always of the same sex. Each twin is enclosed in its own amnion, though portions of the membranes may disappear where the two are in contact. The placenta is almost always single and common.

(2) **Thoracopagi.** If the two rudimental embryos lie near or in contact with each other, a double monster may result. If portions of the trunk, that is of the thorax or abdomen, are coalescent, the monster is described as *Thoracopagus.* As the umbilicus and umbilical cord are single and common, the term *Omphalopagus* is sometimes applied to it. The various forms of this monstrosity are named from the extent to which coalescence is carried.

Xiphopagi are those in which the ensiform processes are united by a cartilaginous bridge. The peritoneum passes for some distance into the connecting structure (the well-known Siamese twins were xiphopagi).

Sternopagi are xiphopagi with a common thoracic cavity. The sternum may be double or single; the heart also double or single, in which latter case it is malformed; the alimentary canal is in part common; the liver double, though the two organs are connected by processes of gland-substance. Two of the upper limbs may be coalescent (*Thoracopagus tribrachius*), or two lower limbs and the pelves (*Th. tripus*). If the heads as well as the breasts and bellies have coalesced, we have a *Prosopo-thoracopagus, Cephalo-thoraco-*

M. I. 3

pagus, or *Syncephalus*. If a face be formed on the posterior aspect of the head as well as on the anterior, the monster is described as Janus-headed or *Janiceps*. Generally one of the faces is a mere rudiment (*Janiceps asymmetros*). The liver of the right-hand twin is usually 'perverted' in position; more rarely this is the case with the other viscera also. Thoracopagi are the commonest kind of double monsters.

(3) **Craniopagus** is a pair of twins whose heads are adherent. They are distinguished as frontal, parietal, or occipital according to the locality of the adhesion. They are rare.

(4) **Ischiopagus** is a monstrosity in which the twins are united only at the pelvis. The spinal column and pelvis is duplicated, but the latter forms but a single wide girdle of bone, in which the two sacra are at opposite sides. This double pelvis carries two or four limbs. The trunks arise distinct and bent away from each other.

In preparing this systematic survey of the double monstrosities use has been made chiefly of AHLFELD's work, *Die Missbildungen des Menschen*. Leipzig 1880, and of the chapter in PERLS's *Allgemeine Pathologie*. Both treatises give references to the literature of the subject.

The genesis of all these double forms seems most easily explained by supposing that two embryonic areas are formed on the surface of a single blastodermic vesicle, and that these as they grow come into contact and coalesce at some part or other of their periphery.

13. Forms in which the development of the **segments** is **unequal**.

These forms fall into two groups. In the first, the nutrition of one twin is somehow cut off, and it dies without alteration of its external form. In the second group, the nutriment of one twin is derived from the other. As a result the form of the first or **parasitic twin** is more or less affected. The parasite may be more or less intimately incorporated with the 'autosite' or host, as the foetus is termed which finds nutriment both for itself and its neighbour. Or again, the parasite may be connected only with the placenta of the autosite. The following varieties have been distinguished.

(1) **Foetus papyraceus**. If the umbilical vessels at their attachment to the common placenta come too close to each other, arterial anastomoses are formed between them; the blood-current in one system may become more powerful than in the other, and thus the main stream is diverted towards the more powerful. The circulation in one of the foetuses is checked, and that foetus sooner or later perishes. The secretion of its liquor amnii ceases at the same time. The dead foetus becomes more and more compressed by the growing one, and may ultimately become reduced to a thin flattened remnant. In other cases, the death of one of the foetuses is determined by haemorrhage into the villi of the chorion, or by torsion, knotting, or compression of the umbilical cord.

(2) **Acardiacus**. This is a monster devoid of a heart; it is always very imperfectly developed. The rudimentary foetus is either free, and connected with the well-developed one only through the placenta; or it is adherent to the well-developed one and blended with it to a greater or less extent (cf. *Teratoma*). In the first case the acardiac twin is in fact an allantoid or placental parasite: its umbilical vessels are connected with those of its host, and its blood is kept in circulation by the host's heart. According to CLAUDIUS, FOERSTER, AHLFELD and others, the monstrosity results from the later development of the allantois in one foetus than in the other. The retarded allantois is prevented from reaching the chorion, and is compelled to insert itself into the expansion of the other allantois. The course of the circulation in the parasite being inverted, its heart is either wanting or rudimentary. The lungs, trachea, pericardium, diaphragm, sternum, vertebral bodies, and ribs, are absent or undeveloped; as are also the liver and the upper limbs. The only organs which are fairly developed are, at most, those of the abdomen and pelvis. We frequently find in such cases an over-development of the subcutaneous connective tissue, giving rise to shapeless unorganised masses or tumours.

The different varieties of acardiac monsters are

(*a*) *Acardiacus amorphus*. This form is rare, and consists of a shapeless lump covered over with skin and containing mere rudiments of organs.

(*b*) *A. acormus*. Head developed; thorax and abdomen absent or rudimentary. Very rare.

(*c*) *A. acephalus*. Head absent; thorax rudimentary; pelvis and attached members developed. This is the commonest variety.

(*d*) *A. anceps*. Trunk well developed; head and limbs rudimentary; heart also rudimentary. Rare.

(3) **Thoracopagus parasiticus**. Should one of the foetuses of a thoracopagous monster be imperfectly developed, it will hang from the other in the form of a mere stunted appendage. The parasite is connected with the autosite by the ensiform cartilage, and the abdominal wall as far as the umbilicus: it is therefore often spoken of as *Epigastrius*. It is seldom completely developed, *i.e.* provided with all its members. In the majority of the cases on record, the parasite has been an *Acardiacus acephalus* or *acormus*, and its vascular system a mere outlying region or extension of the host's. This monstrosity is very rare.

(4) **Epignathus**. This is an amorphous acardiac monster connected with the mouth-cavity of the well-developed twin-foetus. From this cavity protrudes a shapeless skin-covered mass, made up of cartilage, connective tissue, gland-tissue, brain-substance, teeth, bones, intestinal elements, muscles, skin, and foetal down. In very rare instances the epignathus is attached to some other region, such as the orbit.

(5) **Teratoma.** Teratomata are tumour-like formations which are made up of a great variety of very different tissues, and so are distinguished from ordinary new-growths. Some of them contain rudimentary skeletal elements, such as those of the spine, pelvis, &c.; as well as rudiments of various organs, like the brain, intestine, different glands, kidneys, and muscles. Others contain tissue-formations of various kinds, such as muscular tissue, cartilage, skin, bony substance, gland-tissue, cysts, &c.; but no definitely formed masses which can be regarded as representing any special organ or member. The former tumours are undoubtedly to be viewed as remnants of parasitic foetuses which have failed altogether to develope; they are in fact *Acardiaci amorphi* in very close relation with the well-developed twin. With regard to the latter class of tumours, this view is not so certain. It is more likely that they depend in part for their origin on some disturbance or arrest of the development of a single foetus, or on an aberration *in germine* (cf. Aetiology of Tumours, Arts. 178, 179).

Regarded thus, the monstrosities *Epigastrius* and *Epignathus* become teratomata whenever the degree to which they are developed is less than a certain limit. Teratomata occur however most commonly in the form of large tumours attached to the extremity of the coccyx: they are then spoken of as sacral teratomata, or teratoid sacral tumours. If the outward shape suggests that of a foetus or a part of one, it is not hard to diagnose the case as an unequal form of double monstrosity. This is described as *Epipygus* (see Art. 14). When the tumour is of no definite shape, the diagnosis is not so obvious. In this case anatomical examination alone can settle the question, according to the principles just laid down. It is not to be forgotten however that new-born infants are liable to have tumours of the sacral region, which are not unlike teratomata, but which are really of the ordinary fibroid (or it may be the epithelial) kind.

(6) **Inclusio foetalis.** In the form of foetal parasitism just described, it usually happens that the parasite is more or less included and overgrown by some of the tissues of the autosite. This inclusion may be carried to a still greater extent. Teratoid tumours may be so completely enveloped by the body of their host, that they may be scarcely or not at all perceptible upon the exterior. This form of parasitism is spoken of *par excellence* as Inclusion. According to the region in which the teratoma is enclosed we distinguish the varieties:—

(*a*) *Inclusio abdominalis* (or *Engastrius*)

(*b*) *Inclusio subcutanea*

(*c*) *Inclusio mediastinalis*

(*d*) *Inclusio cerebralis* (or *Teratoma glandulae pinealis*)

(*e*) *Inclusio testiculi et ovarii.*

What has above been said of the teratomata applies also to these inclusions. In most cases so described, we have to do not with the enclosure of one foetus by another, but with a pathological growth within the body of a single aberrant foetus.

PERLS has brought together the literature of aeardiac monstrosities in his *Allgemeine Pathologie* Part II, p. 319. The above theory concerning their origin, put forward by CLAUDIUS (*Die Entwickelung der herzlosen Missgeburten* Kiel 1859), and accepted by FOERSTER and AHLFELD, is held by PERLS to be inadequate. He thinks with PANUM (*Virch. Arch.* vol. 72) that one twin-foetus may be seriously mutilated by constricting bands derived from the membranes, or by the funis: that anastomoses may be formed between its umbilical vessels and the placental circulation of the uninjured twin: and that thereupon the latter may, as it were, undertake the nutrition of the mutilated twin, which thus assumes the condition of a parasite. In support of this view he refers to an observation of ORTH'S (*Virch. Arch.* vol. 54), who remarks that even a decapitated foetus has in some such way continued to grow. See also HOUSTON, *Dub. Med. Journ.* 1836.

AHLFELD brings together the literature of *Epignathus* in the *Archiv für Gynäkologie* VII. Since then papers on the subject have been published by SONNENBURG (*Zeitschrift f. Chir.* V); VERNEUIL (*Jahresb. der ges. Med.* 1875); WASSERTHAL (*Epignathus*, Inaug. Diss. Dorpat 1875); and others.

With respect to teratomata the following references may be given—VIRCHOW, *Virch. Arch.* vol. 53 (Terat. of the mediastinum); ARNOLD, *Virch. Arch.* vol. 43 (Terat. of the cranial cavity); WEIGERT, *Virch. Arch.* vol. 65 (Terat. of the pineal gland); BRAUNE, *Doppelbildung und angeborne Geschwülste der Kreuzbeingegend* 1862. With special reference to sacral teratomata see DEPAUL, *Jahresb. der ges. Med.* 1869; REICHEL, *Virch. Arch.* vol. 46; LÜTKEMÜLLER, *Oestreich. med. Jahrb.* 1875; BÖHM, *Berlin. klin. Woch.* 1872; AHLFELD, *Arch. f. Gynäk.* VIII, XII.

β. Partial cleavage of the axial structures.

14. **Duplicitas anterior.** The later the cleavage of the rudimental embryo is in appearing, the less extensive are its consequences. It may thus happen that part at least of the axis of the embryo remains undivided. Cleavages of the cephalic end (*Duplicitas anterior*) are the most common; those of the caudal end are rare. The slightest degree of anterior cleavage is indicated by duplication of the pituitary body. Next in degree come the clefts of the face (*Diprosopus*), of which there are numerous varieties gradually increasing in severity from mere duplication of the mouth-cavity to the formation of two distinct and complete faces (*Diprosopus distomus, diophthalmus, triophthalmus, tetrophthalmus, triotus, tetrotus*).

Dicephalus is a monstrosity consisting in duplication of the head and upper part of the vertebral column, and is either *dibrachius, tribrachius* or *tetrabrachius.* The latter form has two hearts and two pairs of lungs, and is capable of living.

Dicephalus parasiticus is very rare. The stunted foetus has always a part of its vertebral column in common with the full-grown one.

The highest degree of anterior cleavage is called *Pygopagus.* The twins are then united solely by the sacrum and coccyx. The urinary and sexual organs may be either single or double. The equal form of this monstrosity is somewhat uncommon: the twins are capable of living. The unequal form is more common, if we may regard as pygopagi some of the monsters described above (Art. 13) as epipygi and sacral teratomata.

A pair of living pygopagous twins, born in South Carolina in 1851, has been exhibited as "the two-headed nightingale." An anatomical description will be found in the *Brit. Med. Journal* 1869, by SIMPSON, and in the *Berl. klin. Woch.* 1873, by VIRCHOW. The cavities of the pelves were completely distinct, the sacral region alone being common.

15. **Duplicitas posterior.** A monster in which the pelvis and lumbar portion of the spinal column are duplicated is described as *Dipygus*. The duplicated parts are very seldom equally developed; much more commonly one remains rudimentary (*Dipygus parasiticus*). In the slighter cases of this malformation, only individual parts of the pelvic bones or contents are duplicated. The lower extremities are duplicated, or there are but three of them (*Polymelia*). If the rudimentary pelvis is not visible externally, the supernumerary limb looks as if it sprang from a normal pelvis. It is usually very ill developed.

γ. Multiple cleavage, and overgrowth of the entire body.

16. **Homologous triplets** are produced when the rudimental embryo has undergone a complete threefold cleavage, and its subsequent development has been unchecked. They lie inside a single chorion, and the amnion may also be single; though cases occur where each foetus has its own amnion. Frequently one or two of the triplets are malformed (*Acardiacus*). In consequence of a second partial cleavage in an embryo already completely divided, there may be formed a double monster together with a single ordinary foetus—the whole being enclosed in a single chorion. This combination is not infrequent.

Tricephali, or three-headed monsters, arise from a second partial cleavage of an embryo already partially cleft: they are extremely rare. Of multiple cleavage occurring at both extremities of the embryo only a single instance is on record.

If the rudimentary embryo is of abnormal size, and undergoes no form of cleavage, the entire body becomes excessively developed. New-born infants weighing as much as ten kilogrammes (twenty-two pounds) have been met with. In other instances, the abnormally rapid or excessive growth has not begun until after birth.

b. Cleavage affecting the rudiments of particular parts: congenital hypertrophy.

17. Cleavages affecting the rudiments of separate organs, and the multiplication of these organs or their elements which ensues,

vary in significance according to their mode of origin. Some of them must be regarded as conditioned by mechanical influences. Others are demonstrably due to heredity. Others still are referable to atavism, or the tendency of a higher type to revert to the organisation of a lower.

(1) **Duplication in the limbs**. Cleavage of an entire limb, without duplication in the limb-girdle, has not been observed in the human species. Duplication of hands or feet is very rare. On the other hand, the duplication of fingers or toes (*polydactylism*) is a very common occurrence. The additional member is sometimes a mere appendage of skin; in other cases it contains bones, and has the form of a perfect digit. The number of fingers on one hand may be as high as ten. Cleavage affecting the carpal or tarsal bones is rare.

(2) **Duplication of the mammary glands** (*Polymastia*). This occurs not very infrequently, and in men as well as women. The supernumerary mamma may lie close beside the normal one; or it may be remote, having its seat on the abdomen, groin, or shoulder, at times even on the back. Double nipples are less often met with than supernumerary mammae.

See LEICHTENSTERN (*Virch. Arch.* vol. 73), and MITCHELL BRUCE (*Journ. of Anat.* 1879).

(3) **Supernumerary bones and muscles**. These are very common. Extra vertebrae may occur in any region of the spinal column. Connected with the coccyx they may give rise to a tail-like appendage, though all so-called tails are not referable to multiplication of vertebrae.

Multiplication of the ribs (by the formation of cervical or lumbar ribs), and bifurcation of the ribs, are not infrequent.

Multiplication of the teeth is no rare occurrence.

On supernumerary vertebrae and ribs see WELCKER (*Arch. f. Anat.* 1881), STRUTHERS (*Journ. of Anat.* 1875), and TURNER (*Journ. of Anat.* 1870). On so-called tails see ECKER (*Arch. f. Anthrop.* XI), and LEO GERLACH (*Morphol. Jahrb.* VI).

(4) **Duplication** (or multiplication) **of the** thoracic and abdominal **viscera**. This is commonest in the cases of the spleen, pancreas, ureter, and pelvis of the kidney. It is rare in the lungs, ovaries, liver, kidneys, testes, and bladder.

18. **Congenital hypertrophy**, or excessive growth of individual parts. Abnormal enlargement of one side only has more than once been observed. Excessive size of the head without hydrocephalus is rare, whether symmetrical or unilateral. Undue enlargement of one limb or part of a limb is more common. A hand or foot, a finger or toe, may thus grow to an excessive degree and so give rise to very serious deformity. The symptoms of excessive growth are generally apparent at birth. Sometimes the effect

depends on a general hypertrophy of all the elements of the member, sometimes on a mere over-development of adipose tissue.

Like the limbs, other organs also may reach abnormal dimensions by augmentation of their normal elements. This is the case with the thyroid gland, the tongue, the mammae, the kidneys, the bladder, the uterus, the clitoris, the labia pudendi, and the penis.

Full references to the literature of congenital hypertrophy are given in KESSLER'S *Inaugural-Dissertation über einen Fall von Macropodia lipomatosa* Halle 1869. Compare also REID (*Month. Journ. med. science* 1843); CURLING (*Med. chir. Trans.* XXVIII); TRÉLAT and MONOD (*De l'hypertrophie unilatérale, Arch. gén. de méd.* 1869); FRIEDREICH (*Congenital unilateral hypertrophy of the head, Virch. Arch.* vol. 28). Cases of congenital hypertrophy of the limbs are reported by BUSCH (*Arch. f. klin. Chir.* VII); FRIEDBERG (*Virch. Arch.* vol. 40); LITTLE (*Trans. Path. Soc.* 1866); FISCHER (*Der Riesenwuchs, Deutsche Zeitsch. f. Chir.* 1880); ANDERSON (*St. Thom. Hosp. Rep.* London 1882). A good instance of hereditary polydactylism is given by LUCAS, *Guy's Hosp. Rep.* London 1881.

SECTION II.

ANOMALIES IN THE DISTRIBUTION OF THE BLOOD AND OF THE LYMPH.

CHAPTER IV.

ANOMALIES IN THE DISTRIBUTION OF THE BLOOD WITHIN THE VESSELS. HYPERAEMIA AND ANAEMIA.

19. It is the office of the blood to convey nutriment to the organs and tissues. The cells and cellular structures, of which these are built up, cannot long continue to exist unless they are kept supplied with fresh nutriment. For this reason most tissues are furnished with blood-vessels, and those which are not so furnished are in intimate relation with others which are.

The demand for blood on the part of a tissue is not at all times equally great. Hence the supply may also undergo a corresponding increase or diminution, and with the incoming supply varies also the amount of blood actually present in the tissue. If a vascular organ happen thus to contain an unusually large amount of blood it is called **hyperaemic**; if it contains less than usual it is **anaemic.**

The regulation of the amount of blood, which an organ receives under physiological conditions, is effected by modifying the resistances offered by the arterial system. This modification of the resistances again is effected simply by means of changes in the calibre of the arteries. The quantity of blood contained in the entire body is insufficient to fill all the vessels at the same time. It is thus possible to increase the supply to any one organ only by diminishing the amount sent in other directions. The calibre of the arteries is altered by help of the elasticity of their walls and the contractility of their intrinsic non-striated muscles, and this apart from the action of changes in the blood-pressure otherwise conditioned. The intrinsic muscles of the arterial wall constitute the active regulating element. Their activity is dependent partly upon influences which directly affect them, and partly upon nervous impulses. These latter are transmitted to them from centres some of which are intravascular, and some situated in the medulla oblongata. They may act so as to contract the vessels, or to dilate them, as the case may be.

If the amount of blood in an organ deviates beyond the physiological limit from the mean or usual amount; or if there is a deviation dependent on factors other than the physiological ones; or if a deviation persists for an undue length of time, we have to do with a hyperaemia or anaemia which is pathological. Such pathological deviations are produced by agencies only in part identical with those which regulate the normal blood-supply of the organ.

In this book, which deals with pathology, we can only sketch in the broadest outline the general physiology of the circulation. For further details we refer the reader to the chapters on the subject in the classical work of COHNHEIM (*Vorlesungen über allgemeine Pathologie*, 2nd edition, Berlin 1882). Many of the physiological remarks in the text are derived from these chapters. A summary of the main facts will be found in FOSTER'S *Text-book of Physiology*.

20. **Hyperaemia** of an organ shows itself to the eye as a more or less intense reddening and turgescence. The redness will be bright or dark (livid) according as the contained blood is rich or poor in oxygen. In organs which are themselves strongly coloured, the redness may be more or less masked, and its exact tint modified.

The reddening and turgescence are produced simply by the dilatation of the blood-vessels of the part, and their repletion with blood.

Hyperaemia is not easily observed in the dead body: what is seen represents at best but partially the degree of hyperaemia which may have been present during life; and that only in some organs. At death the greater number of the vessels, and especially the arteries and capillaries, empty themselves of their contents. This is partly due to the contraction of their walls; partly to the *rigor mortis* of the tissues in which they have their course. The contraction of *rigor* presses out the blood contained in them much as the pressure of the finger makes a reddened hyperaemic spot become pale.

It may thus come to pass that a membrane, which during life was hyperaemic and red, may after death appear pale and colourless. Or the only reminder of the pre-existing hyperaemia may consist of engorged veins and venules, which, on mucous membranes at least, run in purple branching tree-like courses over the surface.

21. Hyperaemia may be either active (congestive) or passive (mechanical). The first form depends on increased flow of blood to the part, or **congestion**; the second on diminished flow from the part, producing **engorgement**.

Active hyperaemia is either **idiopathic** or **collateral**. The former is the more important, and depends on a relaxation of the muscular fibres of the arteries. This relaxation is brought about by paresis of the vasomotors; or by stimulation of the vasolidators; or it may be by direct weakening or paralysis of the muscular fibres themselves (such for example as is produced by heat, contusion, or atropia). Collateral hyperaemia is merely the consequence of diminished blood-supply to some other part. It ensues first in the immediate neighbourhood of the anaemic part: but afterwards the diverted blood may be conveyed to more remote organs, which happen to stand in need of it.

The causes of **passive hyperaemia** are of a different kind. The veins are normally devoid of tonus. The resistances offered to the venous blood-current are chiefly due to gravitation. They are chiefly overcome by means of the action of the muscles; in part also by the aspiration towards the thorax which takes place during inspiration. When the muscles are inactive and the respiration feeble, these important forces are no longer available: the blood then tends to stagnate in the veins, and collects especially in those parts which are most dependent. This condition is often misnamed hypostasis, or gravitative hyperaemia. Enfeebled action of the heart favours its appearance. Uncompensated valvular disease acts in the same way: the blood is imperfectly propelled into the arteries, and so tends more and more to accumulate in the heart itself and in the venous system.

A further very common cause of passive hyperaemia is the interposition of abnormal resistances in the course of the venous current. Of this nature are obliteration of veins by compression, ligature, coagulation of the contained blood, or thickening of the walls. The forms of engorgement depending on narrowing or obliteration of veins are very various. Often they are scarcely or not at all perceptible, inasmuch as neighbouring veins may dilate sufficiently to provide for the complete drainage of the part. This has however its limits. When, for example, in the arm the greater number of the great veins are occluded; or when in the leg the femoral vein is stopped up at Poupart's ligament; or again when the main renal vein is obliterated, it becomes impossible for the blood to find adequate exit: the current becomes slower and slower, and the blood goes on accumulating in the engorged region. When the process is directly observed in the expanded tongue of the frog, the red blood-cells are seen to become tightly packed together, and to fill completely the lumen of the dilated veins and capillaries. This appearance is due to the fact that, as a consequence of the engorgement, an increased quantity of liquid plasma transudes under pressure from the vessels.

In the systemic circulation the engorgement is confined to the veins and capillaries: the arterial blood-pressure remains unaffected by it. In the pulmonary vessels, on the other hand, where there is no very marked tonus (COHNHEIM), the engorgement is propagated through the arteries to the right heart, and there gives rise to increased blood-pressure.

Congested tissues are bright red in colour, engorged tissues on the other hand are dark purple or livid; though it must not be forgotten that if air be allowed access the livid colour may speedily change to a brighter red.

True hyperaemia must of course not be confounded with post-mortem staining of the tissues. The arteries after death squeeze out by the contraction of their walls the greater part of the blood they contain. This passes into the veins, and, being affected by gravity, most readily into the parts that are lowest. Such a pseudo-hyperaemia is called a **hypostasis**. Reddened patches on the skin due to such post-mortem movement of the blood are called **livores**. They appear three hours or more after death, and commonly upon the back and sides of the trunk and the posterior surfaces of the limbs and neck. If there be already an ante-mortem engorgement of these parts, it will appear more intensely after death.

In order to observe the process of engorgement which ensues when the circulation is disturbed, we may conveniently make use of the tongue or the foot-web of a frog which has been curarised (COHNHEIM, *Virch. Arch.* vol. 40). The object must be spread out under the microscope on a proper holder. For example, the tongue may very simply be arranged by turning it out over a cork ring glued to the stage of the instrument, and stretching it with common pins stuck into the cork. When the circulation is normal the pulsating arterial stream, as well as the continuous venous stream, are seen to be bordered by a zone of plasma. If now engorgement be induced by ligature of the efferent vein of the tongue, the stream becomes slower—the zone of plasma in the veins disappears—and both veins and capillaries become tightly crammed and dilated with the red blood-cells as they accumulate. After a time the tongue begins to swell up, as it becomes infiltrated with the transuded liquid.

The frog's tongue and foot-web are also very well adapted for studying the changes of the circulation in congestive hyperaemia, and in anaemia.

22. Pathological **anaemia** is dependent upon **oligaemia**, or upon **ischaemia**. In oligaemia there is a general deficiency of blood throughout the body: the anaemia of the several organs is due less to defective distribution by the vessels than to the inadequate quantity of blood they contain. Ischaemia on the other hand can give rise only to local anaemia: it always implies a diminution of the blood-supply to the affected part. Ischaemia may of course coexist with oligaemia.

Pathological diminution of the blood-supply to an organ is often due simply to an abnormal increase of the normal resistance offered by the arterial channels; in other words, to powerful contraction of the circular muscular fibres of the arteries. In other cases, the resistances are pathological in character: such are, for example, compression, diminution of the lumen owing to morbid changes in the vessel wall, deposits on the inner surface of the vessel, &c.

The result of diminishing the calibre of an artery is, in the first instance, to slow and to weaken the blood-current behind the constricted point. If the artery be completely occluded, the circulation behind the obstacle comes at once to a standstill. Yet the later consequences of such obstructions to the circulation are by no means always identical. Everything depends on the question whether the arteries behind the point of obstruction have anastomoses of fair size connecting them with other arteries; whether in fact a collateral circulation is possible. If it be possible, the disturbance of the circulation at first produced is quickly compensated by an increased blood-supply through the collateral arteries. The compensation will be the more rapid and complete as the collaterals are larger and more dilatable.

The case is different however when the obstructed artery has no arterial anastomoses beyond the obstruction, when it is terminal, as it is called. The diminution of the current beyond the obstruction cannot be compensated for, and the affected region becomes in the first instance nearly or wholly deprived of blood. This state of things may alter after a time, however. When the movement and pressure of the blood beyond the obstruction have sunk to a minimum, the propelling forces become at length insufficient to maintain the flow. The specifically heavier red blood-cells become stationary, and accumulate in the capillaries and veins. In this way the anaemic region becomes again filled with blood, but with blood which is stagnating, not circulating. The same thing happens when a terminal artery is completely occluded. The blood from the anastomosing capillaries is slowly urged backwards under slight pressure into the anaemic region. Finally, there may be a reflux from the veins themselves sufficient to give rise to an accumulation of blood in the vessels of the anaemic region. This reflux will occur when in the latter vessels the blood-pressure has sunk to zero, and the usual resistances to reversed flow in the veins (such as gravity, or the presence of valves) are not in action.

A further cause of anaemia in an organ may be the excessive determination of blood to other organs. The entire amount of blood available may thus be inadequate to supply the non-congested organs. This is described as **collateral anaemia**.

All anaemic tissues are pale. At the same time they are limp and non-turgescent, and any proper colour which they may possess becomes well marked.

CHAPTER V.

ANOMALIES IN THE DISTRIBUTION OF THE LYMPH. OEDEMA AND DROPSY.

23. The **lymph** which bathes the tissues is merely a transudation from the blood, mingled with the products of tissue-change. The transuded liquid is taken up by the lymphatics from the lymph-spaces of the tissues, and carried back into the venous system through the thoracic duct. Every change in the circulation, which determines an increased transudation of liquid from the blood, leads by consequence to an increased saturation of the tissues. This increased saturation is generally balanced by an increased discharge through the lymph-channels. But this compensating action has its limits. If the transudation from the blood-vessels still increases, there at last comes a time when the saturation of the tissues with liquid can no longer be kept down, and so it rises above the normal degree. The condition in which fluid collects in the substance of the tissues is called **oedema**. When the fluid collects in the greater cavities of the body we have **hydrops** or **dropsy**. The liquid transudation in oedema and dropsy has never the same composition as blood-plasma: it is always markedly poorer in albumen.

Tissues which are the seat of oedema swell up; but the degree of swelling depends in great measure upon the structure of the tissue. The skin and subcutaneous cellular tissue may in virtue of their structure undergo extreme distension: an oedematous limb may thus become enormously swollen. It looks pale, is doughy to the touch, and 'pits' on pressure with the finger. It is customary to describe oedema of the integumentary structures as **anasarca**. If an anasarcous part be cut into, the fibrous bundles of the tissue are seen to be separated from each other by clear liquid, which trickles away from the cut surfaces.

Other structures, like the kidney, are much less capable of containing large quantities of liquid than are the integuments.

When an oedematous kidney, therefore, is cut into, very little liquid flows from it; but the cut surface looks moist and glistening.

The lung can hold a very considerable quantity of liquid. Owing to its narrow accommodation in the thorax, it cannot of course become very greatly distended. But it has within it a multitude of air-cavities, and these fill with liquid when oedema invades it. From these the liquid, generally frothy with air-bubbles, may be squeezed when the lung is cut.

The amount of blood contained in oedematous tissues is variable, and so therefore are their colour and appearance.

Cavities which are the seat of a dropsical effusion contain a greater or less quantity of a clear, generally pale-yellowish, seldom quite colourless, liquid. It has an alkaline reaction, and at times curds of fibrin may be found in it (Art. 35).

Compressible organs situate in the dropsical cavity may be flattened, and the cavity itself enlarged.

If the effusion of liquid be general throughout the body we speak of it as **general dropsy**: if limited to the abdominal cavity it is called **ascites.**

24. Three varieties of oedema may be distinguished, according to their mode of origin: these are—the oedema of engorgement, inflammatory oedema, and hydraemic oedema.

The **oedema of engorgement**, as the name implies, depends upon a disturbance of the circulation. If from any cause the outflow of blood from the veins is hindered, the blood tends to accumulate in the capillaries and venules (Art. 21). If the degree of obstruction exceeds a certain limit, the plasma seeks a lateral exit and escapes from the vessels. The amount of liquid thus escaping is proportionate to the discrepancy existing between the inflow and the outflow.

The escaped liquid is always poor in albumen, poorer even than the normal lymph. It contains however a certain proportion of red blood-cells, depending on the intensity of the engorgement.

The immediate consequence of increased transudation is an increased flow through the lymphatics. Often enough this may be quite sufficient to convey away all the liquid which escapes. If it is insufficient the liquid collects in the tissues and the result is oedema or dropsy.

Obstruction to the outflow through the lymphatics does not usually bring about oedema; direct experiments have demonstrated this. In the first place, the lymphatics of most parts of the body possess ample anastomoses, so that it is not easy for a stagnation of the lymph to occur. Even when the thoracic duct is occluded collateral channels may be opened up and the circulation restored. Furthermore, when in a limb, for example, the whole of the lymphatic outlets have been closed, if no more than the normal amount of transudation from the blood-vessels goes on, no oedema is produced. The blood-vessels themselves have the power of taking up again the lymph they have produced. If the thoracic duct be completely occluded and no collaterals are opened up, then oedema is the result; it takes the form of ascites. At the same time the larger lymphatics become greatly distended with accumulated lymph.

Though lymphatic engorgement alone is inadequate to produce oedema, it may possibly increase an oedema which has already been produced by increased transudation from the blood-vessels.

25. The quantity and the nature of the liquid which escapes from the capillaries and veins depend not only on the intravascular pressure and the resistances to the flow, but also to a great extent on the character and condition of the vessel-wall. Alterations in the amount of transudation may thus be referable, not to disturbance of the circulation, but to changes in the vessel-wall, and especially in its endothelial lining. The vessel-wall may in fact by various causes be made more permeable by the corpuscular as well as by the liquid constituents of the blood. One of these is long-standing engorgement, involving incomplete renewal of the blood-supply to the vessel. More serious causes of injury are persistent ischaemia, imperfect oxygenation, chemical changes in the blood, very high or very low temperatures, and traumatic lesions. What the exact injuries are which these bring about we are not as yet able to say; but it may fairly be imagined that they amount to a loosening of the connexions between the endothelial cells of the intima (Arts. 96—98). It is in virtue of such alterations in the vessels that inflammatory and hydraemic oedema are produced.

As regards **inflammatory oedema** no doubt can exist that it originates in some vascular change. It occurs as an independent affection, in the form of a more or less local and circumscribed swelling with dropsical effusion: but it may also, as a secondary phenomenon, accompany other processes, like severe inflammation. In the latter case it is often characterised as collateral oedema. Inflammatory oedema is distinguished from the oedema of engorgement by the fact that in the former the exudation is very much richer in albumen and white blood-cells: it is also common for coagulation to take place in the dropsical tissues.

Hydraemic or **cachectic oedema** is very near akin to inflammatory oedema. It was formerly believed that hydraemia, in which the blood is impoverished of its solid constituents, and hydraemic plethora, or over-dilution of the blood with water, might directly give rise to increased transudation from the vessels. It was conceived that the vessel-wall acted like other animal membranes, through which liquids poor in albumen filter more readily than liquids rich in albumen. This is incorrect. COHNHEIM and his pupils have shown that the vessel-wall is not to be regarded as a dead membrane; it is a living organ. When hydraemia is artificially produced it is not followed by oedema. Even hydraemic plethora produced by over-filling the vessels with diluted blood, though it does lead to increased transudation, does not do so till the dilution has been carried to an extreme degree. Even then the oedema does not make its appearance at the parts which are the usual seat of hydraemic oedema in man. We must therefore look for another explanation of the oedema of cachexia and of nephritis (in which disease the function of the kidneys is disturbed). According to COHNHEIM, they owe their origin, as we have said, to a change in the vessel-wall. This change is due to the watery character of the blood, or to some deleterious substance circulating in it.

Hydraemic oedema, we say, is near akin to inflammatory oedema; but it is not identical with it. This appears from the fact already alluded to—that the liquid effused in the former is much poorer in albumen than that in the latter, and that it contains considerably fewer of the corpuscular elements.

The doctrine of oedema in its present form is essentially due to the work of COHNHEIM and his school. This is true as well of the theory of oedema from engorgement as of the theory of hydraemic and inflammatory oedema. It was he who made out the nature of the disturbances of the circulation involved in passive hyperaemia, as well as the conditions which govern the morbid alterations of the vessel-wall. (See COHNHEIM'S *Vorles. üb. allg. Pathologie* Berlin 1882, and his *Untersuchungen über die embolischen Processe* Berlin 1872.) The researches on the consequences of hydraemia and hydraemic plethora were carried out by him in collaboration with LICHTHEIM (*Virch. Arch.* vol. 69). Solutions of common salt were injected into the vascular system of dogs, but no oedema was produced by this dilution of the blood. When the blood-plasma is increased in amount, almost all the secretions (urine, saliva, bile, intestinal juice, etc.) are forthwith increased. The current of lymph in the lymphatics is also increased, but not in all parts; notably not in the limbs. In extreme hydraemic plethora the abdominal organs become oedematous, but never the limbs.

On inflammatory transudation and oedema see also LASSAR (*Virch. Arch.* vol. 69).

CHAPTER VI.

ESCAPE OF THE BLOOD FROM THE VESSELS. HAEMORRHAGE. (THROMBOSIS, EMBOLISM, INFARCTION.)

26. **Haemorrhage** or **extravasation** implies an escape of blood (with all its constituent elements) out of the vessels into a tissue, or upon a free surface. It may be arterial, venous, capillary, or from all the vessels together, in which latter case it is termed 'parenchymatous.' Such an extravasation into a tissue takes on various appearances according to the quantity of blood which has escaped; and special names are given to some of these.

When the quantity is small and forms more or less sharply defined red or brown spots, these are called **petechiae** or **ecchymoses**: when larger and less defined they are **sugillations** or **sanguineous suffusions**. If the affected tissue is completely infiltrated by the escaped blood, we speak of it as a **haemorrhagic infarct**. If the blood forms a tumour or swelling, it is called a **haematoma** or **blood-tumour.**

Haemorrhage in quantity always causes serious changes in the tissue invaded: not infrequently (as in the brain) the tissue is stretched, torn, and disintegrated.

If the bleeding take place from the free surface of an organ, the blood flows away either altogether or into the cavity which is bounded by the free surface.

Certain haemorrhages have received names from the localities in which they occur. Thus bleeding from the nasal mucous membrane constitutes **epistaxis**; vomiting of blood is **haematemesis**; bleeding from the lungs gives rise to **haemoptoë** or **haemoptysis**; from the uterus to **metrorrhagia**; from the urinary organs to **haematuria.**

A collection of blood in the uterus is called **haematometra,** in the pleural cavity **haemothorax,** in the tunica vaginalis of the testicle **haematocele,** in the pericardium **haemopericardium.**

Fresh effusions of blood have the colour characteristic of arterial or of venous blood, as the case may be.

In the course of time the extravasation undergoes certain well-marked changes. Especially remarkable are the changes of colour seen in ecchymoses and sugillations of the skin, which pass through tints of brown, blue, green, and yellow. Ultimately the extravasation is absorbed (Arts. 68 and 112—116).

27. The escape of blood from the vessels occurs in two distinct ways. A large and sudden haemorrhage always implies a solution of continuity in the vessel-wall. This has been distinguished as haemorrhage by **rupture** (*per rhexin, per diabrosin*) or, clinically, as apoplexy. Such solutions of continuity are the only causes of arterial bleeding: but from veins and capillaries bleeding may occur in another way, namely by what is called **diapedesis**. In this process the blood passes through a vessel-wall in which no rent exists. The escape is not sudden but gradual. The blood-cells slip through the vessel-wall one after the other. Liquid escapes at the same time; but it is not simply plasma, for it contains less albumen (Arts. 24, 25). These haemorrhages often remain small and circumscribed; but occasionally the process continues for a longer time, and then the infiltration of the tissue with blood-cells may go on to a serious extent. It must not be supposed that haemorrhage by apoplexy (or rupture) is always large, or haemorrhage by diapedesis always small. A rent in a capillary or a small vein will give rise to no great loss of blood; while the haemorrhage from long-continued diapedesis may reach an alarming magnitude. In a given case it is often by no means easy, often indeed quite impossible, to decide whether haemorrhage has occurred by rupture or by diapedesis.

The process of diapedesis may be observed under the microscope. For this purpose the mesentery or the foot-web of a frog is used (COHNHEIM). If the veins of outflow have first been ligatured, the capillaries and veins of the membrane are seen to be crammed with blood. After a certain time the red blood-corpuscles begin to escape from the capillaries and veins (compare COHNHEIM, *Allgemeine Pathologie* I, and *Virch. Arch.* vol. 41). The process is to be regarded as one of filtration (HERING, *Sitzungsberichte der Wiener Akademie* 57, 1868). As a result of the arrested outflow the blood seeks to escape laterally; it is in fact squeezed through the vessel-wall.

We owe to ARNOLD some very beautiful researches upon the diapedesis of red blood-corpuscles, as well as of other particulate substances introduced into the vessels (*Virch. Arch.* vols. 58, 62, 64). ARNOLD at first thought it must be admitted that at the points of escape of the particles holes or slits occur, which he called *stigmata* and *stomata*: afterwards however he recognised the supposed openings to be merely aggregations of the intercellular or cementing substance of the endothelial cells. Under pathological conditions this substance becomes loose, and readily permits the corpuscular elements of the blood to pass through. Some beautiful physical experiments in illustration of the processes involved in diapedesis have been lately described by HAMILTON (*Proc. Roy. Soc. Edin.* vol. XI). See also SCHKLAREWSKY, *Pflüger's Arch.* vol. I.

28. The cause of rupture of the vessel-wall is either traumatic

injury, or disease of the wall itself. In all so-called spontaneous haemorrhage we must take it for granted that the latter cause is in action. Newly-formed vessels are likewise very easily torn. Increased blood-pressure of course tends towards rupture of the vessel-wall, but it never actually produces it if the vessel be perfectly sound.

Diapedesis comes into play when the pressure is raised in the veins and capillaries, and also when, *caeteris paribus,* the vessel-wall becomes more permeable. It is very rapidly set up by obstructing the outflow of venous blood. The nature of the change in the vessel-wall which results in greater permeability is not yet completely understood; but it is known at least that the exciting cause of the change is a disturbance in tissue-nutrition (Art. 25). Thus it may be produced by temporarily checking the blood-supply of the vessel, or by direct injury to the vessel-wall. Moreover certain poisons introduced into the blood may lead to the change The vessel-wall must, in fact, be directly or indirectly damaged.

Sometimes the defective structure of the vessel-wall is congenital. There are persons who show a great tendency to bleed upon small occasion. These are called '**bleeders**,' and are said to exhibit the **haemorrhagic diathesis** or **haemophilia**.

What we may describe as an acquired haemorrhagic diathesis is exhibited in the diseases known as *morbus maculosus* or purpura, and scurvy; as well as in many of the infectious fevers and toxaemic affections, such as septicaemia, spotted typhus, small-pox, plague, *icterus gravis,* yellow fever, nephritis, phosphorus poisoning, etc. In some cases of *haemophilia neonatorum* and of endocarditis, collections of bacteria have been found to be the originating cause of haemorrhage. Such haemorrhages are sometimes slight, sometimes very serious. They occur chiefly in the skin, mucous membranes, and serous membranes. Similar haemorrhages also occur sometimes in connexion with troubles of the central nervous system, chiefly in the stomach and the lungs.

Full references to the literature of haemophilia are given by LEGG (*Haemophilia* London 1872, and *St Barth. Hosp. Rep.* 1881), and by IMMERMANN (*Ziemssen's Cyclop.* vol. 17).

Haemorrhages occurring in connexion with brain affections have been observed in the human subject and have also been experimentally produced in animals (JEHN, *Allg. Zeitschrift f. Psychiatrie* 1874; CHARCOT, *Leçons sur les maladies du système nerveux* I, 1875, *Diseases of the nervous system* (New Syd. Soc.); EBSTEIN, *Arch. f. exper. Path.* II).

ZIEGLER has twice noted serious haemorrhages of this kind in epileptics. In one case three-fourths of each lung was completely filled with blood. He has likewise met with extensive haemorrhage into the lung in a patient who died of traumatic softening of the brain.

29. The obstruction of arteries and veins plays the chief part in the production of irregularities in the circulation, and of haemorrhages. This obstruction may arise in various ways, from without by ligature or compression, from within not infrequently by

thrombosis. By this term is meant the formation of a coagulum or blood-clot within the vessel during life (Arts. 35 and 252—255). This coagulation occurs for the most part when the circulation is already weakened or arrested, and the vessel-walls diseased. The result is that the lumen of the vessel is first narrowed, and then as coagulation proceeds is blocked altogether. In the former stage the thrombosis is called **concentric** or **incomplete**; in the latter it is **obstructive** or **obliterating**. Thrombi are formed oftenest in the veins, but they occur also in the arteries and in the heart. If a thrombus becomes loosened from the vessel-wall, and so gets into the blood, it is carried on by the current. In this way it may pass from the systemic veins into the pulmonary arteries, or from the heart and greater arteries into the smaller ones. It becomes then wedged in at the point where its size corresponds with the section of the vessel: and then by adapting its form to that of the lumen, or by setting up fresh coagulation on its own surface, it speedily blocks the vessel altogether. A thrombus thus swept into the vessel from a distance is called an **embolus**. It is generally situated at the bifurcation of an artery.

The consequences of embolism are very various. Often enough the tissue concerned is very slightly affected; in other cases it may undergo anaemic necrosis (Art. 33); in others still what is called embolic infarction.

30. The bleeding which sometimes ensues upon thrombosis of a vein is, as we have seen in Arts. 27 and 28, the immediate result of arrested outflow through the natural channels. The consequences of the closure of an artery have already been touched upon in Art. 22. The immediate consequences are these. First of all, the circulation is brought to a standstill, and the region beyond the block becomes anaemic. If the arterial twigs of this region are connected directly with some other unobstructed artery, the latter forthwith dilates and conveys a sufficient quantity of blood to irrigate the starved region. The circulation is thus speedily re-established.

If however the vessels of the region possess no such collateral connexions, the region itself is altogether deprived of fresh blood, and sooner or later perishes (Art. 33).

If the embolised artery be, as COHNHEIM calls it, a terminal artery, having no arterial anastomoses, a scanty influx of blood to the tissues from the contiguous veins and capillaries may still be possible. It is in this way that a **haemorrhagic infarct** is produced. The capillaries of the anaemic region become gradually filled with blood, partly derived from the capillaries of neighbouring regions, partly from slow reflux out of the veins. The blood oozing in from the neighbouring capillaries is under a very low pressure. This pressure is insufficient to propel the blood out of the obstructed capillary system into the corresponding veins again. The blood therefore stagnates, and the capillaries become ever more and more engorged. Of course whatever reflux takes place from the veins can only carry blood into the capillary system; it cannot suffice to drive the blood through the capillaries.

In consequence of this engorgement, due to lack of propelling power, diapedesis is soon established, just as in complete obstructions of the venous outflow. The escape of blood is further aided by the disorganisation of the vessel-wall, set up by the cessation or serious diminution of its supply of nutriment. The ultimate result of the diapedesis is the infiltration of the entire tissue with blood, and the formation of a firm, generally conical, haemorrhagic patch. Embolic infarcts of this kind are found chiefly in the lungs, the spleen, and the kidneys. As to their final fate see Art. 37.

The fundamental experiments on thrombosis and embolism were originally made by VIRCHOW (*Gesammelte Abhandlungen* Frankfurt a. M. 1856).

VIRCHOW referred the production of the embolic infarct to increased flow in the arteries of the contiguous regions, consequent on the ischaemia of the region considered. This involved an increased lateral pressure within the vessels, and so increased tendency for the blood to escape. COHNHEIM (*Untersuchungen über die embolischen Processe* Berlin 1872), examining directly the results of embolism in the frog's tongue, established the existence of the reflux from the veins, the gradual refilling of the capillaries, and the escape of blood by diapedesis. The efficient cause of the diapedesis he considered to be an ischaemic disorganisation of the vessel-wall. LITTEN (*Untersuchungen über den hämorrhagischen Infarct* Berlin 1879) regards the reflux from the veins as non-essential, and refers the refilling of the capillaries to the influx from contiguous regions. Even disorganisation of the vessel-wall is, according to him, unessential to the production of an infarct; inasmuch as diapedesis is completely accounted for by the mere fact of engorgement (as is seen when the veins are obstructed). Diapedesis is for this reason increased when it chances that the blood coagulates in the vein of outflow from the embolised region.

CHAPTER VII.

LYMPHORRHAGIA.

31. **Lymphorrhagia** occurs when a lymphatic vessel is ruptured and the contained lymph is effused into the tissues around. The pressure in the lymphatics is very low, scarcely higher, that is to say, than that in the contiguous tissues. An escape of lymph from the vessel can therefore occur only when a cavity already exists at the place of rupture, or when one is made by the same injury which rent the vessel. Thus in wounds, for example, we see lymph and blood escaping together; but the flow of the lymph can be arrested by interposing a very slight resistance. If the opening in the surface be not closed up after the rupture of a lymphatic, so that lymph continues constantly to escape, as sometimes happens in the case of ulcers, we have lymph-fistulae formed. Such fistulae may lead to the loss of very considerable quantities of lymph. The most important lesion of this kind, as well as the most likely to be dangerous, is **rupture of the thoracic duct**. This has occasionally been observed as a consequence of a wound; but more commonly of engorgement from closure of the lumen of the duct by inflammation or tumour. The lymph escaping into the thoracic or abdominal cavity gives rise to **chylous hydrothorax** or **chylous ascites**.

References:—CURNOW, *Lectures on the Lymphatic System*, *Lancet* 1, 1879; DAY and HILL, *Trans. Clin. Soc.* 1869; CAYLEY, *Trans. Path. Soc.* 1866.

SECTION III.

RETROGRESSIVE DISTURBANCES OF NUTRITION.

CHAPTER VIII.

NECROSIS.

32. Everything that lives comes sooner or later to an end—it dies. Death makes its appearance so soon as the vital energy of the organism, infused into it when it was first engendered, is exhausted in antagonising external resistances.

Besides this death of the organism as a whole, or **somatic death**, we recognise what we must regard as a localised death; a death, that is to say, of individual cells or cell-groups, which we call **necrosis**.

The occurrence of local death or necrosis in a cell-group or entire organ is only in special cases associated with recognisable changes in structure. The slight histological changes the cells undergo in dying are not always enough to indicate with certainty the exact factor which has caused life to cease. The naked-eye appearances of the larger organs do not always betray the fact that some part of them has become necrosed.

Even the cessation of the obvious functions of an organ may leave us in doubt whether, as in necrosis, the cessation is permanent, or whether the functions are merely suppressed for a time.

Thus we can only subject necroses to anatomical examination, when death of the tissue involves change in its structure either consequent or antecedent. The latter occurs only to a limited extent: the former (*i.e.* change consequent on necrosis) on the other hand is invariably found after a longer or shorter interval. The varieties of necrosis are in fact distinguished from each other according to the nature of these consecutive tissue-changes.

33. The injuries which lead to local death are divisible into three groups. The first includes those which destroy the tissue by their **mechanical** or **chemical** action. Thus external violence may crush a finger; sulphuric acid may destroy a patch of skin; and fungous parasites may disorganise the structure of a gland in which they are permitted to grow. A second group of injuries may be classed as **thermal**. If the temperature of a tissue be maintained

at 54°C to 58°C for any time, the tissue is inevitably killed. Higher temperatures act still more rapidly. The lower limit within which life may be maintained is 16°C to 18°C. A third cause of necrosis is **arrest of nutrition**. This produces 'anaemic necrosis,' and occurs very frequently in the human subject.

All causes which seriously interfere with the circulation of a part, and bring about permanent arrest of its movement, or **stasis**, may lead to the death of the affected tissue. Such causes are thrombosis, embolism, closure of the vessels by disease or ligature, pressure on the tissue, inflammation, haemorrhage, etc. The arrest of the circulation need not however be permanent: it is enough if it persists longer than a certain time--necrosis still ensues. It is unimportant whether or not haemorrhage then takes place (Art. 30): this will only affect the external appearance of the part. Haemorrhagic infarction is thus pathologically equivalent to anaemic necrosis *plus* haemorrhage.

It is of course possible that mechanical, chemical, and thermal agencies may act together. Not infrequently they come into play successively in the same case.

The effect of a given injury in producing necrosis depends not merely on the normal character and strength of the tissue, but also to an essential extent upon its condition for the time being. A tissue whose nutrition has suffered in consequence of deficient or vitiated blood-supply, general marasmus, or hydraemia, is much more apt to necrose than when it is in its normal state. Thus in old patients, and in those suffering from uncompensated valvular disease of the heart, very slight injuries are enough to induce necrosis of the limbs. In emaciated typhoid patients the slightest pressure on the skin over the trochanter, elbow, sacrum, or heel, suffices to bring on gangrenous necrosis of the skin and subcutaneous tissues. Such necroses are described as senile or marasmic gangrene, and *decubitus* (bed-sores) or decubital necroses.

The time required to produce necrosis by interruption of the blood-supply is different in different tissues. Brain-tissue, renal epithelium, and intestinal epithelium, die within two hours (COHNHEIM, *Allgem. Pathologie*). Skin, bone, and connective tissue, continue to live over twelve hours. In general it may be laid down—that tissues which exercise special functions die much more quickly than those which, like connective tissue, possess only the faculty of self-conservation, so to speak.

34. The course of the necrosis (*i.e.* the character of the tissue-changes it involves) is influenced by such circumstances as the nature of the tissue, its locality, and the form and cause of the necrosis. Not less important are the amount of blood and proper fluid or juice contained in the tissue, and the access or exclusion of air and of putrefactive ferments.

Moreover there may be antecedent tissue-changes which are not without influence on the necrotic process; such, for example, as fatty degeneration, inflammation, and haemorrhage. We thus see that even if the necrotic process be in itself simple, *i.e.* associated with only slight histological change, the consecutive changes it involves may yet be very manifold. We proceed to discuss the chief forms which have been observed.

A constant result of the death of a portion of a tissue is more or less severe inflammation in the surrounding portions. This is most severe when decomposition sets in in the dead portion. By means of this inflammatory zone, the necrosed region is in a way marked off and isolated from the rest. The inflammation is hence described as **definitive**, and the zone as the **line of demarcation**. The process is more fully treated in Arts. 112—116.

Among the various terminations of necrosis we may distinguish four main types. We exclude special complications, such as the development in the necrosed tissue of specific irritant matters. In the first class, the dead tissue is absorbed and replaced by newly-formed normal tissue (**regeneration**, Arts. 72—80). In the second, the dead tissue is likewise absorbed, but is not replaced by normal tissue; an inflammation *in situ* is followed by the formation of fibrous tissue, which fills up the gap in whole or in part (**scarring or cicatrisation**, Arts. 112—116). In the third, the necrosed tissue is only partially absorbed, a part remaining as a caseous mass; this later on becomes in general calcified and enclosed in a capsule of connective tissue (**caseation** and **calcification**, Arts. 112—116). The fourth issue is the formation of a **cyst**. The dead tissue is absorbed, and in its place there is developed a small amount of fibrous tissue, but only over the boundary of the vacated space. In other cases, this space becomes filled with fluid, which is thus encysted. This happens oftenest in the brain.

a. Coagulative (hyaline or fibrinous) necrosis.

35. Necrosis accompanied by coagulation occurs in two ways. In certain of the vital fluids like the blood and lymph, and in fluids which have escaped from the vessels, granular, fibrous, or homogeneous coagula are formed: that is one kind of necrosis. In the other, cells and cellular structures as they die become solid and firm, and coalesce into peculiar homogeneous or hyaline masses.

The granular, fibrous, and hyaline masses which make their appearance when blood coagulates are albuminoid bodies: and we speak of them in general terms as **fibrin**. This fibrin takes the form of flakes or curds, shreds, lumps, or membranes. If red blood-cells are enclosed in the meshes of the fibrin as it separates, the clots are soft and dark red in colour. If coagulation does not take place in the plasma till this has separated from the red blood-cells, the clots produced are pale yellowish, soft, gelatinous, watery, translucent, and somewhat tenacious: after a time they contract and so become drier and tougher. In lymph, mere flakes only are formed. According to current theories, coagulation of the blood, or of the lymph, occurs when the white corpuscles die and dissolve in the plasma. ALEX. SCHMIDT affirms that the plasma contains fibrinogen only. To bring about coagulation, that is the formation of fibrin, the presence of fibrinoplastin (paraglobulin) and of a ferment is necessary. Both of these are supplied by the white corpuscles as they dissolve in the plasma.

Inflammatory effusions or exudations may coagulate as blood does, and so yield masses containing a large amount of fibrin. These may lie on the surface of the inflamed tissue in the form of **false membranes** (Fig. 1). The fibrinous masses may be made

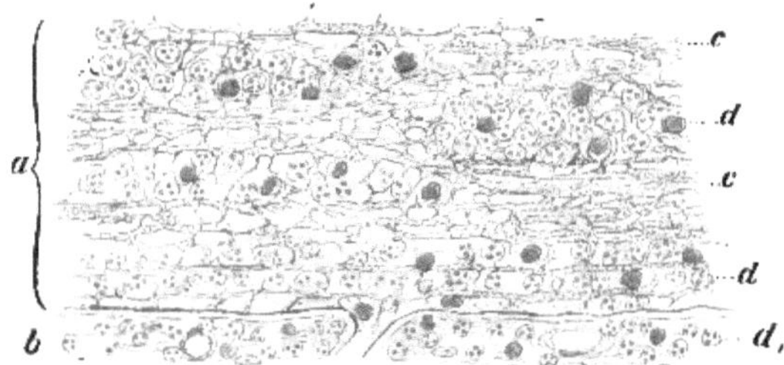

FIG. 1. CROUPOUS (FALSE) MEMBRANE FROM THE TRACHEA. (×250)

a section through the false membrane
b upper layer of the mucous membrane, infiltrated with pus-cells d_1
c fibres and granules of fibrin
d pus-cells

up of granules, of delicate fibres, of a coarse-meshed reticulum (Fig. 1 *c*), or of homogeneous flakes.

ALEXANDER SCHMIDT'S researches on blood-coagulation are to be found in his paper:—*Die Lehre von den fermentativen Gerinnungen* Dorpat 1876. MONTEGAZZA has pursued similar investigations—(*Moleschott's Untersuchungen zur Naturlehre* 1876). For other papers, see GAMGEE'S *Physiological Chemistry* vol. I, chap. 2. WOOLDRIDGE (*Proc. Roy. Soc.* 214, 1881 and *Du Bois-Reymond's Arch.* 1881) has recently published the results of a research conducted in Prof. LUDWIG'S laboratory at Leipzig, in which he seeks to make out that coagulation is mainly due to the action of deleterious liquids on the blood-cells. In shed blood the plasma 'dies' and becomes deleterious in this sense: its action on the cells, especially the white cells, makes them break up and coalesce into a coagulum. A ten per cent. salt solution would have the same effect.

The factors of fibrin are said to be furnished by HAYEM'S haematoblasts, and by BIZZOZERO'S "*Blutplättchen.*" The latter have been recently described (*Centralb. f. d. med. Wiss.* 2, 1882) as small, very transient, delicate, colourless discs. According to BIZZOZERO it is the breaking up of his "*Blutplättchen*" which alone determines coagulation. The true significance of these bodies is not yet determined.

Full discussions on the subject of fibrin and its origin are to be found in VIRCHOW'S *Gesammelte Abhandlungen* 1856. The intra-vascular coagulation of the blood is treated more adequately in Art. 252. It is possible that, in the coagulation of liquids contained in cellular tissues, the fibrinoplastic substance is yielded by the tissue-cells. These latter either dissolve altogether, or they permit their protoplasmic contents to escape in the shape of simple homogeneous masses.

36. In the second form of necrosis with coagulation, the knowledge of which we owe chiefly to WEIGERT, the circumstances and the appearances presented are essentially different from those of the first. Here as before we have to do with the death of tissue occurring under special conditions, and resulting in the formation of coagulated albuminoids: but the coagulation takes place not in a liquid but in the substance of formed tissue-elements, in cells and cellular or intercellular structures.

If by reason of arrested nutrition, or by the action of chemical or thermal agencies, a definite segment of an organ be caused to die, and if then a moderate amount of lymph happen to flow through the necrosed segment, we have the conditions which give rise to coagulation within the tissue. The lymph contains fibrinogen, the cells contain fibrinoplastin; between them fibrin is produced. COHNHEIM introduced the term **coagulative necrosis** to describe this special form of local death. Sometimes at least it may be fitly spoken of as hyaline necrosis. In this process the cells alter their appearance in various ways. The ultimate effect is always the destruction of the cells as such.

The varieties of morphological change observed in coagulating cells and tissues are dependent, partly on diversity of structure in the tissues, partly on the quantity of fibrinogen effused. The manner in which necrosis has been brought about is indifferent; but the dying of the tissue must not be too protracted, or degenerative processes, such as fatty change, may intervene and render the cells non-coagulable.

The chief investigations on this subject of coagulative necrosis are those of WEIGERT. A summary of his results is given in *Virch. Arch.* vol. 79. The proof of the fact—that interfusion of lymph may cause the destruction of cells and the disappearance of their nuclei—was effected by introducing hardened pieces of tissue into the abdominal cavity of rabbits. These tissues were transformed in the manner described.

Similar cell-changes to those produced in coagulative necrosis, and more especially the disappearance of nuclei, may also result from mere putrefaction. Coagulative necrosis may also be found combined with other retrogressive changes, such as fatty degeneration.

37. Among the numerous cases in which coagulative necrosis takes place must be mentioned **embolic infarction**. A certain time after the obstruction of an artery of the kidney or spleen, there is found lying beneath the capsule an opaque yellowish-white conical patch. This patch consists of necrosed kidney- or spleen-tissue, with perhaps fragments of disorganised and completely decolorised blood-clot. If the patch be microscopically examined in unstained sections, its structure will be found almost normal, though paler than the surrounding parts. The difference becomes

however sharply defined when the section is stained, for the necrosed part is incapable of taking up colour. The cells are strikingly pale and transparent, and their nuclei are either gone, or swollen up and unstained. In later stages the outlines of the cells become blurred, the nuclei vanish, and the cell-contents are metamorphosed into a finely-granular fibrinous mass. Later still this mass disintegrates and is absorbed (Art. 115). If the infarct was originally haemorrhagic, the effused blood, like the tissue-elements, is changed into a colourless granular, or it may be homogeneous, mass.

Minute investigations into the nature of haemorrhagic infarction have recently been made by LITTEN (*Untersuchungen über den haem. Infarct* Berlin 1879) and GUILLEBEAU (*Die Histologie d. haem. Infarctes*, In. Diss. Berne 1880). According to LITTEN, renal infarcts are generally anaemic, *i.e.* not accompanied by haemorrhage. GUILLEBEAU on the contrary says that both renal and splenic infarcts are generally haemorrhagic, but become very quickly decolorised. ZIEGLER inclines to the latter view, though he has examined recent infarcts in which he was unable to demonstrate either haemorrhage or its traces.

38. The so-called **waxy degeneration of muscle** (ZENKER) is also an instance of coagulative necrosis. Muscle-fibre invariably coagulates after death, but generally preserves its striation. Under various influences however, as *e.g.* after bruising, forcible extension, raising of the temperature, or febrile disease, the muscle-substance is here and there disintegrated, and the contractile myosin coagulates into a lustrous homogeneous mass (Fig. 2 *b*). This mass breaks up

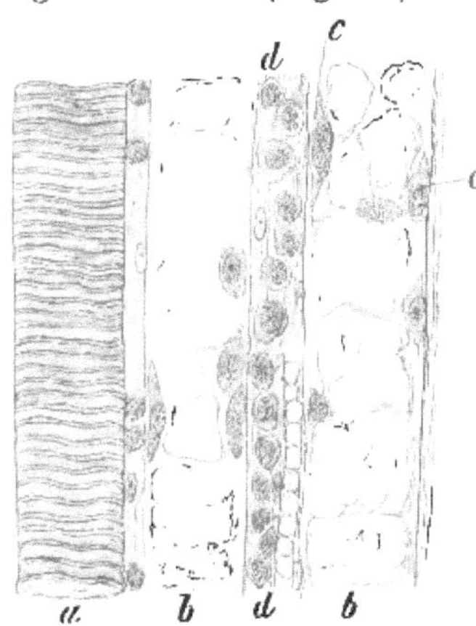

FIG. 2. WAXY DEGENERATION OF MUSCLE. (*From a case of typhoid fever:* × 250)

a normal muscle-fibre
b degenerate muscle-fibre broken up into flaky lumps
c regenerative cells lying inside the sarcolemma
d connective tissue infiltrated with cells

into shining flaky lumps. To the naked eye muscles so affected have a dull semi-opaque lustre, and look not unlike the muscles of fish.

Coagulative necrosis very often occurs in the course of inflammatory processes. It is hardly ever quite absent where there has been copious exudation. In such cases it may take one of two forms. Either the effused fluid dissolves up the contained cells and then coagulates (Art. 35 Fig. 1 and Art. 102); or the tissue-cells themselves coagulate, forming homogeneous lumps or fibrous reticulated masses. To give an example, the ordinary stratified

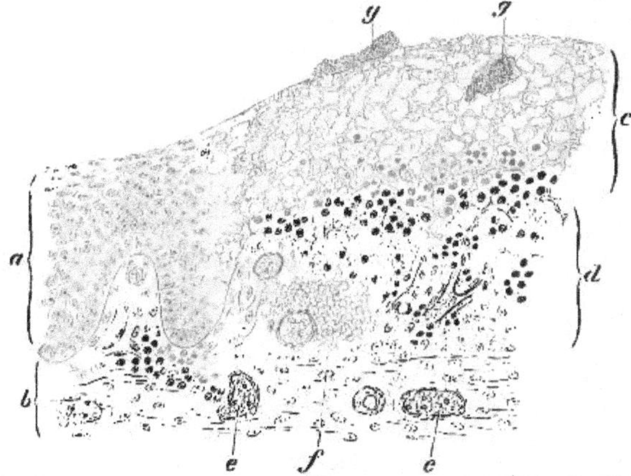

FIG. 3. SECTION THROUGH THE UVULA IN DIPHTHERITIS FAUCIUM.
(*Aniline staining*: ×75)

a normal epithelium
b normal areolar tissue
c necrosed epithelium transformed into a coarse mesh-work
d areolar tissue infiltrated with fibrin and leucocytes
e blood-vessels
f haemorrhage *g* heaps of micrococci

epithelial cells (Fig. 3 *a*) of the pharynx and soft palate in *diphtheritis faucium* (diphtheria) solidify into a peculiarly-formed trabecular mesh-work (Fig. 3 *c*). Similar changes in the epithelium are observed in various cutaneous inflammations, such as small-pox. The aggregations of cells which accumulate in simple inflammation may also solidify into pale hyaline flakes or granular masses. Such solidifications occur, for example, in typhoid infiltration of Peyer's patches and of the lymphatic glands, and in the cellular exudations which fill the pulmonary alveoli in caseous bronchopneumonia. The formation of continuous hyaline masses out of cellular material may be typically seen in diphtheritic desquamation of mucous membranes (Arts. 103 and 425): the entire infiltrated tissue sometimes solidifies in this manner.

The ground-substance of connective tissue, hyaline membranes, the walls of blood-vessels, etc. are all liable to be transfused with coagulable liquid, and then to coagulate into homogeneous masses.

b. Caseation.

39. **Caseation** (or tyrosis) is a pathological transformation of tissue, whose product somewhat resembles in appearance firm new Cheshire cheese on the one hand, or soft cream cheese on the other. The name refers merely to the outward appearance of the product: the process which leads to its formation is by no means always the same.

In the first form of caseation—in which the degenerated tissue is firm, tough, yellowish-white, and somewhat translucent—the process is one of coagulative necrosis. This occurs most frequently in tissues which are rich in cells; for example, in the foci of tuberculous disease, in cellular tumours, and in inflamed lung. A tissue which has become completely caseous is always devoid of nuclei, and is either homogeneous or finely granular. The transformation of a tissue into a firm cheesy mass may occur in one of three ways. The tissue may gradually assume as a whole a more and more homogeneous appearance, losing its nuclei the while. Or detached homogeneous masses may first be formed, which later on fuse together into a continuous mass. Or lastly, the tissue-cells may first dissolve and be replaced by granules and granular fibrils of fibrin; these last then close up and coalesce into a dense uniform mass. The last process is chiefly observed in the caseation of the cellular exudations of pneumonia; the first chiefly in tissues which, in consequence of chronic inflammation or tuberculosis, are the seat of a fibro-cellular hyperplasia. It should be noted that caseating masses originally homogeneous may, by subsequent transformation, take on a more granular appearance.

The softer form of caseation changes the tissue to a dull white. The chief part of the mass is made up of granular fatty and albuminous detritus. Neither cells nor cellular structures are any longer recognisable. This form of caseation is generally the result of a fatty disintegration of cellular tissues or exudations (Arts. 50—54), which have lost water by absorption. The tissue thereupon becomes inspissated. and its opaque appearance is due to the formation in it of minute oil-globules.

The firmer and softer forms of caseous change are not very sharply distinguished. At times both forms may be found together in one organ. It is even possible for the firmer form to be transformed, by processes physical or chemical, into the softer. The ultimate fate of caseous foci is either softening and liquefaction with absorption (Arts. 112—116), or calcification.

c. Colliquative necrosis or Softening.

40. **Colliquative necrosis**, in which the affected tissue becomes as it were liquefied, is closely akin to coagulative necrosis. In each case the necrosed parts become saturated with liquid. Colliquation may thus either precede or follow upon coagulation.

For example, the coagulation of the blood and formation of a clot is preceded by the liquefaction or solution of certain cells contained in the blood. A similar process may be observed in the case of blisters following upon burns.

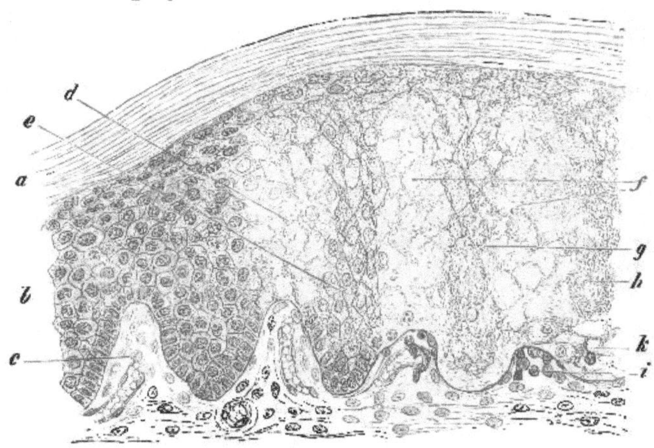

FIG. 4. SECTION THROUGH THE EPIDERMIS AND PAPILLAE AFTER A BURN.
(The preparation (carmine-stained) is from a cat's paw which had been burned with melted sealing-wax: ×250)

- *a* horny layer
- *b* rete Malpighii
- *c* normal papilla
- *d* swollen epithelial cells (in some the nucleus is still visible, in others not)
- *e* interpapillary cells (those below are uninjured, those near the surface are swollen and stretched)
- *f* fibrinous mesh-work (composed of cells and exudation; cell-structure altogether lost)
- *g* swollen cells without nuclei
- *h* interpapillary layer of cells stripped off and destroyed
- *k* subepithelial exudation (coagulated)
- *i* depressed papilla, infiltrated with cells and disappearing

The first change perceived is an enormous swelling up of the epidermal cells overlying the papillae (Fig. 4 *d*); the cells being wholly or in part killed by the action of the heat. This swelling up depends on the absorption by the dead cells of the liquid which transudes from the papillary vessels. It becomes at length so extreme that the cell-substance dissolves completely and the cell-membrane itself disappears. Not until the tumefaction and colliquation have reached a certain point—*i. e.* when the cell is distended to a mere vesicle, or has gone altogether—do the granular fibrils which indicate coagulation begin to appear (*f g h*).

In some tissues this coagulation after colliquation does not occur. Thus in **anaemic necrosis (softening)** of the brain we have simply disintegration and liquefaction of the brain-substance. The several constituents of the tissue break up, and dissolve in the liquid which is poured out from the vessels. They are then absorbed, and the liquid becomes gradually clear again: but there is no coagulation. The reason of this probably is—that brain-substance contains but few coagulable matters, and on the other hand that the effused lymph, not being the result of acute inflammation, contains but little fibrinogen or fibrinoplastin. The same thing is at times to be observed in other tissues, as for instance in so-called 'softening of the heart,' when the muscle-substance has already undergone fatty degeneration. Here the antecedent degeneration has notably diminished the amount of coagulable matter in the muscular tissue.

But colliquation of the tissues may follow upon coagulation as well as precede it. It is a very frequent occurrence for coagulated exudations (as in croupous pneumonia) or thrombi to break down and liquefy. This liquefaction of coagulated masses is always accompanied by certain chemical changes, the efficient causes of which are frequently of the nature of organised ferments (Art. 42).

d. *Dry Gangrene or Mummification.*

41. **Dry gangrene** is commonly the result of necrosis in parts which are exposed to the air.

Typical examples are afforded by the so-called senile gangrene of the extremities, especially of the toes and feet; and likewise by the necroses of the same parts following upon frost-bite. In the first case, the necrosis is determined by defective blood-supply, partly owing to general feebleness of the circulation, and partly to local changes in the blood-vessels.

The affected part is generally engorged with blood when necrosis sets in, and thus exhibits a dark or livid coloration. The engorgement is due to stagnation of the blood-current from mere feebleness of propulsion. After the death of the part, the colouring-matter of the blood transudes and gives the tissues their dark-red appearance. At the same time the tissues begin to dry up by evaporation. This drying process is notably accelerated when the epidermis separates, as happens when the engorgement has been extreme, and in frost-bite. The part becomes first leathery, and then perfectly hard, brittle, and black. Under the microscope the tissue-elements are seen to be shrunken and withered.

Dry gangrene or withering is a physiological process as it affects the stump of the umbilical cord in infants. Between the sound tissue and the gangrenous there is formed an inflammatory zone of demarcation (Art. 115). Dry gangrene may at times occur as a later stage of moist gangrene.

e. *Moist Gangrene or Sphacelus.*

42. **Moist gangrene** is necrosis followed by decomposition and putrefaction of the necrosed tissue. If septic organisms reach a dead tissue which is rich in blood or other liquid, it very soon begins to decompose. The organisms may reach the part either

directly from the air (as in gangrene of the skin or lungs), or through the channel of the circulation (as in gangrene of the testis, or of the foot). Parts which are exposed and abound in blood-vessels, such as the foot, become livid from diffusion of the colouring-matter of the blood. The epidermis frequently rises in blisters and bullae. Soon the putrefying tissue begins to stink, and then to disintegrate. Slight mechanical causes readily give rise to wounds, and in these the tissue is seen to be infiltrated with discoloured blood, and it is brittle or even tinder-like. Corresponding to the obvious naked-eye disintegration of the structure are the profound chemical changes which take place (Arts. 191—192): and the final result is the total destruction of the tissue as such. Not infrequently gases are evolved during the process, giving rise to so-called **gangrenous emphysema** (*gangrène gazeuse*). The rapidity of the destructive process depends greatly on the nature of the affected tissue. Bone preserves its form for a long time in the midst of a gangrenous mass, while the soft parts perish very quickly.

The microscope shews that in this process of decay septic organisms are always present (Arts. 192 *et seq.*). Blood-corpuscles quickly cease to be distinguishable, inasmuch as they break up and dissolve, or here and there become transformed into granular pigmented masses. Other cells become turbid, lose their nuclei, break up, and disappear. Fat-cells disintegrate, and the oil they contain mingles in small globules with the gangrenous mass. The fibres of the connective tissue swell up, grow turbid and ill-defined, and finally dissolve. Elastic tissue, tendon, and cartilage hold out for a long time, but ultimately perish in like manner. In general terms we may put it—that gangrene involves the gradual solution of the solid constituents of the tissue, and results in the formation of a dirty grey, greyish-black, or greyish-yellow, opaque, semi-fluid mass, mixed with shreds and remnants of various structures. The various normal elements of the tissue thus disappear in succession; while new crystalline products of chemical decomposition appear instead, such as fatty needles of margarin, needles of tyrosin, spherules of leucin, 'sarcophagus-crystals' of triple phosphate, and granules of black or brown pigment.

In the later stages of putrefaction, mould-fungi at times make their appearance on parts exposed to the air (Art. 221).

Further details of the tissue-changes in gangrene may be found in DEMME, *Ueber die Veränderungen der Gewebe bei Brand* Frankfort 1857; and in RINDFLEISCH, *Pathological Histology* (Sydenham Society). See also CHAUVEAU, *Nécrobiose et gangrène* Paris 1873; PAGET, *Surgical Pathology*.

Putrid decomposition, and therefore also gangrene, can arise only through the agency of micro-organisms. Furthermore, the presence of a certain proportion of water in the tissue is essential. If the tissue dry up, the development of septic organisms ceases, or is at least seriously retarded; and with it also the process of decomposition. The chemical products of the gangrenous decomposition of the tissues are hydrocarbons, ammonium sulphide, sulphuretted hydrogen, valerianic acid, butyric acid, etc.; and ultimately carbonic acid, ammonia, and water.

CHAPTER IX.

SIMPLE ATROPHY AND PIGMENTARY DEGENERATION.

43. In treating of malformations, we showed that in consequence of arrested development members, organs, or parts of organs may be ill-grown, misformed, or altogether wanting. Or if the plastic energy that determines growth be deficient, the entire organism or some of its parts may be dwarfed and stunted. Defective development of this kind, *i.e.* aplasia or hypoplasia, may occur after birth as well as before it. So long as the organism continues to grow, so long as new parts or organs continue to be formed in it, so long is its growth liable to be checked by external or internal influences.

We may often observe this hypoplasia in the child. At birth it may have been anything but puny, yet under the operation of external causes, such as defective nutrition, various kinds of disease, or others less easily recognized, it later on shows signs of imperfect development in some of its systems or organs. The consequence is a dwarfing of the entire frame or of its parts, very often associated with faulty structure and function of the viscera. This hypoplasia makes itself especially evident when the bones are badly developed, as also when the heart and great vessels, the genital organs, or the central nervous system are under-grown. The association referred to is observed, for example, in cretins, whose bones are generally ill-grown; and in chlorotic females, where with hypoplasia of the vascular system there is also some imperfection of the generative functions.

Now **atrophy** is not to be confounded with such hypoplasias or aplasias. In atrophy we have to do not with defective development, but with retrogressive change in parts originally well-formed and well-grown.

44. The life of an organ, like that of an individual, is limited in its duration. The active cell-growth of the period of development is succeeded by a stage in which the formative activity is less marked. In the latter stage the equilibrium between cell-growth

and cell-decay is maintained with but slight oscillations to one side or the other.

In old age this equilibrium is disturbed, and decay has the upper hand. An involution (the reverse of evolution) of the entire organism and of its parts takes place. Thus a man ultimately dies, even when there is no question of disease, so soon as the advancing involution of his vital organs reaches a stage at which they can no longer efficiently perform their functions.

But besides this general retrogression, or senile decay, there is a physiological retrogression of particular organs, which takes place much earlier in life. The generative organs in woman lose their functional power long before extreme old age. The thymus gland has undergone complete degeneration by the age of adolescence. Various tissues, like the hyaline cartilage which is the first rudiment of bone, are in their very nature temporary structures. The several tissues then, like the organism itself, inherit but a measured lease of life.

Considered anatomically, retrogression shows itself in an organ by diminution of its size: microscopically, by diminution and ultimate disappearance of its constituent elements, especially of the elements which are special to it.

45. An organ, towards the close of its life, undergoes what we have called a physiological retrogression. But analogous retrogressive processes may occur, as it were prematurely, under pathological conditions. Their result we describe as **simple atrophy.**

This pathological atrophy is distinguished, like the other, by shrinking of the organ affected, or by diminution in size and number of its essential elements.

In the case of dense parenchymatous organs like the liver, kidney, heart, or brain, the shrinking is the first thing which is likely to strike us. If the shrinking has been uniform the surface remains smooth: if it has been irregular the surface looks uneven and granular, and the external form of the organ may be altered. On the other hand, atrophy of bone shows itself rather by thinning of the trabeculae and widening of the medullary cavities, than by any general diminution in size. So too in the lungs, we recognise the occurrence of atrophy by the increased size of the air-spaces, and the loss in part of the alveolar septa.

Compared with the shrinking and loss of substance, the **pigmentary change** so often associated with atrophy is of minor importance. It is a secondary, non-essential phenomenon in the process. It depends either on the fact that the normal pigmentation of the tissue becomes more pronounced as the essential elements disappear; or on an actual deposition of pigment associated with the atrophic process; or lastly on some alteration in the amount of blood contained in the tissue.

46. The shrinking of an atrophied organ is due to the fact

that its elements dwindle and disappear. Here, as in the case of senile involution, it is the proper and specific elements of the organ which suffer the most; and the supporting framework of connective tissue the least. It is in fact very frequently observed that the connective structures remain perfectly intact or even increase and grow, while the specific elements have already disappeared. Thus in the illustration (Fig. 5) of a muscle undergoing atrophy, the contractile substance (a) contained within the sarcolemma has distinctly dwindled (b). But the connective tissue separating the fibrillae remains undiminished; the nuclei of its cells seem even to have multiplied.

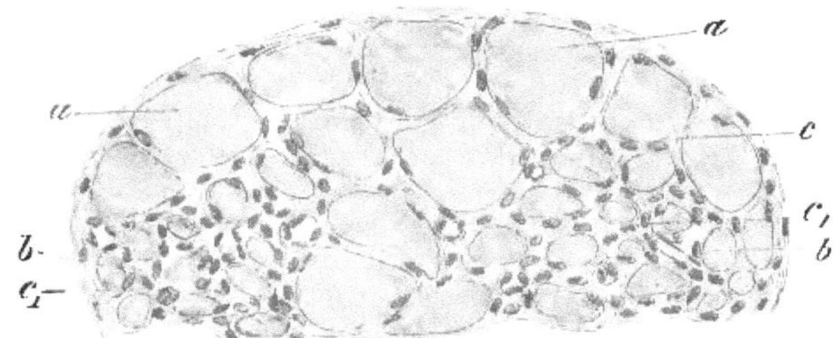

FIG. 5. SECTION OF AN ATROPHIED MUSCLE.

(*From a case of progressive muscular atrophy: Bismarck-brown staining:* × 300)

a normal muscle-fibre b atrophied muscle-fibre

c *perimysium internum*, in which the nuclei as at c_1 are seen to be increased in number

Similar appearances are readily observed in atrophied liver-tissue. There every one of the gland-cells may have vanished, and yet there may be no diminution in the amount of the connective-tissue framework. So too in preparations of brain and spinal cord, the ganglion cells may have altogether disappeared, without any visible change in the neuroglia.

Adipose tissue is peculiar in its mode of atrophy. The fat in the cells breaks up into small oil-globules which are absorbed: the empty cells return to their first condition of ordinary connective-tissue cells. At times the disappearance of the contained fat is followed by multiplication of the nuclei (**atrophic proliferation**). If serum transude into the tissue after the fat has gone, the tissue becomes gelatinous in appearance (**serous atrophy**). If lastly pigment be deposited in the atrophied fat-cells, the tissue becomes yellow or yellowish-brown (**pigmentary atrophy**). See FLEMMING, *Archiv f. mikroskop. Anatomie* VII, and *Virch. Arch.* vol. 52.

47. Atrophy may result from various causes. It has already been indicated (Art. 44) that the tissues may themselves possess inherent properties which determine their retrogression and decay. The efficient cause of this form of atrophy (described as **active atrophy**) is that the cells are no longer able to assimilate properly the nutriment brought to them. Atrophy like this, depending on internal conditions, seldom occurs as a pathological process. Only

the so-called atrophy of inaction and trophoneurotic atrophy should perhaps be classed as pathological.

Atrophy of inaction occurs in organs that are subject to the direct influence of the nervous system, and perform their specific functions in obedience to nervous influence. Such are glands, nerves, and muscles. If a muscle or a gland be condemned to inaction for any length of time, it is apt to undergo atrophy. It is not unnatural to infer that the atrophy depends on the absence of functional activity in the cells, and to frame the hypothesis that nutrition and functional activity go hand in hand and fall off together.

A typical instance of **trophoneurotic atrophy** is seen in the rapid disappearance of the muscles in cases where their proper nerves have been injured, or where there is disease of the anterior horns of grey matter in the cord. It appears that certain ganglion-cells in the anterior horns have a powerful influence on the nutrition of the muscles in connexion with them. The disappearance of these cells, or the severance of their connexion with the muscles, involves inevitably the atrophy of the latter.

Leaving these cases out of account, we may fairly refer all other forms of premature atrophy to defective nutrition. The process of the atrophy is the same whatever be the particular factor underlying the deficiency. This factor may be general anaemia, local change in the nutrient vessels, defective assimilation, or any other disorder of the kind: but it can at most determine the site and extent of the atrophy, not the process. Atrophy of this kind, occasioned by diminished nutrition, is distinguished as **passive atrophy.** Atrophy consequent on pressure is brought about, partly by mechanical hindrance of the cell-functions, partly by direct injury to the tissue, partly by interference with the circulation.

COHNHEIM (*Vorlesung. üb. allgemeinen Pathologie*) includes atrophy of inaction among the passive atrophies, and maintains that it depends on diminished blood-supply. It is not easy to believe that this explanation is in all cases adequate. Without undervaluing the importance of the blood-supply, there seems to be no objection to the theory that the assimilative power of an active working cell may be greater than that of one which is at rest.

CHAPTER X.

CLOUDY SWELLING AND DROPSICAL DEGENERATION.

48. The term **cloudy swelling** or **parenchymatous degeneration** is due to VIRCHOW (*Virch. Arch.* vols. 4, 14). He describes by it a certain swelling up of the elements of a tissue by imbibition or accretion: and defines it as a form of hypertrophy

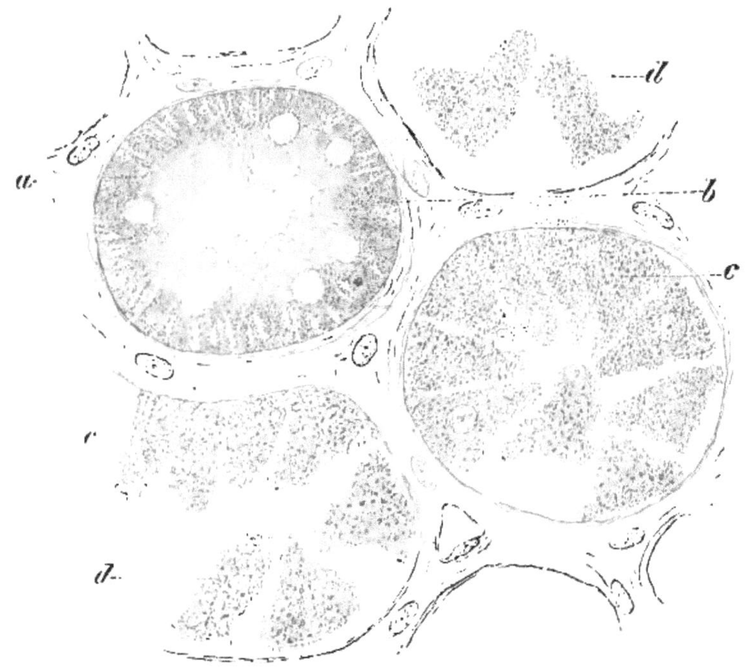

FIG. 6. CLOUDY SWELLING OF THE RENAL EPITHELIUM.
(*Preparation treated with chromic acid and ammonia:* × 800)

a normal epithelium
b cloudy swelling commencing
c advanced degeneration
d loose degenerate epithelium

with a tendency to degeneration. The degenerative side of the process is the more important one. Histological investigation shows that the process consists in the formation of free granules in the substance of the affected cells, which may, for example, be those of the renal epithelium, of the liver, or of the heart-muscle. These free granules are to be regarded, from their microchemical reactions, as albuminoid bodies: they are soluble in acetic acid and insoluble in alkalies or ether. Their presence gives the cell a turbid or cloudy appearance, and its normal form and structure quickly disappear. Thus in cloudy swelling of the renal epithelium (Fig. 6), the cells lose their longitudinal markings and the processes which normally project into the lumen of the tubule (*a*). The cell as it swells becomes rounder, and dark granules appear within it (*b*, *c*). The process depends on a degeneration of the cell-protoplasm. The cell becomes infiltrated with liquid, and a partial separation of its solid and liquid constituents takes place. The degenerative process often ceases when it has reached a certain stage, and the cell returns to its former normal condition. In other cases, the cell-substance perishes and breaks up into granular detritus. Frequently the process is associated with fatty degeneration (Art. 50).

Cloudy or granular degeneration is of very common occurrence. It is found in the parenchymatous organs, such as the liver, kidneys, and heart, in most cases of infectious disease; but chiefly in scarlet fever, typhoid fever, small-pox, erysipelas, diphtheria, septicaemia, etc. The affected organs have a cloudy, dull, often greyish look: in the severer cases they look as if they had been boiled. They contain an abnormally small quantity of blood, and are doughy in consistence. The minuter structure of the organ is blurred or altogether destroyed.

There is a certain morbid change in connective-tissue cells which may be classed under this head. It is frequently observed in oedematous or inflamed connective tissue. The affected cells swell up, and dark spherules form in the nucleus as well as in the cell-protoplasm. These spherules, with which the cells are often tightly crammed, are distinguished by their power of taking up an intense colour when stained, especially with aniline dyes; in this they behave like micrococci. Their significance is not understood, though their formation may probably be regarded as evidence of a retrogressive change.

49. The term **dropsical degeneration** fairly describes a morbid change observed chiefly in epithelial cells. They imbibe liquid and become sodden and swollen. The process is near akin to cloudy swelling and degeneration, though the changes in the dropsical cells are of a somewhat peculiar nature. The imbibed liquid causes the cell to appear translucent (Fig. 7 *e*). The granules of the protoplasm are pushed asunder, and often crowded towards the periphery; so that the cell comes to resemble somewhat a vegetable cell (*f* and *g*). It becomes at the same time vacuolated, the spherical vacuoles containing clear liquid. The nucleus also swells up, and at length appears as a distended vesicle with clear

contents. Changes of this kind may be seen in the cells of dropsical tissues and in inflammation. In inflammation it is chiefly the

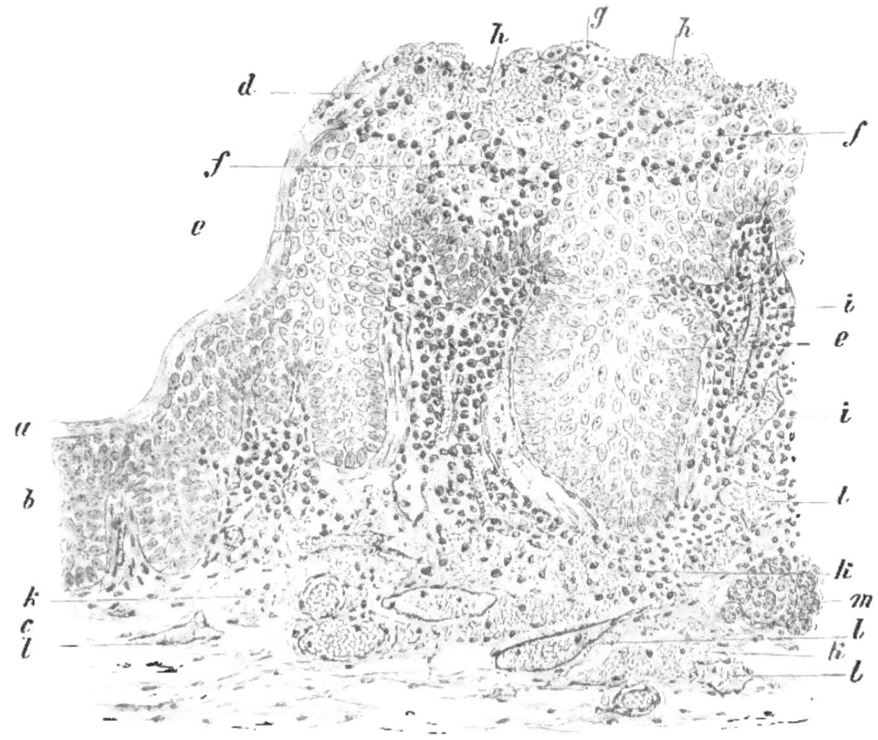

Fig. 7. Section through a 'mucous patch' (*condyloma latum ani*).
(*Aniline-brown staining:* × 100)

a horny layer of the epidermis
b rete Malpighii
c corium
d horny layer swollen up and infiltrated with leucocytes
e swollen cells of the rete Malpighii
f swollen epithelium infiltrated with cells
g degenerate epithelial cells, into which leucocytes have made their way
h granular coagula
i swollen papilla, infiltrated with cells
k corium infiltrated with cells and fibrin
l lymphatic vessel
m sweat-gland

epithelial cells that exhibit marked changes (Fig. 7 *d, e, f, g*). In stained preparations the dropsical cells remain brighter than the healthy ones.

CHAPTER XI.

FATTY DEGENERATION.

50. If parenchymatous degeneration (Art. 48) go beyond a certain point, it often passes into **fatty degeneration**, that is to say, fat-globules form in the disintegrating cells. This variety of fatty degeneration is however of limited occurrence, compared with the other varieties to which the organism is liable.

Fat, as we know, occurs in the body in considerable amount even under normal conditions. Certain regions, and especially certain tissues of the fibrous type, like the subcutaneous and subserous structures, the marrow, etc., are always rich in fat. The fat is as it were stored up in these special regions, being either derived from without, or formed on the spot in the cells of the tissue itself. Increase of the quantity in store, whether due to increased supply or diminished expenditure, does not rightly come under the title of fatty degeneration. We distinguish it as **lipomatosis** (obesity, adiposity). Within limits it must be deemed physiological: when excessive it may pass into the domain of pathology. In such extreme cases, fat is found in cells which normally contain none. The fatty deposit takes the form of oily drops, which soon coalesce into larger spherules; until at length a single large fat-globule occupies the entire cell. Fatty infiltration of this kind affects chiefly the cells of the connective tissue in particular regions, and the liver-cells.

True fatty degeneration must of course be distinguished from lipomatosis or fatty infiltration. The fat which occurs in the former is not fat in store, so to speak: it is fat resulting from the disintegration of albumen in the affected cells. Inasmuch as fat is normally formed from the albumen of the cells, and is consumed as it is formed, we are driven to suppose that in fatty degeneration either the disintegration of albumen is increased, or the consumption of the fat produced is impeded. Both these things may occur, but it is specially to be noticed that in fatty degeneration the lost albumen is not replaced, so that the production of fat is associated with atrophy.

51. A cell undergoing fatty degeneration always shows larger or smaller oil-drops in its interior. These are colourless, bright, dark-contoured, insoluble in acetic acid, soluble in alcohol and in ether. In perosmic acid they stain black. The number and size of the oil-drops in the interior of a cell vary greatly: the size even of the largest is not usually great. Thus, for example, in fatty degeneration of the muscle of the heart, we find more or fewer according to the degree of the degeneration (Fig. 8). But they are all small and seldom coalesce into larger drops: they never form very large ones. In fatty degeneration of the kidney (Fig. 9) the appearances are similar; but the size of the oil-globules is not so regular (*c*, *e*).

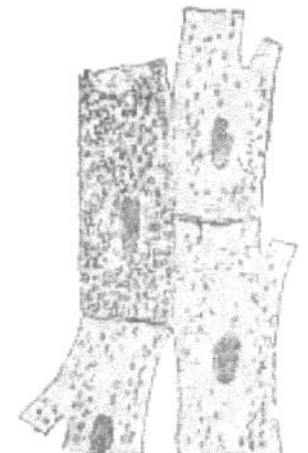

FIG. 8. FATTY DEGENERATION OF THE MUSCLES OF THE HEART (×350)

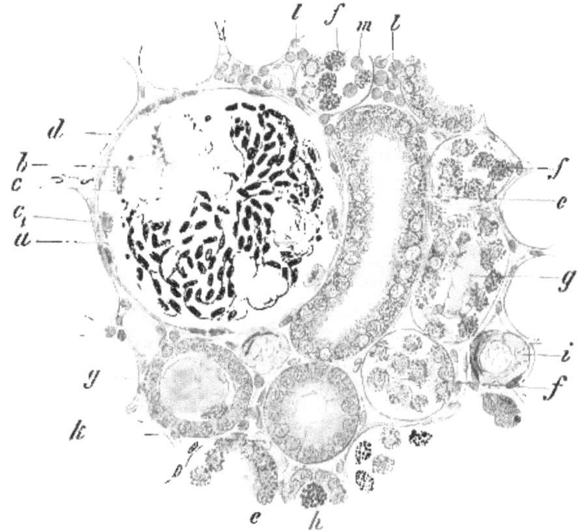

FIG. 9. AMYLOID AND FATTY DEGENERATION OF THE KIDNEY.

(*Preparation treated with Müller's fluid and perosmic acid*: ×300)

a normal capillary loop
b amyloid capillary loop (Art. 57)
c fatty epithelium of the glomerulus
c_1 fatty epithelium of the capsule
d oil-drops on the capillary walls
e fatty epithelial cells *in situ*
f loosened fatty epithelial cells
g hyaline coagula (forming 'casts')
h fatty cast in section
i amyloid artery
k amyloid capillary
l infiltration of connective tissue with leucocytes
m round-cells (leucocytes) inside a uriniferous tubule

When the degeneration becomes more advanced, the fatty epithelial cells are shed and become disintegrated (*f*). The oil-globules they contain are thus set free and accumulate in the tubules (*h*)

Fatty degeneration may occur in connective-tissue cells as well as in epithelial cells. If it affect entire cell-groups or systems, it may be recognised even by the unaided eye; and the more readily as the degeneration is more advanced, the proper colour of the tissue less marked, and the amount of blood present less considerable. Colourless transparent structures, like the intima of the heart (endocardium) and great vessels, take on an opaque white appearance; the cortical tissue of the kidney becomes greyish white or, when the fatty change is greater, opaque yellowish white; the heart-muscle becomes yellowish; and voluntary muscle pale yellowish brown.

If complete disintegration of the tissue follow upon fatty degeneration, and if the mass of detritus lose water and become condensed, the fatty change passes into caseation (Art. 39); and the tissue assumes a dull white cheesy appearance.

Like the cells of solid organs, the cells of organic liquids such as pus, and those of coagulated exudations, very often undergo true fatty degeneration ending in their complete destruction as cells.

In tissues undergoing fatty degeneration, as also in liquids whose cells are degenerating, there are very frequently found cells crammed full of fat-granules. They are referred to as 'fat-granule cells.' Their origin is only in part traceable to fatty degeneration of the cells themselves. They are rather to be looked upon as migratory corpuscles which have taken up the fatty products of disintegration, and so have become transformed into granule-carriers (Art. 114). See REINHARDT, *Virch. Arch.* vol. 1.

52. The **cause** of fatty degeneration is to be sought in an alteration in the constitution of the blood, *i.e.* of the nutriment supplied to the cells. Deficient supply of oxygen plays a chief part in it. To this must be ascribed, on the one hand, the disintegration of albumen and the formation of fat; on the other hand, the fact that the fat produced is not straightway consumed.

If to the lack of oxygen there is added a deficiency of proper nutriment, so that the albumen which is used up by transformation into fat is not replaced, the amount of albumen in the affected part must of course diminish.

Corresponding to the case just indicated, we find fatty degeneration taking place in conditions which are associated with general or local anaemia. For example, if the blood becomes diseased in such a way (anaemia, leukaemia) that its power of taking up oxygen is diminished, and its nutritive value lowered, fatty degeneration is found to occur in the most widely different organs. The same thing comes to pass in particular organs which happen to receive too little blood, either in consequence of disease in the afferent vessels, or because the outflow of blood from them is checked and its renewal hindered. Lastly, organs like the muscles which for any reason are left unexercised, and so fail to undergo an adequate amount of tissue-change, are very apt to become fatty.

Various poisons, such as phosphorus, arsenic, and the ferments which produce fevers, may, like imperfect oxygenation, lead to disintegration of the albumen of the tissues and so to fatty degeneration.

We still seem far distant from an exact understanding of the origin and the ultimate fate of the fat which is formed in the body in physiological and pathological conditions. HOPPE-SEYLER (*Physiolog. Chemie*) inclines to think that fat cannot be formed directly from albumen. He regards it as not unlikely that glycogen is first formed, and from the glycogen fat. VOIT (*Zeitschr. f. Biol.* v, and *Neues Rep. f. Pharmacie* xx), on the other hand, thinks it quite certain that fat may be formed at once from albumen: compare QUAIN, *Med. chir. Trans.* vol. 33. According to HERMANN, it is probable that certain products derived from the disintegration of albumen are normally utilised in regenerative processes. If the oxygen needed for regeneration is wanting, these products cannot be utilised and disintegrate still further: the expenditure of fresh material is thus increased. BINZ and SCHULZ (*Arch. f. exper. Path.* vol. 14) hold that the cells, in their avidity for oxygen, take it up from the blood so long as the blood continues to part with it: when it ceases to do so the cells attack each other, and act as mutual reducing agents. The lateral 'chain' of the albumen-molecule (the chain which includes the nitrogen, on the theory of these chemists) is thus broken: the consequence is increased production of urea and of fat. They explain in this way the fatty changes observed in carbonic oxide poisoning. BENCE JONES (*Lectures on Pathology &c.*) accounts for the proneness of the liver to become fatty in a somewhat similar way. See also RANVIER (*Société anat.* 1868).

On the effect of phosphorus in inducing fatty change, see VOIT and BAUER (*Zeitschr. f. Biol.* VII), LEWIN (*Virch. Arch.* vol. 21), RANVIER (*Soc. de Biologie* 1866).

53. It is generally, though not always, easy to decide whether the fat present in the cells of an organ is a product of degeneration, or simply a deposit by way of storage. It is commonly stated that the fat of degenerative atrophy appears in the form of minute non-coalescent drops; while deposited fat occurs in large drops which readily run together. This is true of most tissues, but not of all. It is true, for example, of striated muscle, heart-muscle, non-striated muscle, neuroglia, &c. But when the renal epithelium becomes fatty, fat-globules of very considerable size are sometimes formed. In the liver again, the fat of degeneration may form either small or large drops (the latter in phosphorus-poisoning).

On the other hand, what we may call storage-fat is, in the first instance, deposited in very minute globules: while the great globules of fatty deposits, when about to undergo re-absorption, break up again into minuter globules.

But if the distinction is not always clear from the histological appearances, we may get more certain information by considering the site in which the fat is found. The appearance of fat-globules in tissue-cells normally free from fat, in circumstances which preclude the idea of a determination of fat to the tissue, is evidence that fat has been formed *in loco* from the cell-albumen, and therefore that the cells have so far become disintegrated. Difficulty can thus arise only in the case of organs, such as the liver, which may normally be the seat of fatty deposit, and on the other hand are prone to fatty degeneration. In such organs it is often hard to say how much of the fat they contain has been produced *in loco*, how much has been brought to them from without. There is a further complication, for the fat of degeneration is sometimes carried away from its original seat, and deposited in other spots in the form of a fatty infiltration, or of storage-fat.

54. When fat is present in considerable quantity it happens not infrequently that crystalline products separate out from it. The so-called 'fat-crystals' appear as feathery needles, grouped together in tufted bunches (Fig. 10 *b*). They are often described as needles of **margaric acid**. Whether they really contain margaric acid is doubtful. It is known that equal parts of palmitic and stearic acid would give a mixture having the same composition as is ascribed to margaric acid: and further that palmitic, stearic, and oleic acids in combination with glycerin (as tripalmitin, tristearin, and triolein) form the chief components of ordinary animal fat. It is therefore doubtful whether margaric acid or trimargarin really exists as a distinct component of animal fat at all. These fat-crystals may form in fatty products of disintegration as well as in normal fat-cells. In the latter case they are only produced *post mortem*.

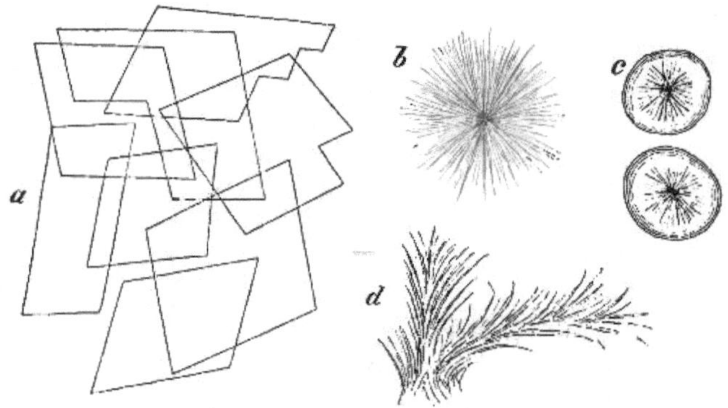

FIG. 10. FAT-CRYSTALS. (× 300)

a cholesterin-tablets *b* free tuft of margarin-needles
c tuft inclosed in fat-cells *d* feathery needles of 'margaric acid' or margarin

In masses of fatty detritus it is very common to find what is called **cholesterin** (properly cholestearin). This forms thin transparent rhombic tablets (Fig. 10 *a*), often notched at the angles. If these tablets are present in quantity, they may often be recognised by their lustre with the naked eye alone. They are soluble in hot alcohol, ether, and chloroform, in oils, and in the sodium compounds of the two bile-acids (glycocholic and taurocholic). Treated with sulphuric acid the crystals become purplish red, rusty, or violet, at their edges. The same coloration appears still better on treatment with iodine. Nothing is known of the mode in which cholesterin is formed. It is said to exist as a normal constituent in the brain (GAMGEE).

SCHULZE and BARBIERI (*Journ. f. prakt. Chem.* 25, 1882) regard cholesterin as an intermediate product of vegetable metabolism and a constant component of vegetable cells. Cholesterins of various composition are known, so that the term seems to indicate rather a chemical *genus* than a definite substance.

CHAPTER XII.

MUCOID AND COLLOID DEGENERATION.

55. The **mucoid degeneration** of the tissues has its physiological type in the mucus-secretion of the mucous membranes and mucous glands.

As is well known, the epithelium of the mucous membranes contains so-called goblet-cells (EIMER). These look like goblets filled to overflowing with a transparent substance. This latter is mucus formed from the cell-protoplasm. The epithelial cells of the mucous glands are similar. They swell up when about to secrete mucus; the central parts become transparent, and the granules of the protoplasm become aggregated into groups or strings. The so-called mucus-corpuscles in the salivary secretion, with their glassy contents and tremulous granules, are merely leucocytes which have undergone mucoid metamorphosis. The mucous substance formed from the protoplasm of the cell may be extruded, and the cell may recover: in other cases the cell perishes.

The same process of mucus-formation takes place under pathological conditions. For example, in catarrh of the mucous membrane we find that the increased secretion of mucus depends on an increased mucus-forming power in the lining epithelial cells, as well as in the cells of the mucous glands. Investigation shows that in cylindrical epithelium the goblet-cells (Fig. 11, 6) are increased in number. In the secretion also we may find cells in a state of complete mucoid degeneration; they are transformed into glassy masses containing a few scattered granules (3 and 5). In other cells (7) the mucus may take the form of lumps of various sizes, enclosed within the unchanged cell-protoplasm.

The epithelia of pathological tissues may like the normal ones undergo mucoid change. Typical goblet-cells are occasionally found in the epithelial lining of ovarian and intestinal cysts. In certain forms of cancer, the majority of the epithelial cells undergo mucoid degeneration.

The fibrous tissues, like the epithelia, are also liable to undergo mucoid degeneration. Thus connective tissue, cartilage, bone,

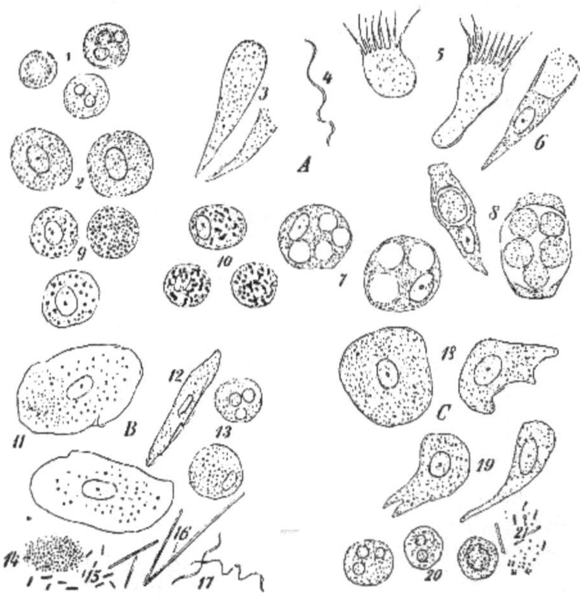

FIG. 11. CATARRHAL SECRETIONS FROM VARIOUS MUCOUS MEMBRANES. (× 400)

A from cylindrical epithelium, *B* from the mouth, *C* from the bladder. 1, round-cells (pus corpuscles). 2, large round-cells with clear nuclei from the nose. 3, mucoid cylindrical cells from the nose. 4, *Spirillum* from the nose. 5, mucoid ciliated cells from the nose. 6, goblet-cell from the trachea. 7, round-cells with mucus-masses from the nose. 8, epithelial cells containing pus corpuscles from the nose. 9, fatty cells in chronic laryngeal and pharyngeal catarrh. 10, cells from sputum containing soot-pigment. 11 and 12, squamous epithelium from the mouth. 13, mucus-corpuscles. 14, micrococci. 15, *Bacterium termo*. 16, *Leptothrix buccalis*. 17, *Spirochaeta denticola*. 18, superficial cells from the bladder; 19, deeper layer. 20, pus corpuscles. 21, *Schizomycetes* or bacteria.

adipose tissue, marrow, sarcomatous tissue, may all become mucoid, and so assume a jelly-like translucent appearance. In these tissues it is usually the ground-substance which is transformed. The fibrous constituents lose their structure and become homogeneous. The tissue-cells may persist, or become fatty, or they may take part in the mucoid change. The final product is a hyaline mass recalling the original tissue only by virtue of a few stray fibrous shreds, or single cells, or groups of cells, scattered through it.

Mucus swells up readily in water; acetic acid makes it coagulate; alcohol makes it turbid, white and opaque.

56. **Colloid degeneration** is closely akin to mucoid degeneration; for here too the essence of the process is the metamorphosis of an albuminoid substance. The details of the chemical changes which occur are not known. The material which constitutes the colloid substance is derived from the epithelial cells. In aged persons, a certain amount of colloid change in the thyroid gland may be regarded as physiological. The parenchyma of the gland is full of large and small spherules, which on section have a translucent sago-like appearance. They are generally yellowish or brownish in colour, and of the consistence of firm jelly. If the colloid change has gone on to a pathological extent, this translucent substance may form the greater part of the mass of the gland. It may even lead to a marked increase in its size, forming a colloidal goître. Microscopic examination shows that the colloid mass is homogeneous. It encloses but few cellular elements, and these for the most part at the periphery, where the colloid change is in progress. Sometimes a large continuous patch of degenerate tissue may be produced by the coalescence of smaller ones. The formation of the colloid substance is indicated by the appearance of minute homogeneous spherules in the cells of the acini. These spherules escape from the cells, or become free when the cells themselves break up. When they come into contact, they coalesce to form the homogeneous colloid substance.

Colloid spherules, exactly like those just described, are found in the tubules of morbidly altered kidneys. At times large masses of coalescent spherules occur in cystic degeneration of the tubules. In the prostate gland similar formations also occur.

Colloid substance is distinguishable from mucus by the fact that acetic acid does not induce coagulation, while alcohol and chromic acid produce no turbidity.

In VIRCHOW's opinion, the homogeneous spherules, while contained in the cells, are not actually composed of true colloid substance. The latter is formed from them after they run together, in virtue of a special chemical transformation. VIRCHOW describes the spherules as modified protoplasm. Colloid substance is probably a resultant of several albuminoid bodies. See VIRCHOW (*Virch. Arch.* vol. 1), WAGNER (*Arch. f. phys. Heilk.* 1856, 1866), EBERTH (*Virch. Arch.* vol. 21).

CHAPTER XIII.

AMYLOID DEGENERATION AND AMYLOID CONCRETIONS.

57. **Amyloid degeneration** is a peculiar degenerative process, which is apt to affect the connective tissues, and is progressive in character. It leads to the deposit of a special albuminoid body (the amyloid substance) in the affected tissues: these therefore increase in bulk and assume under the microscope a peculiar uniform semi-translucent appearance. The affection may occur in any of the organs, but it is specially common in the spleen, liver, kidneys, intestines, and lymphatic glands.

When sufficiently intense the morbid change is recognisable with the naked eye; the part looks semi-translucent, so that it is described as 'waxy' or 'lardaceous', *i.e.* like the fat of fried bacon. If the change is confined to scattered patches, as it often is in the spleen, these look like grains of boiled sago or tapioca: hence the name 'sago-spleen'. In other cases, the process affects the spleen-tissue uniformly. The whole organ grows large and firm to the touch; while the section presents the peculiar translucent lardaceous appearance. Like appearances are found in the liver. The kidneys too may undergo considerable increase in size, and present in patches or throughout the lardaceous character, becoming at the same time firmer in consistence. In other cases the translucent patches are so small as not to be readily noticed; the possible presence of amyloid substance is however often indicated by changes of another kind, such as fatty degeneration. In the intestine the degeneration is seldom recognisable without optical or chemical examination. The same is true of the organs that are less liable to the change, such as the heart, the great vessels, the thyroid gland, &c.

58. The amyloid substance so deposited in the tissues in uniform shiny patches exhibits a peculiar reaction with iodine, and with some of the aniline colours. A solution of iodine in water, or better in potassium iodide and water, when poured on

the tissue to be tested, stains the amyloid substance a dark brownish red or mahogany colour. If added to a section under the microscope the staining is a bright brownish red, while the unaffected tissue remains pale yellow. Where the degeneration is extreme the tissue may become almost woody in consistence, and then the staining may be violet or blue or greenish. If the ordinary iodine-stained tissue be treated with very dilute sulphuric acid, the amyloid patches take on a darker brown, or become violet, blue, or greenish: but the reaction is generally imperfect. Methyl-aniline or aniline-violet stain the amyloid substance bright ruby-red, and the healthy tissue blue or dark indigo.

The peculiar iodine-reaction was first observed by VIRCHOW, the discoverer of the amyloid substance. This reaction led him to consider the amyloid substance as a non-nitrogenous body allied to cellulose and starch. Cellulose, when treated with iodine and strong sulphuric acid, is stained bright blue. Starch with iodine alone gives an ultramarine tint. For this reason VIRCHOW called the new body 'amyloid'. It was not until some years later that FRIEDREICH and KEKULÉ proved the amyloid substance to be nitrogenous, to be in fact an albuminoid body. The special reaction of the amyloid substance enables us to detect its presence in the tissues, even when to the eye it is not differentiated from them. In examining fresh specimens in a cursory way, the only precaution necessary is to see that the surface is washed free from blood: the red colour of the blood blended with the yellow of the iodine may simulate the characteristic brownish-red staining.

The amyloid substance is very slightly acted on by acids or alkalies. Alcohol and chromic acid do not alter it at all: and it has the power of withstanding putrid decomposition for a long time. It is not dissolved by gastric juice at the temperature of the body.

Amyloid degeneration was not altogether unknown before VIRCHOW'S researches. ROKITANSKY had previously introduced the names bacon-liver or lardaceous liver, waxy liver, bacon-spleen, sago-spleen. But it was VIRCHOW who first investigated the nature of the amyloid substance, first of all in amyloid concretions (Art. 61), afterwards in degenerated tissues; and he discovered the iodine reaction (*Virch. Arch.* vols. 6, 8). FRIEDREICH and KEKULÉ first showed that the substance was nitrogenous (*Virch. Arch.* vol. 16), which was confirmed by RUDNEFF and KUEHNE (*Virch. Arch.* vol. 33). The literature of the subject is fully given by KYBER, who has also made numerous additions to our knowledge regarding its occurrence (*Die amyloide Degeneration* Dorpat 1871, and *Virch. Arch.* vol. 81). JÜRGENS first described the colour-reaction with iodised methyl-aniline (*Virch. Arch.* vol. 65); CORNIL studied the reactions with other aniline colours (*Arch. de physiol.* 1874). DICKINSON showed that a characteristic blue colour is imparted to the amyloid substance by sulphate of indigo.

59. The amyloid substance is either formed or deposited in the fibrous textures of the blood-vessels, and in the walls of the smaller vessels especially.

If a microscopic section of an amyloid liver be so treated as to bring out the minuter changes in its structure, it is not hard to show that the seat of the affection is in the capillary walls, that is, in the periendothelial fibrous tissue. The endothelium is thickly coated on its outer aspect with a uniform glassy layer, here and there broken up into lumps (Fig. 12); this is the amyloid deposit. The liver-cells may remain unchanged between the amyloid masses, or they may be misshapen and partly atrophied. They very often contain fat.

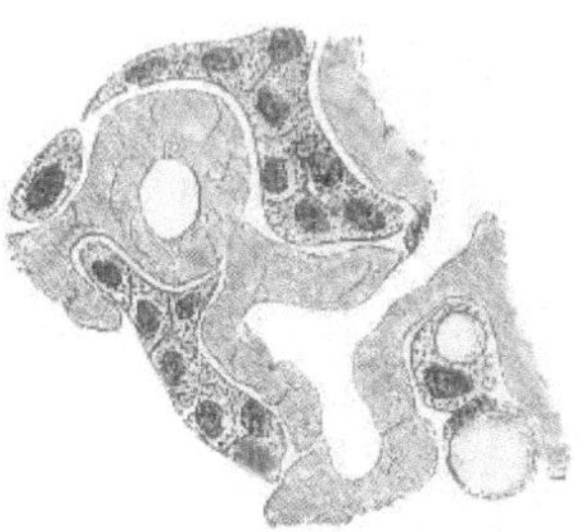

FIG. 12. AMYLOID DEGENERATION OF LIVER CAPILLARIES. (*Section treated with perosmic acid:* × 300)

If the afferent vessels be examined, it will be found that they too exhibit amyloid patches, especially in their middle coat.

The appearances in an amyloid kidney are exactly similar (Fig. 13). A good section shows as before that the formation of the homogeneous deposit occurs mainly in the vessel-walls. The

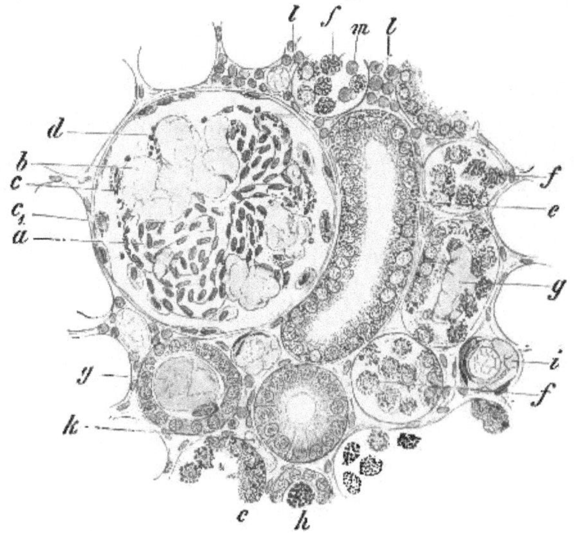

FIG. 13. SECTION OF AN AMYLOID KIDNEY.
(*Treated with Müller's fluid and perosmic acid:* × 300)

- *a* normal capillary loop
- *b* amyloid capillary loop
- *c* fatty epithelium of the glomerulus
- c_1 fatty epithelium of the capsule
- *d* oil-drops on the capillary wall
- *e* fatty epithelial cell *in situ*
- *f* loosened fatty epithelial cells
- *g* hyaline coagula (forming 'casts')
- *h* fatty cast in section
- *i* amyloid artery
- *k* amyloid capillary
- *l* infiltration of connective tissue with leucocytes
- *m* round-cells (leucocytes) inside a uriniferous tubule

walls of the vascular loops in the glomeruli (*b*) are greatly swollen and homogeneous in structure, and the arteries (*i*), veins, and capillaries (*k*) of the parenchyma show traces of amyloid deposit.

In other parts, such as the intestinal mucous membrane, the appearances are of the same kind. The vascular system however is not invariably the chief seat of deposit; the connective tissue is often chiefly and directly affected. In the lymphatic glands and the spleen (EBERTH), it is the fibrous trabecular network which suffers most; in striated muscles the *perimysium internum* and the sarcolemma (ZIEGLER). In glandular organs with a *tunica propria* (*e.g.* the mucous glands and kidneys), this latter may undergo degeneration and become greatly thickened.

The above account of the common seat of amyloid deposit differs essentially from that given in various text-books (*e.g.* RINDFLEISCH's) and memoirs. Most authors assert that in glandular organs the chief seat of amyloid formation is in the gland-cells, that is, in the epithelial elements. ZIEGLER has not succeeded in convincing himself that this is the case. In no one of seven specimens of amyloid liver could he find, on the carefullest examination, that the liver-cells had undergone amyloid degeneration. The cells were always recognisable, though at times greatly atrophied and compressed by the interposed deposits. The examination of mucous glands and kidneys yielded like results. He is therefore constrained to agree with WAGNER (*Arch. d. Heilkunde* II 1861), EBERTH (*Virch. Arch.* vol. 80), HESCHL (*Wiener Sitzungsberichte* vol. 74), and others—who regard the connective tissue as the primary seat of amyloid formation, and deny that the epithelium is commonly concerned in it. ZIEGLER does not go so far as to say that epithelial cells are incapable of amyloid change; but he is sure that even in extreme cases of amyloid disease they may remain unaffected. The notion that the liver-cells are commonly affected is due to the fact that they have been overlooked among the amyloid flakes and patches which surround them. The iodine method is probably to be blamed for this, for it fails to bring the liver-cells distinctly into view. Ordinary staining-reagents and perosmic acid are much more useful in this respect than iodine.

ZIEGLER had recently an opportunity of examining a very interesting case of amyloid disease. The patient was a woman of about fifty, who had died of heart-failure. On post-mortem examination it was found that the heart, all the mucous membranes, the peritoneum, tongue, and lungs were amyloid. The pericardium and endocardium were everywhere thickened and beset with numerous translucent gristly nodules as large as millet-seeds. Similar nodules in vast numbers were found in the peritoneum, and in lesser number in the heart-muscle, the *muscularis mucosae* of the intestine, the *mucosa* and *submucosa* of many of the mucous membranes, and in the lungs. In addition to these nodules the heart-wall (and especially that of the auricles) was traversed by thick seemingly fibrous bands. The *submucosa* of the small intestine was for the most part transformed into a firm bacon-like tissue. The nodules and also the dense thickenings were composed of a uniform substance, either structureless or showing traces of coalescent homogeneous blocks. This was deposited in the walls of the vessels, and in the connective tissue. The vessel-walls were in some places thickened ten- to twenty-fold. When the margins of the affected patches were examined microscopically, it seemed as if the homogeneous substance had been directly produced from the ground-substance of the connective tissue, by a process of swelling and condensation. Some of the homogeneous masses yielded the iodine reaction, others did not.

60. The consequences of amyloid degeneration, as regards the functional efficiency and general condition of the affected organ,

show themselves in two ways. On the one hand the structure is profoundly altered, on the other the epithelial elements of the organ become secondarily diseased. Amyloid change is essentially a degeneration. The connective tissues are permanently altered, for the amyloid substance being but slightly soluble does not disappear again when once deposited. It is obvious that a foreign element of this kind must seriously interfere with the functions of the affected organs, such as the kidney, or intestine.

The morbid change in the vessel-wall often leads to narrowing and closure of the vessel, and so to permanent disturbance of the circulation. These are not without effect on the epithelial elements: they speedily become fatty. And inasmuch as the fibrous framework of the organ is at the same time increasing in size and volume, the gland-cells are compressed and so tend to disappear altogether. In the liver such misshapen and atrophied cells, as well as others in a state of fatty degeneration, are very often met with. In the kidney the fatty changes in the epithelium (Fig. 13 *e, f*) form a striking and characteristic accompaniment of amyloid degeneration.

In the spleen and lymphatic glands the lymphoid cells are likewise apt to perish, atrophied and fatty, under the pressure of the swollen and altered trabecular network. In muscle the contractile substance vanishes, as the amyloid masses in the connective tissue increase and multiply.

61. Amyloid degeneration, as above described, is generally a process affecting several organs at the same time; or when it happens to affect only one, it takes the form of a change extending throughout the entire organ. But in addition to this diffused form we find a more local one, presenting the appearance either of circumscribed foci of degeneration, or of **amyloid concretions.**

These localised amyloid formations occur, so far as we know, only in tissues which have already undergone morbid change. They are especially apt to follow in the wake of inflammations, either early in the process of granulation, or later when cicatricial tissue has been formed. They are also found in tumours which are undergoing retrogressive change. Small single foci may be formed in the affected tissue, or they may be confined to the walls of the vessels. In other cases the greater part of the tissue degenerates together; nodular patches are formed, consisting almost wholly of amyloid substance, and often assuming a woody hardness of texture. Such formations have been observed in the conjunctiva when altered by old inflammation, in syphilitic scars of the tongue and larynx, in diseased lymphatic glands, in ulcers of the leg, in tumours of the larynx and stomach, and in cartilage in the course of degeneration (VIRCHOW).

In many cases homogeneous bodies exhibiting the amyloid reaction are obviously formed in the exudation-products of inflammation or haemorrhage. For example, the so-called tube-casts of the kidney, formed in the tubules by a singular transformation of transuded liquid and shed epithelium, show not infrequently the amyloid reaction if they have lain long *in situ*. In the remains of old haemorrhages amyloid bodies have often been found (Fig. 14 *b*).

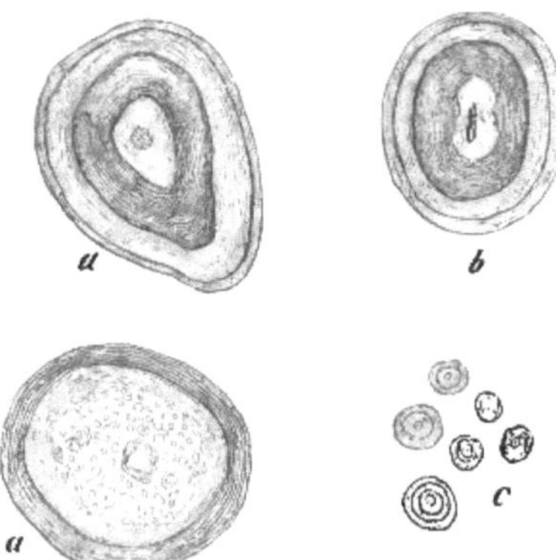

FIG. 14. *CORPORA AMYLACEA.*

a stratified concretion from the prostate
b *corpus amylaceum* from an old haemorrhagic infarct of the lung
c *corpora amylacea* from the spinal cord (× 400)

They often enclose a foreign substance, such as a crystal of haematoidin. These bodies are called amyloid concretions or *corpora amylacea*. They are found under normal conditions in the central nervous system, especially in the ependyma of the ventricles. It was here that VIRCHOW first discovered them. They take the form of small more or less clearly stratified spherules (Fig. 14 *c*). At times they may be found abundantly in morbidly altered brain-substance, and in cerebral tumours. Corpora amylacea are also very common in the prostate gland. They lie in the lumen of the acini and are of considerable size: often indeed they may be recognised by the naked eye as brown grains upon the surface of a section. They are distinctly stratified (Fig. 14 *a*), except towards the centre.

These localised amyloid formations, and especially those originating in tube-casts and old extravasations of blood (Fig. 14 *b*), serve to prove that amyloid substance may arise from a direct metamorphosis of the albumen of blood and of epithelium. The prostatic concretions, when they really are amyloid (and this is not always the case), are probably to be regarded as modified cell-products.

A large number of memoirs have dealt with the question of localised amyloid change. KYBER (*loc. cit.*), LEBER (*Arch. für Ophthalm.* XIX, XXV), HIPPEL (*ibid.* XXV), VON BECKER (*Amyl. degen. tarsi* Helsingfors 1876) refer to amyloid formations in the eyelid. FRIEDREICH (*Virch. Arch.* vols. 9, 10) and ZAHN (*ibid.* vol. 72) found amyloid bodies in the lung; LANGHANS in cancer-nodules (*ibid.* vol. 38); BUROW (*Langenbeck's Arch.* XVIII) in tumours of the larynx, &c. On prostatic concretions see PAULIZKY (*Virch. Arch.* vol. 16).

ZIEGLER discovered amyloid bodies in syphilitic scars (*Virch. Arch.* vol. 65), in a haemorrhagic infarct of the lung which had healed, and in a cancer of the stomach.

62. As to the **causes** and the nature **of amyloid degeneration**, there is little to say that is quite definite or quite certain. We know of course in what circumstances it is apt to occur, namely in cachectic conditions of the system. On the other hand, we do not know to what alterations in normal metabolism the morbid process owes its special character. The forms of cachexia which lead to extensive amyloid change are in particular tuberculosis, syphilis, chronic destructive ostitis or periostitis, chronic dysentery (coeliac flux), and leukaemia; while the cancerous cachexia seldom tends to favour it. Amyloid degeneration may however occur without previous disease. Some of COHNHEIM'S researches show (*Virch. Arch.* vol. 54) that the degeneration may become developed in two to three months.

Amyloid change extending to several organs is a local disorder conditioned by general causes. The amyloid substance does not exist in the blood, yet the material out of which it is developed is derived from the blood. It would appear that reduced vital activity of the tissues dependent on general cachexia favours the formation of the substance. We may perhaps provisionally picture to ourselves the formation of this peculiar substance, as due to a combination of an albuminoid body from the blood with certain components of the tissues: or we may regard it as a modification of the albumen of the blood, separating out from the latter in consequence of some abnormal metabolism in the cachectic patient.

In local amyloid formations, the substances metamorphosed are partly albumen from the blood (concretions formed in extravasations), partly albumen derived from epithelial cells (tube-casts and prostatic concretions). In the latter case the special metamorphosis is effected, without the co-operation of living tissue, in albumen which has lain for a time in the tissues without being of them. Here the conditions must be of a purely local nature.

VIRCHOW (*Cellular Pathology*) and KYBER (*Virch. Arch.* vol. 81) have compared the amyloid degeneration of tissues to the process of chalky deposit, and the comparison seems a good one. In both cases we probably have a tissue whose nutrition is somehow lowered; a substance brought to the tissue by the blood; and an intimate combination between this substance and a substance pre-existing *in loco*. WAGNER (*Handbuch d. allgem. Pathologie* 1874 p. 417) considers the lardaceous material we have described to be due to a retrogressive metamorphosis of albuminoids, forming in fact an intermediate stage between these bodies and fat. DICKINSON argues that it is of the nature of fibrin (blood-albumen) 'modified by loss of alkali or gain of acid' (*Trans. Path. Soc.* 1879).

A statistical analysis of the causes of amyloid degeneration is given by HENNINGS (Inaug. Diss. Kiel 1880). He makes out that phthisis and suppuration of bone hold the first rank among the aetiological conditions. The spleen is oftenest diseased; after that follow in order the kidneys, liver, intestine, stomach, suprarenal capsules, pancreas, lymphatic glands, thyroid gland, aorta, lungs, ovaries, uterus. Somewhat similar analyses are given by FAGGE (*Trans. Path. Soc.* 1876) and TURNER (*ibid.* 1879).

CHAPTER XIV.

HYALINE DEGENERATION OF THE FIBROUS TISSUES.

63. **Hyaline** (or vitreous) **degeneration** of the fibrous tissues resembles amyloid degeneration in its superficial appearance as well as in its seat; but it does not give the special and peculiar reactions of the amyloid substance. It occurs chiefly in the adventitious tissue of the arteries. The adventitia becomes transformed into a shining, translucent, strongly-refracting substance, increasing at the same time in thickness. Water has no effect on this substance; iodine stains it pale yellow; ether and chloroform give no reaction. It thus resembles in many respects the colloid substance. It is specially common in the vessels of the brain and of the lymphatic glands (WIEGER). Apart from the blood-vessels a hyaline thickening is also observed in the stroma of tumours, in inflammatory hyperplasias, especially in those of hereditary syphilis (such as occur in the liver, for example) and in structureless membranes like the hyaloid membrane of the eye. As to the nature of the change nothing is known. Disturbances of the circulation (WIEGER), and inflammations of the affected regions, have been mentioned as exciting causes.

WIEGER under the guidance of VON RECKLINGHAUSEN has lately examined and described the hyaline degeneration of the lymphatic glands (*Virch. Arch.* vol. 78). It seems to be very common in these organs. Memoirs on the hyaline degeneration of the cerebral vessels have been published by ARNDT (*Virch. Arch.* vol. 41), NEELSEN (*Arch. d. Heilkunde* XVII), EPPINGER (*Vierteljahrsschrift f. pract. Heilk.* Prague 1875), LUBIMOFF (*Arch. f. Psychiatrie* 1874), and others. The degeneration is found in the central nervous system in connexion with various disorders.

PETERS has quite recently (*Virch. Arch.* vol. 87) made a series of researches in VON RECKLINGHAUSEN'S laboratory on hyaline degeneration, and he manages to bring under this head all sorts of diverse changes and processes. Thus he includes under it inflammatory coagulations within and without the blood-vessels, coagulative necrosis of the epithelia in diphtheritic inflammation, homogeneous coagulation in exuded fluids, the formation of false membranes, the mucoid metamorphoses of the epithelial cells of mucous membrane, and thrombi in lymphatic vessels,—in brief everything that has a hyaline look. This is a mere uncritical agglomeration of things that have nothing in common. We may perhaps be unable to distinguish with certainty the exact chemical and physical processes which lead to the formation of homogeneous masses in the various tissues and liquids; but this does not justify us in affirming that no distinction is at all possible.

The case referred to in Art. 59 has great interest, as bearing on the discrimination of hyaline degeneration in fibrous tissues. It shows that hyaline change is near akin to amyloid change; and that in the former as in the latter an albuminoid may be deposited in the tissues in the form of solid lustrous masses. Whether the hyaline degeneration of the vessel-walls, observed in various conditions, has always the same significance—is as yet an open question.

GULL and SUTTON (*Med. chir. Trans.* 1872) have described a 'hyalin-fibrous' degeneration of the blood-vessels in connection with chronic renal disease. KLEIN (*Trans. Path. Soc.* 1877) has described and figured hyaline changes in the arterioles in typhoid fever and in scarlatina.

CHAPTER XV.

INFILTRATION OF THE TISSUES WITH SALTS.

64. **Petrification** or **incrustation** is a process of transformation characterised by the deposit in a tissue of various salts derived ultimately from the blood.

In by far the greater number of cases the deposit consists of carbonates and phosphates of calcium, with a small quantity of the magnesium salts: it is in fact calcareous or chalky.

As we know, calcareous deposition takes place in special regions as a normal physiological process. The formation of true bone is always preceded by the deposit of calcareous salts in the cartilaginous structures first laid down. This deposit takes the form of minute granules, which on magnification look like grains of dust or irregular crumbs, and they are seen to lie chiefly in the matrix-substance and cell-capsules of the cartilage. If the grains lie thick together, they give the part a whitish colour and a firm consistence.

In the same way as under normal conditions, but in the most various regions of the body, we may have a morbid deposition or precipitation of calcareous salts in the tissues. Experience shows that the tissues affected are either already necrosed, as in the case of caseous lymphatic glands, dead parasites, thrombi, and dead foetuses (lithopaedia),—or have been seriously stinted in their nutrition. This latter is the case in fatty degeneration of the tunica media of the arteries, or in fatty degeneration of tumours such as uterine fibroids. The cause of calcareous deposits is thus a local one. The calcium-salts dissolved in the blood are not simply precipitated and retained by the tissue, but they proceed to form solid compounds with the albuminoids.

Commencing calcification is not recognisable by the naked eye. When the deposit becomes more dense the tissue turns white. At the same time it often becomes extremely hard and cannot be cut with the knife. In other cases it becomes in colour and consistence more like mortar.

LITTEN affirms (*Der haemorrhagische Infarct* 1879) that calcification depends on a necrotic modification of albumen, possessing a special chemical affinity for lime-salts. KYBER asserts (*Virch. Arch.* vol. 81) that the lime-salts combine with the fatty acids, as well as with the albuminoids.

65. Calcification invades the cells of a tissue as well as the ground-substance. Thus ganglion-cells (Fig. 15) which have ceased to live in consequence of some brain-affection may become impregnated with lime-salts. Shining calcareous spherules are formed, which fill out the contour of the cell and its prolongations.

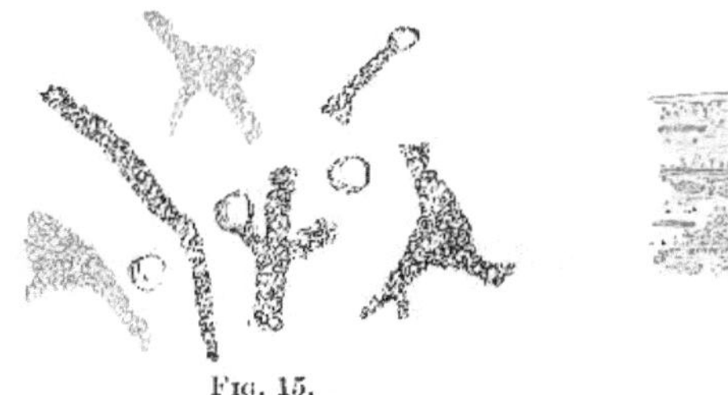

FIG. 15.

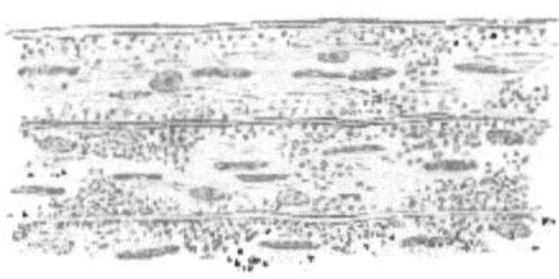

FIG. 16.

FIG. 15. CALCIFIED GANGLION-CELLS.
(*From the brain of a hemiplegic idiot with unilateral hydrocephalus.*)

FIG. 16. CALCIFICATION OF THE TUNICA MEDIA OF THE AORTA.

When an artery is affected, the cells as well as the ground-substance become calcified. Small shining granules are deposited in the latter, which at length thickly infiltrate the tissue (Fig. 16). Simple calcification does not produce any alteration in the apparent structure. The tissue is petrified as it stands, so to speak, without destruction or transformation of its form and texture. It is thus easy to distinguish histologically between calcification and ossification.

In tissues altered by inflammation, such as tuberculous lymphatic glands, fibrous false membranes or adhesions, as well as in certain tumours of the brain (psammomata), we find at times so-called **chalky concretions**. They are stratified bodies having an organic basis, in which lime-salts have been deposited. Fig. 17 represents some of these concretions: *a* comes from an omentum thickened and deformed, and adherent, in consequence of chronic inflammation; *b* from a tuberculous lymphatic gland. The several layers of the stratified concretion have a uniform shining appearance.

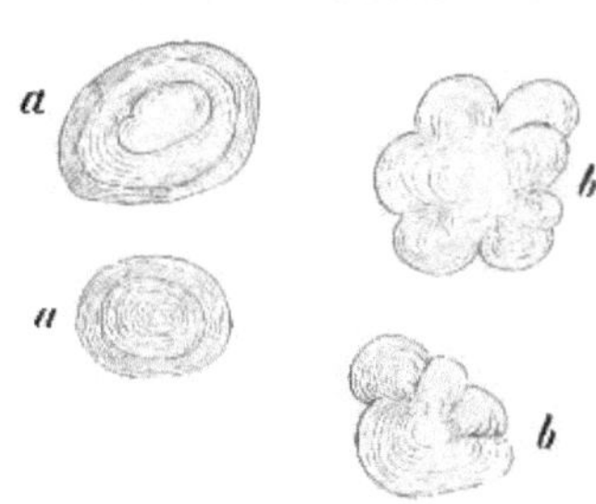

FIG. 17. CHALKY CONCRETIONS.
a concretions from an inflamed omentum
b from a lymphatic gland altered by inflammation

66. In **gout** we find deposits of urates, chiefly of urate of sodium, together with carbonates and phosphates. The deposition is apt to occur paroxysmally, especially in the metatarso-phalangeal joint of the great toe, but not infrequently in other joints also. Shining white masses (chalk-stones or tophi) are thus formed in the ligaments and cartilages of the joints, and even in the bones. These may also occur in the arteries, endocardium, skin, and kidneys. The deposit is usually in the form of needle-like crystals (RINDFLEISCH), or amorphous granules. It is said that the cells are the first to exhibit the deposit, the ground-substance being invaded secondarily (CORNIL and RANVIER).

CHAPTER XVI.

FORMATION OF PIGMENT IN THE TISSUES.

67. The fibrous as well as the epithelial tissues, in certain regions, contain a **normal pigment**. It lies within the cells in the form of yellow, brownish, or black granules; or the cells may seem more or less uniformly impregnated and stained. Of the pigmented epithelia the best examples are the deepest layer of the rete Malpighii, and the retinal epithelium. In the former the granules are mostly yellow or brown, in the latter they are black (melanin). When the coloration of the skin is more marked, pigment is found in the other cellular layers of the rete. Among fibrous tissues the pia mater, the choroid, the sclerotic, and the cutis are the most frequently pigmented: and brown or yellow granules are likewise found in the connective-tissue cells of the heart-muscle.

These pigmentations may become more marked under pathological conditions. Thus in Addison's disease, in the course of a general disorder leading to profound cachexia and associated as a rule with changes in the supra-renal bodies, the normal pigment of the skin increases and the consequent colour-changes are very pronounced (*cutis aenea* or bronzing). So too in atrophic conditions of the heart, the normal pigment is markedly increased. In the voluntary muscles also when they pass into atrophy, yellow pigment is frequently discoverable.

The highest degree of pathological pigmentation is met with in morbid new growths, such as tumours (naevi, melano-carcinomata, melano-sarcomata). The amount of pigment may become so great that the tissue looks uniformly and intensely black.

The pigment lies usually within the cells of the tissue, less often in the intercellular substance. In either case, as above remarked, it may take the form of yellow, brown, or even black granules; or of diffuse staining of the protoplasm. Of its mode of formation we know nothing. It is possible that the colouring-matter is derived from the blood, but we are unable to determine in what way the derivation is effected.

7—2

LAYCOCK (*Med. chir. Review* I, 1861) discusses and classifies the various forms of morbid pigmentation: he gives full references to previous papers on the subject.

GUSSENBAUER has lately attempted (*Virch. Arch.* vol. 63) to refer the production of melanin in pigmented tumours to a modification of the colouring-matter of the blood. He thinks the blood-vessels of the tumour become here and there thrombosed; the colouring-matter of the blood escapes from them by diffusion, saturates the tissue, and is ultimately precipitated in granular form. LANGHANS (*Virch. Arch.* vol. 49) had previously sought to derive the pigment of tumours from cells containing blood-corpuscles (Art. 68).

According to KUNKEL (*Sitzungsb. der phys. med. Gesell. Würzburg* 1881), it is possible to isolate from melanotic tumours a pigment containing iron. This argues that the pigment is derived from the blood; but we cannot as yet say by what process it is produced. It is not related to haematin, bilirubin, or hydrobilirubin, as the spectroscope shows. It seems doubtful whether the escape of the colouring-matter from the blood-vessels always occurs in the way described by GUSSENBAUER. The diffused staining of individual cells may perhaps suggest that the colouring-matter first infiltrates the cell, and then breaks up into granules.

68. **Haematogenous pigments** are such as are demonstrably derived from the colouring-matter of the blood. They generally originate in blood which has escaped from the vessels. More rarely the change to pigment occurs in blood which is still circulating. As is well-known, the colour-changes recognisable by the eye take place very quickly in small extravasations as well as large. In the skin, such extravasations become first brown, then blue, then green, then yellow. Where small haemorrhages have occurred in the deeper tissues, such as the peritoneum, pleura, or lungs, we find even long afterwards brown, or grey, or black spots and patches. Larger haemorrhages (apoplexies) into the substance of the brain or lungs take on after a time a rusty brown colour; and still later leave only a dirty yellow or yellowish brown staining. All these colour-changes correspond to definite chemical and physical transformations of haemoglobin.

Wherever in the tissues or in a cavity of the body a haemorrhage may have occurred, there ensues a series of changes in the escaped blood of which the following are the most important.

One part of the blood, including red cells as well as plasma, may be re-absorbed by the lymphatics and carried off unchanged.

Another portion of the corpuscles may become in a way dissolved; their haemoglobin diffuses from them into the surrounding tissues, and the pale residual stroma breaks up and disappears. It is this diffused and altered colouring-matter (or haematin) which gives rise to the colour-changes in cutaneous extravasations, as it passes through various transformations. The transformed pigments (which are similar to the biliary colouring-matters) are partially re-absorbed and at length excreted in the urine (urobilinuria): another part crystallises in the tissues, and forms the orange or ruby-red rhombic tablets and needles known as haematoidin-crystals (Fig. 18 *B*). These are very frequently found as the residue of old haemorrhages, such as occur in the brain: they may remain a long time in the tissues without change.

A third portion of the corpuscles shrink up or crumble down into brown granular masses. This is especially the case in the large extravasations forming so-called haematomata. These masses become in part transformed into brown amorphous pigment. This lies free in the tissues, and often becomes darker in colour with age.

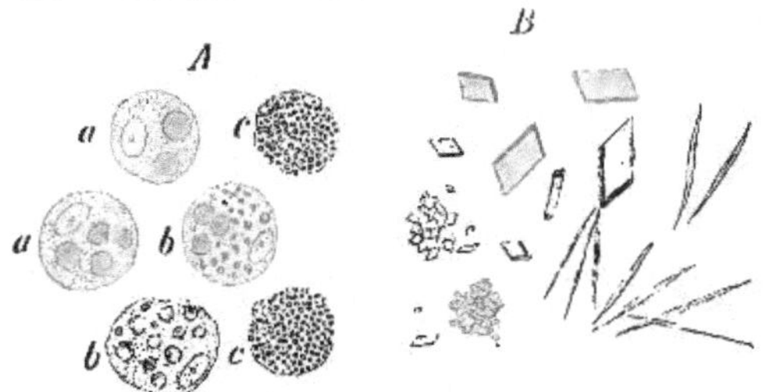

FIG. 18. (× 500)

A CELLS CONTAINING RED BLOOD-CORPUSCLES: in *a* the fragments are few but large, in *b* and *c* they are numerous and minute

B RHOMBIC TABLETS AND NEEDLES OF HAEMATOIDIN

A fourth and that the greater portion of the corpuscles and the products of their disintegration is taken up by leucocytes (Art. 114), which gather in large numbers round the seat of extravasation and even penetrate into it. The cells become in this way corpuscle- and pigment-carriers (Fig. 18 *A a* and *b*). The transformation of the haematin into brown pigment is completed within these cells, the corpuscles breaking up into minute granules (Fig. 18 *A b* and *c*). The pigment may be set free again by the disintegration of the carrier-cells. Probably the cells have also the power of eliminating it, without themselves perishing.

These various modes of transformation of the blood-corpuscles very frequently go on at the same time in the same extravasation. Their ultimate result is, in the first instance, a local discoloration, due to pigment partly amorphous and partly crystalline in character. Secondary pigmentation of remote organs such as the lymphatic glands, the spleen, and the liver, may follow upon this, owing to absorption of the pigment by the lymphatics.

The formation of pigment in blood which is actually circulating is not carried beyond the first stage (the breaking up of the red corpuscles) within the vessels (Arts. 262 and 268): the completion of the process is effected outside the vessels. The pigments just described are only in part organic derivatives of the colouring-matter of the blood (like haematin and haematoidin). A considerable part is composed of an inorganic iron-compound; namely, the hydrated sesquioxide (KUNKEL). This is especially the case in large extravasations, where the haemoglobin is decomposed on the spot. The contained iron being thereupon set free in the form of oxide, remains where it is and forms yellow or brownish flakes.

It may be of use to mention that *haemoglobin* is the unchanged colouring-matter of the blood as it exists in the living corpuscles. *Haematin* is the coloured constituent obtained when haemoglobin is decomposed (*e.g.* by boiling); the other constituent being a proteid body. *Haematoidin* is formed when the decomposition is carried still further; it is identical with bilirubin (see GAMGEE, *Physiol. Chem.* I, 2).

The first exact researches into the nature of the blood-pigments were made by VIRCHOW (*Virch. Arch.* vols. 1, 2, 4 and 6, and *Cellular Pathology*). He sought to show that haematoidin is to be regarded as the typical final resultant of the transformations of haemoglobin within the human body. He assumed that the haemoglobin escaped into the tissues unchanged, and was then by a secondary process transformed into granules and crystals, either within or without the cells. LANGHANS (*Virch. Arch.* vol. 49), on the other hand, maintained that the transformation of the red corpuscles into pigment could only take place inside the carrier-cells. CORDUA (*Ueber den Resorptionsmechanismus von Blutergüssen* Berlin 1877) has convinced himself by his investigations that the formation of pigment from haemoglobin may take place partly outside the carrier-cells, partly within them. ZIEGLER's researches, carried out upon specimens from dead bodies and upon extravasations experimentally produced, lead him to agree with VIRCHOW and CORDUA.

PERLS pointed out (*Virch. Arch.* vol. 39) that the haematogenous pigments all yield the reaction of ferric oxide when treated with ferrocyanide of potassium and hydrochloric acid. Even when the pigment has become black it still exhibits the reaction. KUNKEL was the first to show (*Virch. Arch.* vol. 81 and *Zeitschr. f. phys. Chemie* IV, V) that the brownish red flakes found in old extravasations are not always composed of haematoidin. Sometimes these flakes contain no organic colouring-matter at all, but consist entirely of hydrated ferric oxide. The urobilin (hydrobilirubin), which appears in the urine when free absorption of large extravasations takes place, is derived either directly from haemoglobin, or from haematoidin. Further details on the disintegration of the blood under normal and pathological conditions, and the pigmentations connected therewith, are to be found in the Special Pathological Anatomy Arts. 262 and 268.

A distinction must be made between the true slate-coloured pigmentation of the tissues dependent on certain blood-pigments, and the slaty discolorations seen in corpses (pseudo-melanosis), chiefly in the intestinal canal and its neighbourhood. These discolorations, usually in the form of indefinite and diffused grey patches, are due to the formation of ferrous sulphide: combination takes place between the iron of the haemoglobin present and the sulphuretted hydrogen evolved in commencing decomposition.

69. **Biliary pigmentations**. If the excretion of bile be in any way hindered, it passes over into the general circulation, and biliary pigments are thus carried to the various organs. The yellow staining of the tissues so brought about is called **icterus** or **jaundice**. When jaundice persists for some time the tint becomes olive-green or dirty greyish green. The bile in the tissues is usually diffused through them indefinitely; more rarely granules and ruby-red crystals occur. Crystals are chiefly found in the tissues in the so-called **icterus neonatorum**, or jaundice appearing within a few days of birth. These crystals take the form of ruby-red rhombic tablets, and are composed of bilirubin; they are identical with haematoidin-crystals. In the jaundice of adults crystals are seldom found: generally the pigment is more granular, and yellow or brown. This is especially the case when it occurs in the cells of the liver, and in the uriniferous tubules. In addition to the hepatogenous jaundice which depends on re-absorption of

bile, there is said to occur also a haematogenous form resulting from a disintegration of blood within the blood-vessels: this is however disputed by many observers.

The hypothesis of a haematogenous jaundice was based on certain experimental phenomena by KÜHNE (*Virch. Arch.* vol. 14). He injected dog's blood, in which the corpuscles had becomed dissolved, into the vessels and then found bile-pigments in the urine. KUNKEL (*Virch. Arch.* vol. 79) questions the decisiveness of these experiments. Since bile-pigments are formed in the liver by the disintegration of red corpuscles, the process of pigment-formation would be intensified by KÜHNE's injections, and the surplus bile produced might in part pass into the blood again. ORTH has a paper (*Virch. Arch.* vol. 63) on the deposition of bilirubin-crystals in the jaundice of infants.

The most various theories have been started from time to time to account for *icterus neonatorum*. BIRCH-HIRSCHFELD has recently (*Virch. Arch.* vol. 87) treated the question afresh. He maintains that the benign form of jaundice (*i.e.* jaundice not depending on septic infection or profound anatomical change in the liver) is the result of oedema of the capsule of Glisson. This oedema arises in consequence of venous engorgement in the region of the remnant of the umbilical vein and vena portae. This explanation seems somewhat far-fetched. May not the jaundice simply depend on an over-great resorption of bile from the meconium?

70. **Pigmentation** of the tissues **by extraneous substances**. Any substance optically distinguishable from a tissue, which becomes in any way incorporated with it and remains for a time unchanged, may give rise to a special coloration of the tissue. The number of such substances is of course large, and the manner of their incorporation various. The commonest avenues of entrance are surface-wounds, the air-passages, and the alimentary canal.

The most familiar instance of wound-staining is **tatooing**, common among civilised peoples as well as among savages. The way in which the coloured tatoo-marks are produced is this:—the skin is first wounded by scratches or punctures, and then insoluble granular colouring-matters such as charcoal, cinnabar, &c. are well rubbed in. Where the skin is broken the coloured particles penetrate and infiltrate the cutaneous tissues. One part remains where it is, so that the skin continues permanently pigmented: another part is carried off to the lymphatic glands, which also become pigmented.

The lungs and their lymphatic glands may become very deeply pigmented by the long-continued inhalation of foreign matters, such as coal-dust, soot, particles of iron or rust, &c. In consequence of prolonged inhalation of coal-dust, for example, the lung-tissue may become perfectly black (**miner's lung**).

Among the pigmentations arising from matters taken up in the alimentary canal, we must mention the so-called **argyrism** (*argyria*). This is a staining of the tissues consequent upon long-continued internal use of salts of silver. The skin in such cases may assume an intense brownish grey colour; and the internal organs may also be more or less discoloured. The silver is deposited as fine granules in the ground-substance of the different tissues.

CHAPTER XVII.

THE FORMATION OF CYSTS.

71. A **cyst** is an excavation bounded by an envelope of fibrous tissue or other more complex structure, and enclosing contents distinguishable from the envelope. According to its mode of origin the inner surface of the envelope may be lined with epithelium or with endothelium.

Epithelial cysts arise by the dilatation of pre-existing epithelial cavities. The commonest instance of this is the glandular cyst, which ensues upon closure of the gland-duct. The secretion collects behind the obstruction, and the gland dilates to a cyst filled with altered secretion. **Cysts of retention**, as these are called, are chiefly met with in the uterus, intestine, mamma, kidney, and skin.

In the case of ductless organs, like the Graafian follicles and the thyroid, dilatation of the cavities ensues whenever the secretion is morbidly increased. Cysts may also be formed in glandular structures occurring in morbid new growths. Various canals moreover, which are normally clothed with epithelium, may in consequence of obstruction and local dilatation develope into epithelial cysts. Such canals are, for example, the bile-duct, congenital cervical fistulae, the vermiform appendix, and the ureter.

Endothelial cysts arise primarily by dilatation of pre-existing cavities in the connective tissues, such as bursae, tendon-sheaths, obstructed lymphatics, &c. In other cases they are owing to the collection of fluid in new-formed or false membranes. The contents of these cysts vary with their mode of origin, but consist generally of mere lymph. These might also be described as cysts of retention, in a special sense of the term; they are really exudation-cysts.

The cavities which are formed in the substance of a solid organ by softening and disintegration of a defined region are very frequently described as cysts. Such cysts occur, for example, in the brain, and they usually contain semi-liquid detritus of the brain-substance. Similar cavities arising in tumours by the same process are also called cysts. In order to emphasise the difference between such cysts and cysts of retention, the former may be spoken of as **cysts of disintegration.**

Lastly, a species of cyst may be formed around a foreign body which has become lodged in the tissues; round a parasite like a hydatid, for example (Art. 245). It is the result of a new tissue-formation in the neighbourhood of the foreign body.

The student should consult the admirable lectures on *Cysts* in PAGET'S *Surgical Pathology;* they contain many references of value.

To the varieties in the text we might add—**cysts of extravasation,** or blood-cysts, resulting from haemorrhage into closed cavities (*e.g.* haematoma, haematocele): and **dermoid cysts,** which are congenital (Art. 178). The various neoplastic cysts or cystoid tumours will be referred to under their proper headings in Section VI.; and, so far as they affect particular organs, in the Special Pathological Anatomy.

SECTION IV.

PROGRESSIVE OR FORMATIVE DISTURBANCES OF NUTRITION.

CHAPTER XVIII.

THE CELLULAR PROCESSES CONCERNED IN HYPERTROPHY, HYPERPLASIA, AND REGENERATION.

72. In treating of the malformations, we had occasion to speak of excessive development of the organism as a whole, and of its constituent parts—of over-size and over-growth. When a tissue manifests an abnormal tendency to overgrowth, it is said to **hypertrophy.** This term tacitly implies that the structure of the overgrown tissue continues to correspond with that of the normal.

The overgrowth first described implies an excessive development of the organism, or organ, in the embryonic stage of existence. Such forms of overgrowth form however but a part of the class of tissue-changes described as hypertrophies. In adult life, as in infancy, certain organs are very apt to hypertrophy, that is to increase abnormally in size while preserving their normal structure. Such hypertrophies are to be met with in the voluntary muscles, the heart-muscle, the unstriped muscles of the alimentary canal, bladder, and ureters, in the kidneys, thyroid gland, skin, &c.

The increased size of a hypertrophied organ depends on two factors. The several elements of the organ may increase in size, or they may increase in number. With VIRCHOW we may distinguish between **simple hypertrophy**, *i.e.* elementary overgrowth in the stricter sense of the term, and **numerical hypertrophy** or **hyperplasia**, *i.e.* an increase in the number of constituent cells or cellular structures in the organ or tissue. Thus a muscle may very greatly increase in bulk by mere increase in size of each fibre of it; while the number of fibres remains the same. Of course hypertrophy and hyperplasia may go hand in hand in the same tissue; indeed it is hard to conceive of a hyperplasia which has not been preceded by a hypertrophy, at least of some of the cells.

When an increase in the number of cellular elements occurs at a part where tissue has already been destroyed by some retrogressive process, we speak of it as **regeneration**. We assume that the formation of new tissue does not go on beyond the normal limit, but suffices merely to replace what has been lost.

73. Hypertrophy, hyperplasia, and regeneration are dependent ultimately upon certain cellular processes. The formation of new tissue can only take place through the agency of the cells. The intercellular substance, unaided by the cells themselves, has no power or potency to produce new tissue. The cells which go to form new tissue arise by subdivision from pre-existing cells. New cells are never generated from plastic exudations, as was formerly supposed.

Hypertrophy, *i.e.* increased size of a cell, is in general consistent with the maintenance of the properties of the cell. The formative process which results in hypertrophy is confined to the addition of new constituents similar in kind to those already present; the cell simply grows. We know but little of the structural changes which this growth involves. It is however sometimes noticed that the cell-protoplasm becomes more granular; or that the granulation alters as its amount increases: the nucleus also changes more or less its appearance.

Our knowledge concerning the process of cell-multiplication, or **proliferation** (as it is called, though the term is not a happy one), is more minute. Researches, most of them very recent, have shown that multiplication is attended by peculiar changes in the structure of the cell and of its nucleus, which affect the disposition of their several constituents. Movements within the nucleus are usually the first sign that cell-division is about to take place. These issue in subdivision of the nucleus. Then sooner or later the protoplasm as a whole is set in motion, and this ends in the complete subdivision of the cell itself.

74. The fully-developed nucleus of a cell is not homogeneous, but possesses a very peculiar structure. This is clearly to be made out, by appropriate handling, under the higher powers of the microscope. A resting nucleus, *i.e.* one which is not about to subdivide, consists of an external capsule or membrane (FLEMMING *Virch. Arch.* vol. 77), and certain contents. The latter are divisible into a denser highly-refractive nuclear substance, and a rarer colourless nuclear juice, or intermediate substance. The nuclear substance contains—first, certain nucleoli or nucleolar corpuscles, and secondly, scattered granules and filaments. Frequently the filaments are aggregated into a framework or network (Fig. 19 *a*), which may be brought out very distinctly by proper reagents.

When the cell is about to subdivide the nuclear network undergoes a series of typical changes of form, ending in the division of the nucleus into two equal portions.

According to FLEMMING, the first stage of **nucleus-division** is the solution and disappearance of the nucleoli; while the nuclear substance takes the form of a ravelled coil of sinuous filaments

(Fig. 19 *b*): this is the 'coil-form' of the mother-nucleus. The nuclear membrane itself seems to break up and furnish filaments

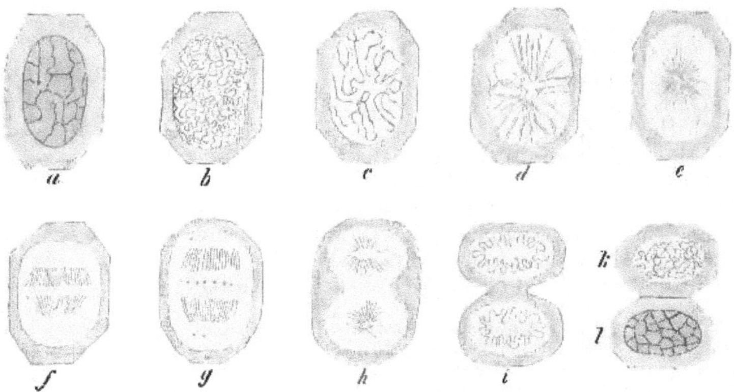

FIG. 19. INDIRECT CELL-DIVISION (*from* FLEMMING: *diagrammatic*)

a cell with resting nucleus
b coil-form of mother-nucleus
c wreath-form showing the central and peripheral loops, some of them broken through
d star-form with free rays, showing the filaments in the act of splitting
e fine-rayed star-form
f nucleus with equatorial plate; division into polar segments
g half-barrel or half-spindle form; the points in the middle are STRASBURGER'S equatorial cell-plate
h star-form of daughter-nucleus
i wreath-form
k coil-form
l resting nucleus with network

to the coil. From this stage onwards the nuclear figure alone takes up the staining reagent (hence the nuclear substance is sometimes spoken of as chromatin).

The filaments then become thicker and the coil looser; its continuity is broken here and there, and at length it passes into the 'wreath-form' (*c*). In this the filaments are arranged in a loose series of central and peripheral loopings, the centre of the figure being unoccupied. From this is fashioned a 'star-form,' or *aster* (*d*), with free double rays, the peripheral loops of the wreath-form dividing at their ends. The double rays next divide longitudinally, and the whole star-form contracts. The filaments of the single-rayed star (*e*) thus formed next gather into an equatorial group, which soon divides into two equal polar segments (*f*). This division is effected by the development of a transparent equatorial plate (*g*) often studded with fine points (STRASBURGER'S cell-plate). The two segments, which are the rudiments of the daughter-nuclei, move asunder towards opposite poles and form the 'half-barrel' or 'half-spindle' figure (EBERTH'S and MAIZEL'S 'creel-form,' or 'basket-form'). The half-spindle form of the daughter-nucleus passes into a star-form (*h*), and this into a wreath-form (*i*) by the fusion of the ray-ends. The wreath-form shrinks and its filaments become more ravelled, till at length it takes the coil-form (*k*). This becomes looser and more regular, and so finally the daughter-nucleus fashions itself a nuclear network (*l*), and passes into the resting state corresponding to the resting state of the mother-nucleus.

In the stage of the star-form and the wreath-form of the daughter-nucleus, constriction of the cell-protoplasm commences (*i*), and ends with the completion of the coil-form (*k*). During the active stages of the subdividing process the nuclear juice or intermediate substance does not stain, though it stains in the resting state. During subdivision the nucleus is surrounded by a clear areola. The whole process takes place rapidly: it ends with the complete constriction and severance of the cell-protoplasm. The above mode of subdivision is called indirect or **karyokinetic** (*καρυον*, a kernel).

According to a recent communication of FLEMMING'S (*Arch. f. mikrosk. Anat.* XX), the intermediate substance of the nucleus contains (in stained preparations, and presumably also in the living state) a delicate prolongation or continuation of the nuclear network. The fine granulation observed in the intermediate substance with lower magnifying powers is really but an optical section of the meshes and filaments of the finer network. The nuclear membrane is merely the peripheral expansion of the nuclear network.

Most important and valuable researches on the changes in cells and nuclei during subdivision have been made by FLEMMING (*Arch. f. mikrosk. Anat.* XVI—XX) and STRASBURGER (*Zellbildung und Zelltheilung* Jena 1880). The former has worked upon animal cells, the latter upon vegetable cells. STRASBURGER'S description of the process of nucleus-division is not quite the same as FLEMMING'S. He distinguishes a nuclear substance (chromatin), and a nuclear juice (achromatin). The capsule or nuclear membrane, as well as the granules, network, and nucleoli which lie in the interior, belong to the nuclear substance. When the nucleus sets about subdividing, its granulation becomes coarser, and the granules run together into convoluted filaments; the nucleolar corpuscles and capsule also take part in forming the filaments. These filaments have the power of stretching or streaming out into the cell-protoplasm. Then follows an elongation of the nucleus and, at the same time, of the filaments, so that the whole assumes a spindle-like shape, and two poles become distinguishable. The filaments shrink up towards the equator, and so form the nuclear disc, the entire nuclear substance going to make it. From this account it appears that the nuclear disc consists entirely of shortened rodlets or filaments. On both sides of this equatorial disc appear slender striae or filaments, the so-called spindle-filaments, and these together with the nuclear disc make up a secondary spindle-form of which the disc constitutes the equatorial zone. The spindle-filaments converge at the poles, or end freely. The material of which they are made is furnished by the cell-protoplasm. They are not taken up by the nuclear substance; indeed they are eliminated again as the subdivision proceeds. The daughter-nuclei originate in the nuclear disc. This parts asunder at the equator, and the two halves draw apart towards the poles. These halves become the daughter-nuclei: they are still connected by a few fine spindle-filaments. A row of granules now makes its appearance in the equatorial plane; this is the cell-plate, and in this the new cell-wall is formed. Protoplasm appears on each side of it, in which the spindle-filaments are merged—and thus the process of division is completed.

STRASBURGER'S account of cell-division in the vegetable kingdom would seem to indicate that a certain difference exists between that and the animal kingdom. FLEMMING however has shown in a recent paper that the physical processes involved in karyokinetic subdivision are in all cases essentially the same, at least in so far as they are to be made out optically. He thinks the apparent differences are not so great as STRASBURGER conceives them to be.

It is of great interest to note the fact established by FLEMMING—that in the segmentation of the ovum the process of nucleus-division follows throughout that which we have described as the karyokinetic mode (BALFOUR, *Comp. Embryology* I, 3).

This mode of nucleus-division has often been observed and described as occurring in pathological proliferations. The chief memoirs are by EBERTH (*Virch. Arch.* vol. 67), ARNOLD (*Virch. Arch.* vols. 77, 78, 93), FLEMMING (*loc. cit.*), MARTIN (*Virch. Arch.* vol. 86), DRASCH (*Wiener Sitzungsber.* 1881), KLEIN (*Quart. Journ. Micr. Science* 1878 and 1879). PRIESTLEY gives a summary of the early researches in *Q. Journ. M. S.* 1876; CUNNINGHAM reviews the more recent ones in the same journal, Jan. 1882.

75. These structural changes in the nucleus point unmistakeably to the energetic internal motions which affect its molecules in the process of growth. Our knowledge of the molecular changes in the cell-protoplasm is unfortunately more meagre and incomplete. Here however it is also possible to make out by proper means—that the protoplasm assumes a special structure, and that various movements and transmutations of form occur amongst its component elements. Thus in certain cases nucleus-division is accompanied by lively rotary movements in the protoplasm. Such transformations and transpositions explain certain phenomena which are frequently observed—for example, the formation of a transparent areola round the subdividing nucleus, of radiating lines of granules making up the so-called 'karyolytic' figure, &c. Such radiating lines of granules have especially been seen in the process of impregnation of the ovum. They occur in the neighbourhood of the male and female pronuclei, and have been described as the *aster* (BALFOUR, *Comp. Embryology* vol. I, ch. 3). FLEMMING, as well as STRASBURGER, assigns to the cell-protoplasm an essential part in the process of subdivision. STRASBURGER even asserts that it is the penetration of the protoplasm into the nucleus which calls forth a reciprocal activity in the latter, and so gives it an impulse towards subdivision. Whether this be true or not we cannot at present decide, inasmuch as no penetration of the protoplasm into the nucleus has ever been directly observed. The ordering of the granules into radiate figures, like the other movements of the protoplasm hitherto observed, takes place as a rule simultaneously with the process of nucleus-division. In some cases however it may precede, in others it may succeed, the latter. Thus, according to GRUBER (*Zool. Anzeiger* 1880) the infusorian *Euglypha alveolata* first gives rise to a daughter-cell, then the nucleus becomes subdivided and migrates into the daughter-cell; while at the same time active movements become visible in the cell-protoplasm.

A special form of cell-division is that which takes place after an antecedent conjugation. It is common among the infusorians.

In order to make out the nuclear figures, the cell must be examined either in the living state or after treatment while still living with a rapidly fixing solution. If this is not done the process of subdivision is completed as the cell gradually dies. There is no general rule of proceeding which will apply to the examination of all cells.

76. The indirect process of cell-division just described will serve as a pattern of the processes which occur in pathological cell-formation. No satisfactory demonstration has been given of the theory that cell-division may occur in another way, namely by direct constriction of the cell without interior structural change. Nor has it been certainly established that a nucleus or cell can arise *de novo* out of an indifferent blastema (or homogeneous matrix), at any rate within the domain of pathological cell-formation. VIRCHOW'S aphorism "*Omnis cellula e cellulâ*" is, in this domain at least, most fully and completely confirmed.

But though we maintain that, so far as we know, cell-division is always indirect, never direct, we do not imply that every cell-division proceeds exactly according to the scheme we have indicated. On the contrary, the examination of different specimens shows that the form and construction of the nuclear figures are by no means always the same: deviations within certain limits may occur.

But while the figures formed by the nuclear filaments may differ considerably, the principle and plan of the process is fundamentally the same. Even the simultaneous formation and development of three or four daughter-nuclei is but a modification of the general process.

The subdivision of the cell-protoplasm usually follows immediately upon the division of the nucleus; but the connexion of the two processes is by no means inevitable. Not infrequently the nucleus subdivides while the cell does not. The result is the formation of binucleated, or finally of multinucleated cells, the so-called **giant-cells**. These giant-cells may afterwards break up into uninucleated cells, the protoplasm gathering itself around the several nuclei and dividing along the boundaries of the regions so defined. Sometimes this happens in a peculiar way. The protoplasm of the daughter-cell separates from that of the mother-cell, but in such wise that it remains surrounded by the latter on all sides: the one cell includes the other. VIRCHOW has called such cells **brood-cells**. They do not occur frequently. They have been thought commoner than they really are—inasmuch as leucocytes which have penetrated into a large ordinary cell have been taken for a brood of daughter-cells. The process of cell-division takes a peculiar form also in the formation of cell-buds, or **gemmation**. The mother-cell shoots out a longer or shorter process; this then receives a nucleus; and lastly divides off from the parent (see under New Blood-vessels Art. 86). The peculiarity is chiefly in this—that the movements of the protoplasm (evidenced by the protrusion of the bud) precede the nucleus-division. The new nucleus, derived as in all other cases by subdivision from the mother-nucleus, migrates into the bud after it is already marked off from the parent.

Until quite lately the process of nucleus-division was described (after REMAK) somewhat in this fashion:—The nucleus lengthens out, becomes indented and constricted in the middle, and at last divides (compare RINDFLEISCH, *Pathological Histology*, vol. I, p. 71; CORNIL and RANVIER, *Manual of Path. Hist.* vol. I, pp. 9, 83). The constricted bean-shaped nuclei found in some preparations were regarded as in the preliminary stages of subdivision; and the multiplication of the nucleoli was regarded as the first step in the actual process. This view must now be given up. The various shapes of the nuclei depend partly on actual contractions, partly on shrinkage during the hardening process. Increased size of the nucleus may perhaps have a relation to its imminent subdivision: the mere multiplication of its nucleoli has certainly no such relation.

The older theories of direct nucleus-division have been discredited by the latest researches; so also have the still older views concerning the formation *de novo* of cells and nuclei. (See STRASBURGER *op. cit.*, where full references to the literature of this subject are given.)

The question whether or not the white blood-cells subdivide is as yet unsettled. Indirect nucleus-division has not been observed in them. See KLEIN, *Centralb. med. Wiss.* 1869, *Q. Journ. Mic. Sc.* 1875 and *Handb. of Phys. Lab.*; RANVIER, *Traité technique d'histologie* p. 161.

On 'endogenous gemmation,' by which brood-cells are produced, see VIRCHOW, *Cellular Pathology*; and KLEIN, *Wiener Sitzungsber.* 1871 and *Anatomy of Lymphatic System* vol. I London 1875.

77. The formation of new cells is the first step towards hyperplasia as well as towards regeneration. They yield the formative tissue out of which the definitive structures are developed. As the processes of cell-division in pathological new-formations are closely analogous with those of normal multiplication, so also do the succeeding formative processes run parallel with those of normal growth. If epithelium or fibrous tissue is to be fashioned out of the indifferent tissue which results from cell-division, the process of transformation is exactly the same as occurs in the normal development of the organism from embryonic tissue.

So far as investigation in this region has yet extended, we find the law of the **specific nature of the tissues** to be everywhere obeyed. The cell-progeny of the embryonic cells which went to form any given layer of the blastoderm can go to build up such tissues only as are normally derived from that layer. An epithelial cell can in no possible circumstances form bone or cartilage: a connective-tissue corpuscle cannot bring forth an epithelial cell or a gland-cell. This law has frequently been called in question: the specific distinction between the various tissues was formerly not recognised or not accepted. Thus VIRCHOW, to whom we owe the fundamental principles of cellular pathology as regards new-formations, held that connective tissue might serve for the matrix of the most various structures. This view is no longer tenable: observed facts constrain us to believe that a tissue cannot give rise to new tissue other than of its own kind or kindred.

Epithelial tissues are, generally speaking, built up by the

cementing together of formative cells in a way which is characteristic of epithelium everywhere: the cells are in juxtaposition, the intercellular cementing substance is subordinate. In fibrous tissue on the other hand, the intercellular material derived from the cells is the chief constituent, and gives to the tissue its characteristic properties.

78. A morbid growth is the product of various factors. If a cell is to grow and multiply it must first be endowed with the faculties necessary to growth and reproduction. In other words it must have the power to take up from the blood a greater quantity of nutriment, to assimilate this, and apply it to the formation of new protoplasm. This property of the cell VIRCHOW has called the nutritive and formative excitability (*Irritabilität*): a term which implies that it is some stimulus or excitation from without which stirs up the cell to increased assimilation.

We must therefore begin by enquiring of what kind the stimuli must be that can thus excite the cell to intenser activity.

When, in embryonic development, a part or organ grows to an abnormal size and thus becomes so to speak gigantic, we may refer the phenomenon to several possible originating causes. The primary rudiment of the part may have been unusually large: the embryonic cells may have been endowed with an abnormal share of vital energy: they may have had specially favourable chances of nutrition: the resistances to proliferation may have been abnormally slight. It is not in general an easy task to decide which of these factors has in a given case determined the result. It is of course always possible that several factors have been working together.

In the hypertrophies of later life (including the hyperplasias and regenerations), which are demonstrably conditioned from without, and so do not depend on pre-existing or embryonic factors, the question of aetiology is so far simplified. We must direct our attention to the other possible factors, namely increased vital energy, increased supply of nutriment, or diminished resistance to growth. It is however not to be forgotten—that the cause of the increased activity of the cell may be of the nature of a stimulus from without, which acting directly upon the cell excites it to more intense productiveness. We may assert then in general terms that, when the nutritive and formative activities of a cell are morbidly increased, the effect is due to augmentation of the physiological stimuli or diminution of the physiological resistances to growth, or to the direct influence of external stimuli.

79. Experience has shown that many tissue-cells, even when they seem, by their close connexion with their neighbours, to be as it were firmly built into the tissue of which they form a part, still retain for a time the power of growth and subdivision, or in other words, of multiplication. This is especially the case with cells whose

protoplasm has not undergone any serious metamorphosis. As to the conditions governing such multiplication, experience alone can inform us.

Many observers (STRICKER, BOETTCHER, NEUMANN, &c.) assert that extrinsic stimuli, that is to say physically or chemically active substances, have the power of exciting the cell to proliferate. Thus caustics and the actual cautery applied to tissues are said to induce in them cell-multiplication by direct action. There seems to be no certain observation which either establishes or confirms the assertion. Researches made in this direction have shown that the action of such external agencies is in the first instance destructive: that in caustic corrosion, for example, not only does the tissue which is directly attacked perish, but that in its neighbourhood undergoes secondary degeneration as well. It has furthermore been uniformly observed that formative changes do not begin to appear until a certain time after the injury; it is therefore very unlikely that they are directly brought about by it. Lastly, they do not commence at the injured spot, but in its neighbourhood.

From these considerations it appears that the proposition, often enunciated as if it were self-evident,—'The stronger the external stimulus, the greater the proliferation'—cannot be accepted as true. We can at most admit that very slight stimuli, sufficient merely to excite the cell without injuring it, may perhaps call into play its power of multiplication: but nothing has been experimentally established concerning the nature, the action, or the mode of application, of such stimuli.

The researches on the reaction of cells to external stimuli have been made chiefly with the view of determining the source of the migratory cells in inflammation (Art. 99). STRICKER and his pupils affirm that the stimulus of inflammation excites the affected cells to rapid multiplication. The tissue-cells and their appendages swell up (it is said) under this excitation, and subdivide into new cells and non-nucleated lumps of protoplasm (STRICKER'S *Vorles. über allg. Pathol.* Vienna 1878; and *Pathology of Inflam., Internat. Encyclop. of Surgery* vol. I, 1882). COHNHEIM (*Lehrb. d. allg. Pathol.*), KEY, RETZIUS, EBERTH, and others have failed to make out any such consequence of inflammatory irritation.

Even if the meaning of the word *stimulus* be extended to include any mechanical or chemical agency which can influence the cell, we cannot adduce any undoubted observation serving to establish STRICKER'S view.

80. If then it be true that external injurious agencies are not competent to induce multiplication in cells, we must have recourse to the normal vital stimuli if we are to explain the process of pathological cell-growth. For the due growth and multiplication of a cell certain external conditions must be fulfilled. Above all it is necessary to provide for a certain degree of warmth, and a certain modicum of proper nutritive material. In addition to this there must be no obstacle in the way of multiplication. These are the external requirements. The internal condition is the inherent faculty of the cell to assimilate the nutriment offered to it.

In a tissue not undergoing transformation, the factors favouring proliferation and those which inhibit it must be in a state of balance. If this balance be disturbed toward the side of the proliferous forces, the cells proceed to grow and to multiply. The factors in question resolve themselves on analysis into three.

In the first place, it is conceivable that the capacity of the cell to assimilate nutriment may be increased. Such increase can only be conditioned by an increase in the normal stimuli required for the preservation of the cell. Such stimuli are warmth, for many cells light, for the muscles motor impulses, for glands special excitations from the nervous system, &c. Increased stimulation of this kind may as a fact lead not only to intensified functional metabolism in the tissue concerned, but even to hypertrophy of its elements. Such hypertrophies, which we may call functional hypertrophies or hypertrophies of action, are specially common and remarkable in muscles and glands (heart-muscles, bladder-muscles, kidneys, &c.). As we have said, they are referable in part at least to increased vital activity in the cells, consequent upon increased physiological stimulation.

A second possible factor is increase in the supply of nutriment. This plays a chief part in hyperplastic processes, at any rate.

A third is the removal of the normal checks to growth. Its effect is most evident in the processes described as regenerative.

If we attempt in particular cases to make out to which of these factors cell-multiplication is due, we are led to see that it is rare for any one factor alone to be the efficient cause. The remarkable regulating mechanism of the vessels is so adjusted, that when the function of a tissue is increased its blood-supply is increased to correspond. In like manner when the smallest fragment of tissue is removed, the slight loosening of the surrounding texture is enough to augment the stream of transudation from the vessels. In consequence of these adjustments, increased supply of nutriment plays a great part in all the formative disturbances of nutrition.

COHNHEIM, in his *Allgemeine Pathologie*, has insisted on the importance of increased supply of nutriment even more strongly than we have done. According to his view it is the sole influential factor, compared with which the intrinsic activity of the cell is quite secondary. We are unwilling to condemn the cell to play so passive a part, but rather agree with VIRCHOW, who (*Cellular Pathology*) lays it down that—'the cell is not nourished, but nourishes itself.' Functional hypertrophy is therefore not to be looked upon as the mere consequence of the increased blood-supply to the active organ. If the assimilative activity of the cells were not augmented, the mere presence of a greater supply of nutriment would be valueless. See SAMUEL'S *Allg. Path.* 1879; PAGET'S *Surgical Pathology* Lect. 3.

81. We shall more readily comprehend the activity of the tissue-cells, *i.e.* their behaviour under various conditions, and the changes they pass through—now at rest, and now manifesting intense formative energy—if we consider first the vital manifestations of an organism that is unicellular. In later chapters we shall have

frequently to speak of unicellular micro-organisms, of bacteria and yeast-plants, and their mode of life. If we reflect on the conditions essential for the multiplication of such organisms, we note that the nature of the nutrient fluid is (next after the adjustment of the temperature) the factor of highest importance. In suitably-composed fluids the fungi develope much more luxuriantly than in those that are ill-suited. But we are not thereby justified in assuming that the cell plays a merely passive part, that all it has to do is to take up the nutriment offered to it. The cell is on the contrary active, and its activity has a special influence on the liquid itself. It has the power to induce certain chemical changes in the liquid, to decompose certain substances contained in it, and to change their condition so as to adapt them for assimilation by itself. The cell does not merely take in and give out material: it acts 'catalytically' on its environment. This is proof at least that the cell possesses a high degree of spontaneity—that it has the power of making more available for its own sustenance the various forms of nutriment that come in its way.

It is also of great interest to remark that the cell is ultimately limited in its formative activity by its own products. When the amount of nutriment present is abundant, the activity of the cell comes to an end, not through the exhaustion of the supply, but through its contamination with certain products of cell-metabolism. Many of the substances engendered in fermenting liquids by the action of fungi tend to check the growth and multiplication of the fungi themselves: when present in quantity they may put a stop to multiplication altogether. The alcoholic fermentation, and the multiplication of the yeast-plant which produces it, come to an end when a certain proportion of alcohol has been generated in the fermenting liquid. In septic putrefaction the bacteria generate compounds, such as carbolic acid, which are destructive to themselves. If we may apply these facts of fungus-physiology to the cell-physiology of higher organisms, we find that they illustrate first of all this principle—that the quantity and quality of the nutritive material at the disposal of the cell have a profound influence upon its behaviour. And secondly, this other,—that the cell has nevertheless an intrinsic power of utilising this material, and of appropriating what is suitable to itself out of various combinations. Lastly, the limits imposed on the multiplication of fungi by the products of their own activity may help us to understand how the formative activity of the cells of complex organisms may be temporarily checked. We cannot indeed regard the intercellular substance of the connective tissues as equivalent in significance to the products of the chemical changes induced by the bacteria. Yet the comparison may at least enable us to conceive how cell-growth may tend to limit and to check itself, without the interposition of extrinsic resistances. In the connective tissues the formation of the intercellular substance is the limiting factor, in the epithelia it is the cohesion or cementation of the individual cells into a firm and single whole; just as in yeast-fermentation it is the formation of alcohol. When the alcohol is withdrawn in the latter case the multiplication of the yeast-fungus goes on again. So likewise if the intercellular substance be dissolved away from a connective tissue, or if the continuity of the epithelial mosaic be loosened or interrupted, the faculty of multiplication is again awakened in the constituent cells; or if (as in the epithelia) it has never been dormant, it is at once intensified.

In the human organism temperature is not a factor of such importance as it is in regard to unicellular organisms. In the former the temperature is approximately uniform: change of temperature cannot therefore play any great part in promoting cell-growth. Even changes in the quality of the cell-nutriment can have but a small part of the significance here that it has in the case of fungi living in a nutrient solution: such grave changes as may be artificially produced in the character of the solution do not occur in the body. Quantitative variations are thus of the greater importance.

82. It often happens in an organ which is the seat of hyperplastic proliferation that the different elements do not take an equal share in the process. Thus an enlarged gland may in one case owe its increase in size entirely to additions of gland-substance, in another to increase in the fibrous constituents. We may have a glandular hyperplasia, or a fibrous hyperplasia. This may happen in any organ which is composed of more than one kind of tissue. The inequality in the relation of the two tissues may be so extreme, that while one is highly hyperplastic the other may not merely fail to increase but may even undergo atrophy. In the latter case it is generally the specific elements (ganglion-cells, nerves, gland-cells, muscles, &c.) which atrophy, while the fibrous elements increase and multiply. A very frequent cause of such unsymmetrical hyperplasia of the fibrous tissue is inflammation (which see). Inflammation plays a chief part in pathology; only too frequently its disastrous result is **fibrous hyperplasia** of the affected organs, involving atrophy of their essential elements.

What is true of hyperplasia, holds also for regeneration. When part of a tissue has been destroyed, the regeneration which ensues is by no means always complete and perfect. In the human organism at least, the power of restoring or regenerating a lost part is very limited. Parts of any appreciable size when once lost are never replaced. This is true for example of a limb, a finger, a piece of liver, or of brain-substance. All highly-specialised structures, and their specific elements, show but slight traces of regenerative power. Thus in adults it is highly probable that ganglion-cells are never reproduced, if once destroyed. Glandular epithelium is only restored when the loss is very trifling, and when some of the essential cells still remain intact within the gland-unit (acinus or tubule). When a gland is wounded and its texture broken into ever so little, the wound in healing fills up not with gland-substance but with fibrous tissue. Pathological vicarious tissue of this kind is described as **cicatricial** or **scar tissue**. It is the result of an inflammatory process (Art. 108), or of multiplication among the connective-tissue cells.

With nerves and muscles the case is much the same. Deficiencies of any size are filled up with scar-tissue.

The connective and epithelial tissues are more favourably circumstanced. The latter especially have the power of reproducing wide areas of lost surface. Among the fibrous tissues, the periosteum is remarkable for its regenerative power; while cartilage is replaced very imperfectly if at all.

83. When by a process of proliferation a new tissue is produced whose elements are normal in type, though the type is not that of the matrix-tissue, we speak of the formation as a **heteroplasia**. In one sense a cicatrix in an organ like the liver is a heteroplasia, inasmuch as fibrous tissue replaces the proper liver-tissue. And even when the fibrous tissue of the cicatrix is compared with that of the liver, we must still regard the cicatrix as heteroplastic: the characters of the two tissues are markedly different. This is true of fibrous hyperplasias in general, and in particular of those consequent on inflammation. Owing to the generic resemblance of the normal and pathological tissues, however, it is not usual to reckon these among the heteroplasias.

The special field of heteroplastic formations lies among the tumours or morbid growths. A tumour, in the limited sense of the term, is a formation of new tissue. It may resemble more or less the matrix-tissue from which it grows, but it always possesses certain characteristics which distinguish it from the surrounding structures, and which justify us in speaking of it as heteroplastic.

CHAPTER XIX.

HYPERPLASIA AND REGENERATION IN PARTICULAR TISSUES.

84. The morphological changes which take place in the hyperplasia and regeneration of the epithelia are comparatively simple.

Epithelium can arise only from epithelium: the several varieties even do not usually pass into each other. EBERTH's researches (*Virch. Arch.* vol. 67) have shown that the nuclear transformations in epithelial cells during their reproduction are quite analogous to those figured in FLEMMING's scheme. The disappearance of the nucleoli and nuclear membrane, the formation of filaments, of two semi-spindle forms (or as EBERTH calls them 'creel-forms'), of star-forms, &c., are all observed in the epithelial cell, within a clear areola of cell-protoplasm. The star-forms likewise, as they move asunder polewards, become transformed into nuclear networks in the midst of the clear intermediate substance of the daughter-nuclei. ARNOLD describes (*Virch. Arch.* vol. 78) nuclear figures observed in tumour-cells, which in details seem rather to correspond with STRASBURGER's version of the phenomena. The subdivision of the cell-protoplasm occurs either during the later stages of nucleus-division, or after it is complete. In other cases processes are first thrown out by the subdividing epithelial cell, and into these daughter-nuclei then migrate. The budded processes become independent cells by separation from the mother-cell.

Small losses of lining epithelium are in general replaced quickly by means of regenerative multiplication. Glandular epithelium, like that of the kidney, may also be quickly reproduced when lost, provided only the structure of the basis-tissue (from which the cells derive their sustenance) is not altered or destroyed. Hyperplastic multiplication of epithelial cells is very common, especially in tumours.

Epithelial cells have also the power of remaining alive for a time when separated from their proper matrix. They may in this way be transferred from one basis-tissue to another. Thus epithelial cells from the skin of one person may be transplanted to the surface of a granulating wound in another, and there grow and multiply (REVERDIN'S skin-grafting). This is a simple and convincing proof of the independence or autonomy of the cell, and of the importance of its inherent powers in reference to its nutritive and formative activity.

The regeneration of epithelium has of late years been made the subject of numerous researches. Most observers agree that epithelium can arise only from epithelium: only a small number like BURKHARD (*Virch. Arch.* vol. 17), CORNIL and RANVIER (*Man. Path. Hist.* vol. I), and RINDFLEISCH (*Gewebelehre*, 4th ed. p. 128; *Pathological Histology* vol. I, p. 106) assert that epithelium may be formed from connective-tissue cells. No convincing proof of the assertion is alleged; while the fact that cutaneous wounds begin to skin over only at spots where epidermal cells still remain tells strongly against it.

ARNOLD (*Virch. Arch.* vol. 46) believes that in epithelial regeneration a plasma is effused into which nuclei subsequently migrate. KLEBS (*Arch. f. exper. Path.* III), VON WYSS (*Virch. Arch.* vol. 69), COHNHEIM (*Virch. Arch.* vol. 61), and EBERTH (*loc. cit.*) have failed to confirm this, but found on the other hand that regeneration was effected by subdivision of the old epithelial cells. KLEBS observed in the young cells phenomena suggesting contractility and the power of locomotion: WALDEYER has made a like observation in the case of epithelial tumour-cells. The first communication on epithelial transplantation and skin-grafting was made by REVERDIN (*Soc. de chirurgie*, 13 Dec. 1869; *Brit. Med. Journ.* 2, 1870; *Arch. gén. de méd.* 1872). His method has since been extensively employed with a view to the speedier skinning over of wounded surfaces (*Int. Ency. of Surgery* vol. I). SCHWENINGER has shown (*Ueber Transplant. von Haaren* Munich 1875) that the mere laying on of hairs, which have been plucked out with the outer root-sheath adhering, suffices to set up epithelial proliferation on granulating surfaces.

GRIFFINI (*Virch. Jahresber.* 1876) has shown that, when ciliated cylindrical epithelium is lost, it is first replaced by ciliated squamous epithelium: this is then gradually transformed into the cylindrical variety.

85. New **fibrous tissue** is invariably developed from cells, and the process is the same as that by which normal fibrous tissue is formed. The formative cells have been named **fibroblasts**. They are derived by proliferation either from the stationary cells of the connective tissue, or from migratory leucocytes, *i.e.* white blood-cells which have escaped from the vessels. The development of the latter will be treated when we discuss inflammatory new-formations.

Fibroblasts are cells with large vesicular nuclei and nucleoli, and are capable of active subdivision and multiplication. By proper handling it is possible to make out the nuclear figures, but the subject has not been sufficiently investigated to afford means for a detailed description of the process of subdivision. The cell-protoplasm is pale and highly granular: the size of the cells varies, on the average it is about that of an ordinary squamous epithelial cell. They are often described as epithelioid cells. Not infrequently multinuclear cells are met with, the so-called giant-cells. The form of the fibroblasts is extremely variable. In the earlier stages they are rounded, later on they become club-shaped, spindle-shaped, star-shaped: in short they assume every possible shape and form.

When they have accumulated in any spot and begin to address themselves to the formation of tissue, they become connected with each other by means of their processes and projections; or they arrange themselves in a compact mass of densely-packed multiform cells.

The intercellular substance which gives the fibrous tissues their characteristic texture is derived from the cell-protoplasm. The ends and lateral borders of the cells become fibrillated; or the boundaries between the cells disappearing a homogeneous mass of protoplasm is formed, and in this fibrils are afterwards developed. A great many of the formative cells are used up in this way: some however retain their nucleus and a part of their protoplasm, and form the fixed connective-tissue corpuscles of the new tissue. (Cf. Art. 108.)

According to the greater or less compactness with which the formative cells are deposited and grouped, the new tissue is firm and dense, or loose and reticular. Fibrous tissue, rather than areolar, is that most commonly developed, especially as a consequence of inflammation. It may become hyperplastic, either by itself, or accompanied by hyperplasia of contiguous tissues such as the epithelia. In respect of the diffusion or extension of the hyperplastic process it is of some importance to distinguish between diffuse or indefinite hyperplasia, and that which is limited to definite areas: the latter leads to tissue-formations which resemble tumours. (See under Tumours, Sect. VII.)

Adipose tissue is formed from normal or pathologically developed connective tissue, or from mucous tissue, by the deposition of fat in the interior of the cells.

Mucous tissue, characterised by the mucous consistence of its ground-substance, is generally derived from an existing tissue by metaplasia (Art. 90): it may also be formed from new proliferating cells.

Neuroglia is developed by the multiplication of the neuroglia-cells.

The structure and development of the connective tissues, both normal and pathological, have been the subject of many researches. The origin of the ground-substance has given rise to controversy. Some consider it to arise outside the cells, others from within them. A third theory again, while admitting its external origin, supposes that the fibrils are produced in it by the formative power of the cell as if they were a kind of plastic secretion. The view of the text only applies to the formation of fibrous tissue from new-formed embryonic or indifferent tissue. It does not apply, for example, to the formation of fibrous tissue by metamorphosis of the basis-substance of a different tissue, such as bone (see under Metaplasia Arts. 90—92). For further details the reader is referred to the following:—VIRCHOW (*Virch. Arch.* vol. 13), NEUMANN (*Arch. für Heilk.* 1869), AUFRECHT (*Wiener med. Wochenschr.*

1868), RINDFLEISCH (*Pathological Histology* vol. I, p. 92), ZIEGLER (*Untersuch. über path. Bindegewebs- und Gefässneubildung*), PERLS (*Handbuch d. allg. Path.* I), TILLMANNS (*Virch. Arch.* vol. 78).

86. The formation of **new blood-vessels** plays a chief part in hyperplasias of every kind. Wherever fibrous tissue, bone-tissue, gland-tissue, or any other is produced in quantity, new blood-vessels must of necessity be developed. In no other way is it possible to keep the new-formed tissue adequately supplied with nutriment. For this reason new blood-vessels begin to be formed at a very early stage in all new growths, and they must be regarded as the chief factors in the formative process.

New blood-vessels are developed out of off-shoots which start from the walls of existing blood-vessels.

The first change observed is the formation of a conical sprout or projection on the outer surface of some capillary vessel. From the top of this runs off a fine filament of protoplasm, which gradually lengthens. The granular mass forming the projection increases in size, growing out into an irregular process or off-shoot. This is at first solid; but nuclei soon begin to appear among its granules.

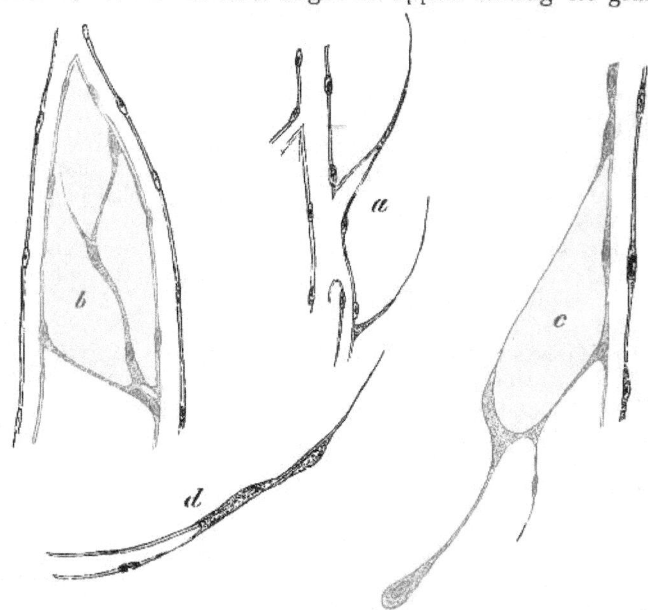

FIG. 20. DEVELOPMENT OF BLOOD-VESSELS BY SPROUTS AND OFF-SHOOTS.

(*From preparations of inflammatory granulation-tissue.*)

a b c d various forms of vascular off-shoots; some solid (*b, c*), others in process of excavation (*a, b, d*); some single (*a, d*), others branched (*b, c*); some with nuclei (*b, c*), others without (*a, d*). Formative cells from without have attached themselves to the off-shoot *d*.

The off-shoot may become attached to another vessel; it may unite with a second off-shoot; or it may return back into the vessel from which it starts, forming an arch of protoplasm (Fig. 20 *c*). From the solid off-shoot other secondary off-shoots may start (Fig. 20 *b*, *c*). Sometimes their extremities become club-shaped (*c*). The originally solid off-shoot becomes by and by excavated, by liquefaction of its central parts. The excavation quickly becomes continuous with the lumen of the vessel (*a*), or the wall of the latter bulges into the excavation. In either case the blood from the parent vessel penetrates the new one, and distends it. The excavation proceeds and extends onward to the point of junction of the new vessel with another, so that at length a new pervious capillary loop is formed.

The off-shoot as it starts from the wall of the parent vessel is in effect a sprouted bud from an endothelial cell: when it subsequently receives a nucleus it becomes an independent cell. The new blood-vessels are therefore intracellular channels, produced by the excavation of elongated or filamentous cells.

For a short time after the opening up of the new capillary channel the vessel-wall remains homogeneous in structure. Soon the protoplasm begins to gather round the nuclei of the wall, which in the meantime have been multiplying by subdivision. Cells become in this way distinguishable, and presently the capillary-wall appears in its perfected form as a mosaic of flat endothelial cells. (As ARNOLD and others showed, the boundaries between the cells may be rendered apparent by injecting the vessels with solution of nitrate of silver.) By this time the wall has generally reached a considerable thickness. This is in part owing to the fact that ordinary formative cells attach themselves in numbers to the vessel-wall; they then dispose themselves along its length, and thus tend to give it needed strength (Fig. 20 *d*).

So far as we have been able to make out, the process of forming new blood-vessels nearly always passes through the stages described. It is only at times that another stage is interpolated in which spindle-shaped, club-shaped, or branching formative cells become connected with the off-shoots from the capillary-walls, and develope into new vessels by central excavation in the same way as the off-shoots themselves develope.

The subject of the formation of new vessels has a special interest in reference to the theory of cell-multiplication. We have in this case to do not with symmetrical subdivision, but with gemmation: and moreover the initial movement is set up not as usual in the nucleus, but in the cell-protoplasm. The protoplasm of the endothelial wall-cells throws out a non-nucleated process: the subdivision and migration of the nucleus is subsequent to the movement in the protoplasm.

The author has verified the above account in the course of his researches on granulation-tissue and on tumours (ZIEGLER, *Ueber path. Bindegewebs- und Gefässneubildung* Würzburg 1876). STRICKER (*Wiener Sitzungsberichte* 1865—1866), GOLUBEW (*Arch. f. mikro. Anat.* 1869), and ARNOLD (*Virch. Arch.* vols. 53, 54) have described the above mode of development of new vessels as observed in tadpoles' tails, TRAVERS in the foot-web of the frog (*On inflammation* &c.). It is the only mode which certainly occurs in pathological formations. For this reason we have not given the customary enumeration of the primary, secondary, and tertiary modes formulated by BILLROTH (*Untersuch. ü. d. Entwick. d. Blutgef.* Berlin 1856) and RINDFLEISCH (*Pathological Histology* vol. I, p. 89). In the primary mode the embryonic cells become directly transformed into red blood-cells on one hand, and into the parietal cells of a vessel on the other. The embryonic cells in fact arrange themselves into cords: the axial ones become blood-cells, the peripheral ones cohere as elements of the containing vessel-wall. This process takes place in the mesoblast of the embryo, but not in pathological formations (KLEIN, *Wiener Sitzungsberichte* 1871, *Q. Journ. M. Sc.* 1872; BALFOUR, *Comp. Embryology* vol. II).

In the secondary mode (BILLROTH, O. WEBER, RINDFLEISCH) spindle-shaped cells cohere to form cylinders in such wise as to enclose a continuous canal. This notion seems to rest on a mistake, occasioned by the fact that in granulation-tissue, for example, the vascular off-shoots are very quickly surrounded and wrapped about with spindle-shaped formative cells: and this gives the off-shoots the appearance of strings of cells.

The so-called tertiary mode is that given in the text. Compare the description by PAGET (*Surgical Path.* Lect. 10).

87. Proliferation in **cartilage** may be either a regenerative or a hyperplastic process. The reproduction of cartilage-cells at the margin of a breach is effected by the cells first enlarging, and then undergoing subdivision of nucleus and protoplasm. Nuclear figures are observed. In this process many of the cells attain to great dimensions and may contain as many as twelve nuclei apiece (EWETZKY). The cells are rounded or branched, stellate or spinous. The capsular membranes disappear as the cells enlarge and multiply. Later on the cells or cell-groups become surrounded by the characteristic hyaline matrix-substance.

In hyperplastic proliferation the process is similar. The cells multiply and stretch the capsules, or cause them to give way and disappear: in like manner the intercellular matrix is distended or destroyed. Subsequently the new-formed cells generate for themselves fresh capsules and matrix-substance.

When a breach in cartilage is not repaired by multiplication of the cartilage-cells, fibrous tissue, developed from fibroblasts, usually fills up the gap. In other cases bony tissue is developed as well.

Cartilage may arise not only from cartilage, but from other allied tissues, such as growing periosteum in particular, perichondrium, marrow, bone, fibrous tissue, and epithelium. The metamorphosis is sometimes effected directly, as from perichondrium or marrow, sometimes through the intermediate stage of granulation. In the latter case an indifferent tissue is first formed, which is rich in single cells: these then become transformed into hyaline matrix-substance and cartilage-cells. Cartilaginous new growths are most commonly found in connexion with the skeletal structures: in other regions they are rare.

Memoirs on the formation and proliferation of cartilage have been published by VIRCHOW (*Onkologie* I), GOODSIR (*Anat. and Path. Obs.* 1845), REDFERN

(*Month. Journ. med. science* 1851), EWETZKY (*Entzündungs-versuche am Knorpel*, EBERTH'S *Arbeiten* III), WARTMANN (*Recherches sur l'enchondrome* Geneva 1880), KASSOWITZ (*Die normale Ossification* Vienna 1881). Further details will be given in the section on the Special Pathological Anatomy of the Bones.

88. The **bones** have a very marked power of regeneration and of hyperplastic proliferation. The seat of this power is not so much in the osseous tissue itself as in those tissues which normally possess the power of bone-production; these are the periosteum in particular, and in a less degree the marrow. In very many cases the periosteum alone performs the office of replacing a loss of bony substance. Many osseous hyperplasias are essentially the work of the periosteum. Cartilage has also some power of reproducing bone.

Fibrous tissues unconnected with the skeleton very rarely give rise to bony tissue. Such abnormal bone-formation is however not unknown in certain cartilaginous and fibrous structures, such as the dura mater, the laryngeal cartilages, the intermuscular septa, and inflammatory fibrous tissues.

The formation of new bone may occur in various ways, but it follows in general the lines of the normal process of ossification. The simplest mode is perhaps that in which the periosteum (or medullary tissue) gives rise to **osteoblasts** (*i.e.* large multinuclear formative cells resembling fibroblasts). These come into contact and cohere, and then imbibing calcareous salts are transformed partly into homogeneous matrix-tissue, partly into bone-corpuscles. In other cases the formation of bone is preceded or accompanied by the formation of granulation-tissue. Owing to this the exact mode in which the bone-substance is generated may be somewhat masked; but close investigation shows that here also osteoblasts are produced in the first instance, and that these are afterwards transformed into bone. The proliferating periosteum very often produces cartilage to begin with. Part of this cartilage may then pass directly into bone by a peculiar transformation. Or the cartilage may be replaced by a medullary tissue abounding in cells; and from this, by the agency of osteoblasts, the bone-substance may ultimately be produced.

Normal cartilage behaves in the same way as that produced by proliferation of the periosteum. Like the latter it may be transformed into medullary tissue and bone-trabeculae. We have thus, in addition to the osteoblastic mode of bone-formation, a second or metaplastic mode, by which an already existing tissue is transformed into bone. As we have said, this occurs most frequently in cartilage; but other fibrous and sarcomatous tissues, by taking up calcareous salts, may in like manner be changed into bone. Their basis-substance is transformed into bony matrix-tissue, and their cells into bone-corpuscles (Arts. 90—92).

Further discussion of the subject of pathological bone-formation will be found in the Special Pathological Anatomy. The recent memoirs of the following authors will serve to illustrate the main questions—KÖLLIKER (*Die normale Resorption des Knochengewebes* Leipzig 1873), STEUDENER (*Beiträge zur Lehre von der Knochenentwickelung* Halle 1875), STRELZOFF (*Die Histogenese der Knochen* Zürich 1873), MAAS (*Ueber Wachsthum und Regeneration der Röhrenknochen, Langenbeck's Arch.* XX), ZIEGLER (*Virch. Arch.* vol. 73), WOLFF (*Unters. üb. d. Entwick. d. Knoch.* Leipzig 1875), BUSCH (*Deut. Zeitschr. f. Chir.* vol. 8), KASSOWITZ (*Die Ossification* Vienna 1881), MACEWEN (*Proc. Roy. Soc.* vol. xxxii).

89. In **muscular fibre,** striated and non-striated, regeneration and hyperplasia start primarily from the existing muscle-cells. Non-striated muscular fibres may possibly be developed from connective-tissue cells also. New muscular cells are produced by ordinary nucleus- and cell-division. In striated muscle, the so-called muscle-corpuscles grow into large cells, losing meanwhile their contractile substance, and multiplying their nuclei. They become elongated and spindle-shaped, and then become converted into striated fibres. It is highly probable that no other cells have the power of generating striated muscle-cells, but on this point opinions differ. Wounds in muscle are filled up by cicatricial tissue, when the superficial muscle-corpuscles have been destroyed.

Nerves and **nerve-cells** have but slight power of reproduction. It is very questionable whether ganglion-cells can be regenerated at all in adult individuals. We have no knowledge of ganglionic hyperplasia.

In the case of nerves themselves, both regeneration and abnormal multiplication occur, though only to a slight extent. In nerve-regeneration the axis-cylinder and sheath of Schwann are the first to be formed, and then the medullary sheath. New nerves are developed only from existing nerves: at any rate very serious doubts attach to the statements which have been made in the opposite sense. Opinions differ as to the part played by the cells of the neurilemma and by the existing axis-cylinder.

The statement that non-striated muscular fibres may be developed from connective-tissue cells has been made by more than one observer (J. ARNOLD, *Virch. Arch.* vol. 39; E. NEUMANN, *Arch. d. Heilkunde* X). It appears certain that cells having at least the structure and appearance of non-striated muscle-cells are so developed; but no proof has been given that they have corresponding physiological properties.

With regard to striated muscle and its regeneration, KRASKE, the latest writer on the subject, asserts positively that new muscle is produced only from existing muscle-elements. ZIEGLER's observations are in accordance with this. An embryological argument may be brought against the possibility of deriving voluntary muscle from connective tissue. According to the HERTWIGS (*Die Coelomtheorie* Jena 1881) the striated muscle-fibres of vertebrates are of epithelial origin: they arise from the epithelia of the body-cavities. They are thus in their genesis and descent distinct from the connective tissues. (Cf. BALFOUR, *Comp. Embryology*, vol. II, ch. xxii.) On the striated muscle-cells of tumours see Art. 153. On the repair of nerves see PAGET, *Surg. Path.* Lect. 11; and RANVIER, *Hist. d. Syst. nerv.* 1878.

CHAPTER XX.

METAPLASIA.

90. A tissue is said to undergo **metaplasia** when it is transformed into another of a diverse kind; and that without passing through an indifferent blastema stage, with the characters of embryonic or formative tissue.

In the foregoing chapter we have more than once pointed out that, of the several tissues belonging to the connective group, one may pass into another by simple modifications, partly affecting the cellular elements, partly the ground-substance. Such modifications are of the nature of metaplasias. They are confined to the connective tissues:—fibrous tissue, cartilage, bone, mucous tissue, and adipose tissue, are so to speak potentially convertible. No such relation holds between fibrous tissue and epithelium or muscle.

The processes involved in metaplasia have their physiological and embryological prototypes. Hyaline cartilage for example is specially prone to transformation: its matrix-substance often undergoes a mucoid softening on the one hand, or a change to fibrous tissue on the other. Hyaline cartilage is in fact at best a transitory structure in man: it disappears in ossification, partly by retrogressive changes, partly by transformation into other tissues such as medullary tissue and true bone. Simple areolar and adipose tissue are likewise prone to change: the *panniculus adiposus* or subcutaneous fat of the adult is in the foetus a mucoid tissue.

Pathological metaplasias are however still more common than such physiological metamorphoses.

The term metaplasia is due to VIRCHOW, who has also fully investigated the significance of the processes included under it (*Virch. Arch.* vols. 8, 79; *Gesammelte Abhandlungen* 1856 pp. 500, 509; *Cellular Pathology*, and 4th German ed., p. 70). The subject seems to have awakened but little attention: it well deserves it, however, for metaplasia plays no small part in pathological change.

91. One of the commonest metaplasias of a connective tissue is that by which cartilage is transformed into mucoid tissue or into areolar tissue.

The first step in the process is the liquefaction or dissolution of the matrix into a mucous or limpid mass (Fig. 21). The capsules

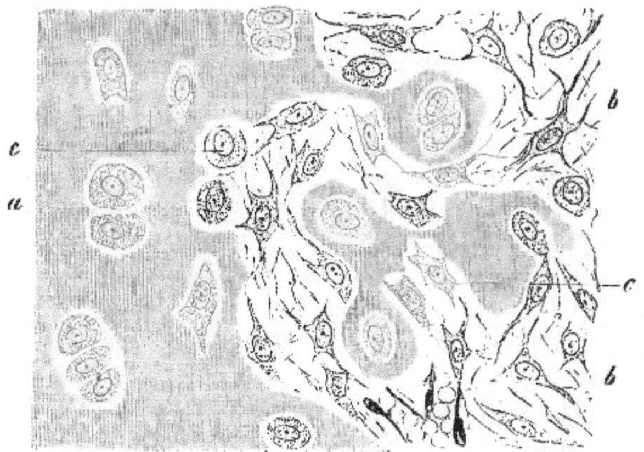

FIG. 21. METAPLASIA OF CARTILAGE INTO AREOLAR TISSUE.
(*From a case of fungous arthritis; haematoxylin staining:* × 100)

a hyaline cartilage *b* tissue made up of branching cells
c cartilage-cells, set free by dissolution of the matrix, becoming converted into connective-tissue corpuscles

also dissolve away and the cartilage-cells are set free (*c*). These change their form (*b*), becoming spindle-shaped or branching; and they then cohere into a cellular reticulum such as is met with in mucous tissue. The matrix-substance does not always become true mucus; it may pass into a liquid of different composition. Such changes are met with in the cartilages of diseased joints. The areolar tissue may subsequently become filled with marrow-cells or with simple fat; in the last case the tissue is transformed into mere adipose tissue (*e.g.* in rheumatic polyarthritis).

Cartilage also changes very readily into osseous tissue. Part of it becomes transformed into bony trabeculae, part into medullary tissue. The latter is effected through the intermediate stage of areolar tissue: the former by the deposition of calcareous salts in the matrix, itself simultaneously undergoing change into gelatin; while the cartilage-cells pass into osteoblasts and bone-corpuscles. It often happens that the cartilage-cells proliferate abundantly during this process; it is not then strictly speaking a pure metaplasia.

Fibrous tissue, like cartilage, may also be transformed into mucoid tissue and bone. The changes in this case are similar to those described in the other. The fibres and fibrillae disappear as the tissue becomes mucoid tissue: when it becomes bone, calcareous salts are deposited in the ground-substance. Here too cell-multiplication is not uncommon.

9—2

Conversely, osseous tissue may pass into fibrous tissue or cartilage, especially the former, as happens very frequently in senile bone-affections. The ground-substance of the bone becomes decalcified and fibrillated, while the bone-corpuscles become connective-tissue cells.

The fibrous structures found in tumours are, like the normal ones, liable to metamorphosis into others of the same class. The metaplastic processes resemble those in normal tissues. The highly cellular sarcomatous tissue is very prone to transformations; and these are generally such as to show that it is allied to the connective-tissue group.

92. Metaplasia is to be distinguished from the simple degenerations as well as from the proliferative processes. In degeneration no new tissue is formed, and what exists perishes. In proliferation new tissue is formed from a cellular matrix or blastema, which is the result of cell-multiplication. Metaplasia stands in a measure between these. New tissue is formed; but there is no cell-multiplication, or if there is it is quite subordinate.

From many points of view metaplasia seems related to the retrogressive processes. The transformation of a tissue into mucoid tissue is near akin to mucoid degeneration. The new or transformed tissue is moreover not infrequently an unstable and perishable one. On the other hand, proliferation is no uncommon accompaniment of metaplasia, which is thus brought into relation with the progressive or formative disturbances of nutrition. The factor of greatest importance, as regards the further development of the transformed tissue, is the behaviour of the blood-vessels. If good vascularisation is effected, the tissue continues to live and grow: if not, then retrogressive changes are apt to set in.

SECTION V.

INFLAMMATION AND INFLAMMATORY GROWTHS.

CHAPTER XXI.

THE EARLY STAGES OF INFLAMMATION. EXUDATION.

93. **Inflammation** is a term implying a whole series of processes partly vascular and partly textural; and these processes admit of a great variety of combinations. Inflammation being thus a complex of many elements, we are unable to give a definition of it that shall be brief and at the same time exact. We might say indeed that one or other element (such as that relating to the vessels) is characteristic of inflammation: but the whole content of the term cannot be fully indicated without describing the processes to which the term is applied.

From the time of CELSUS, *i.e.* from the first century A.D., four cardinal symptoms of inflammation have been recognised; namely '*rubor, tumor, dolor, calor*'—or redness, swelling, pain, and heat. To these we may generally add a fifth, the *functio laesa, i.e.* impairment or arrest of the function of the inflamed part.

These cardinal symptoms are, as a fact, very easily and very frequently to be made out; especially in cases where the inflammation is sudden and intense. In other cases, and especially in chronic inflammations, one or other of the symptoms is generally absent, or beyond the reach of observation. The constitution of the inflamed tissue may also modify the symptoms: its texture and composition may be such that the redness, for instance, or the pain, or the swelling, may be absent.

94. GALEN rightly attributed the redness to an increased afflux of blood, and the swelling to an increased exudation from the vessels. The vascular changes, which thus take the form of hyperaemia, have been the subject of special attention during the last twenty or thirty years. Many investigators indeed have regarded the vascular changes as constituting the essential feature of the inflammatory process.

ANDRAL defined inflammation simply as hyperaemia. HENLE, STILLING, VACCA, LUBBOCK, and others referred the dilatation of the vessels, the accumulation of blood in them, and the resulting exudation, to paralysis of the vessel-walls from excitation of the sensory nerves (the neuroparalytic theory); HOFFMANN, EISENMANN, JOS. HEINE, BUDGE, BRUECKE, CULLEN, and others, to spasmodic contraction of the vessels (the neurospastic theory). In the latter case, the contraction of the arteries and the consequent slowing of the blood-current were supposed to lead to an afflux of blood through the neighbouring vessels, but in an inverse direction. The result of this vascular disturbance was engorgement and exudation.

In opposition to these neuropathic theories, some authors, like HALLER, VOGEL, KOCH, EMMERT, SIMON, PAGET, &c., explain the inflammatory disturbance of circulation and nutrition by supposing that the normal attraction of the tissues for the blood is somehow intensified. VIRCHOW has formulated this 'theory of attraction' with the greatest precision. In his view, the tissue-cells are excited by the 'inflammatory stimulus' to increased activity: they thereupon attract to themselves more nutriment, and so are impelled to grow and multiply. The hyperaemia and vascular dilatation are the result of this intenser attraction. The essential and efficient factor in inflammation is thus the application of a 'stimulus' to the cells, which excites them to increased activity.

Numerous experimental researches during the last twenty years (amongst which those by COHNHEIM are perhaps the most fundamentally important) have shown that neither the neuropathic nor the attraction theory can be maintained. Mere dilatation or mere contraction of the vessels does not bring about the disturbances of the circulation characteristic of inflammation. The changes observed in the tissue-cells at the beginning of inflammation do not bear the character of productive or formative disorders of nutrition. There is no evidence of any influence exerted by the tissues on the vessels and the blood, which is at all of the nature of attraction. The changes in the tissue-cells are partly concomitant with those in the circulation, partly antecedent to them, and partly subsequent. The vascular disturbance is not dependent on any peculiar influence exerted upon the vessels; it is the result of injury or deterioration (SAMUEL) of the vessel-walls, with or without an actual lesion of the tissues. To simplify the explanation of the entire process of inflammation, it will therefore be well to consider separately the vascular changes, and the textural changes.

For an account of the contributions which English pathologists (notably HUNTER, GOODSIR, BOWMAN, LISTER, and BURDON SANDERSON) have made to our present knowledge of Inflammation the student should consult PAGET (*Surgical Pathology* Lects. 13–18), SIMON and BURDON SANDERSON (Arts. on *Inflammation*, *Holmes's Syst. of Surgery*, vols. 1 and 5), and BURDON SANDERSON (*Lectures*, *Lancet* 1, 1876 and *Lumleian Lectures*, *Lancet* 1, 1882). References to the work of others will be found below.

95. **The vascular changes**. COHNHEIM'S researches were the first to make us accurately acquainted with the vascular disturbances connected with inflammation. He showed that these disturb-

ances may be directly studied under the microscope. The object is usually some transparent vascular membrane belonging to a living animal. The most convenient is the frog's mesentery, which from its fineness is well adapted for microscopic examination. The frog, paralysed with curare, is laid on its back on a large object-stage. The abdominal cavity is opened by means of a cut along the left side, and a loop of intestine is carefully drawn out. This is then spread over a thin circular cover-glass (10—12 mm. in diameter) surrounded by a thin ring of cork stuck to the stage with Canada balsam. The intestine is readily fixed to the cork ring by means of fine pins. If it is not desired to make a protracted examination, it is enough to fasten a cork ring (4—6 mm. thick) to a large object-stage with sealing-wax, and to spread out the intestine over that. The preparation need not be covered with a cover-glass. If no strain is thrown on the mesentery, and it as well as the frog is kept properly moist, the vascular changes may be observed for hours together.

Further details of the method are given by COHNHEIM in his various memoirs on inflammation and embolism (*Virch. Arch.* vol. 40; *Neue Untersuch. üb. Entzünd.* Berlin 1873; *Untersuch. üb. d. embol. Processe* Berlin 1872). The foot-web and tongue of the frog are also very convenient objects. The latter is to be turned out, spread over a cork ring, and fastened down with fine pins. Inflammation is then produced by a drop of acid, or by clipping out a fragment with the scissors.

For the study of the inflammatory process on a large scale the rabbit's ear is well adapted. Inflammation may be set up by rubbing it with croton oil (SAMUEL, *Berl. klin. Woch.* 24, 1866, and *Der Entzündungsprocess* Leipzig 1873). The mesentery or omentum of a warm-blooded animal may also be employed, if proper precautions are taken to maintain the body-heat, &c. See STRICKER and SANDERSON, *Handbook for Phys. Lab.* 1870; THOMA, *Virch. Arch.* vol. 74.

96. The exposure of the mesentery to atmospheric air quickly sets up inflammation. The earliest vascular change is a general **dilatation** of the vessels, first of the arteries, then of the capillaries and veins. The **flow** of the blood through the widened channels at first becomes **more rapid**; but sooner or later the speed diminishes, and at length the flow becomes **slower** than the normal. The individual blood-cells, which at first were indistinctly seen as they hurried past, become recognisable, especially in the veins and capillaries. In these latter the blood begins to accumulate more and more as the current slows. In the veins the peripheral layer of the current, usually containing plasma only, begins to be filled with white blood-cells. These have left the axial stream, and float slowly on with the slower peripheral current; or, fastening themselves to the wall, they remain immoveable or oscillate to and fro. This is described as the marginal or **peripheral disposition** of the white blood-cells (Fig. 22 *d*). At this stage the red cells take the place of the white in the capillaries.

Before long the peripheral disposition of the cells is associated with another appearance. Here and there white blood-cells throw out processes which pass into the vessel-wall (*e*). Soon the processes appear outside the vessel (*e*), and thereupon the whole

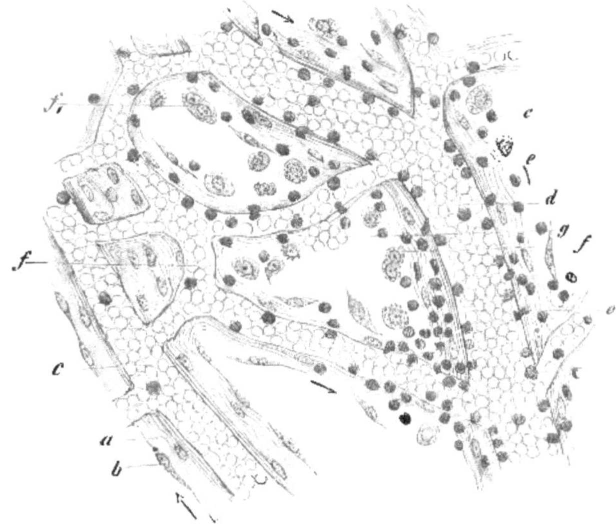

FIG. 22. INFLAMED OMENTUM FROM THE HUMAN SUBJECT.

a normal fibrous trabecula
b normal endothelium
c small artery
d vein with white blood-cells peripherally disposed
e white blood-cells migrated or migrating
f desquamated endothelium
f_1 multinuclear cell
g migrated red blood-cells

protoplasmic mass of the cell passes through the wall. The white cells in this way escape, migrate, or extravasate from the vessel (vein or capillary) by **diapedesis.**

The first white blood-cells which migrate are quickly followed by others, and in six to eight hours the veins and capillaries are surrounded by a multitude of white cells, or leucocytes, which gradually distribute themselves through the tissue by active locomotion.

From the capillaries, in which the circulation becomes very irregular and often stops altogether, there escape red blood-cells (*g*), as well as white. If the mesentery be slightly strained so that the circulation is brought to a stand-still (stasis) at some point, the migration ceases there. Blood-cells do not escape from the arteries.

Associated with the escape of the formed elements of the blood, there is always an **escape of liquid.** This is not in general directly perceptible, but is evidenced by the accumulation of liquid which takes place in the substance and on the surface of the mesentery.

This escaped liquid is comparatively rich in albumen, and thus differs essentially from the exudation which follows upon simple vascular engorgement. Moreover it coagulates readily, especially when it is effused on the surface of the mesentery.

This description of the inflammatory process as observed in the mesentery applies also to that produced elsewhere, as in the frog's tongue, by caustics. In the latter case the process is not observed in the cauterised piece (which is in fact dead), but in its neighbourhood. THOMA (*Virch. Arch.* vol. 74) has shown that the process in warm-blooded animals is identical with that in cold-blooded animals.

W. ADDISON (*Trans. Prov. Med. Ass.* 1842—5) observed the escape of the white blood-cells from the vessels so early as 1842. WALLER (*Phil. Mag.* vol. 29) described the phenomenon more fully in 1846. The discovery was however completely forgotten until COHNHEIM made it anew in 1867. CATON (*Journ. Anat. Phys.* 1871) showed that the white cells escape even from healthy vessels, at least in the amphibia.

The peripheral disposition of the white blood-cells is a purely mechanical phenomenon (WEIGERT, Article *Entzündung*, *Realencyclopädie der ges. Heilkunde*). It was first observed by WILLIAMS (*Gulstonian Lect.* 1841). SCHKLAREWSKY (*Pflüg. Arch.* vol. 1) has shown that a similar effect is produced when a slow stream of liquid, containing fine powders of various densities in suspension, is made to pass through a narrow tube. When the stream flows at a certain rate the lighter particles cling to the periphery, the heavier ones are hurried on by the axial current. This is what happens in the case of blood. When the current is slowed to a certain extent, the white cells go to the periphery: when it becomes still slower (as in engorgement) the red cells go there also. (See also APPERT, *Virch. Arch.* vol. 71; HAMILTON, *Proc. Roy. Soc. Edin.* vol. XI.)

The chemical composition of inflammatory exudations and inflammatory lymph has been investigated by HOPPE-SEYLER (*Virch. Arch.* vol. 9), REUSS (*Deutsch. Arch. f. klin. Med.* XXIV), F. A. HOFFMANN (*Virch. Arch.* vol. 78), and LASSAR (*Virch. Arch.* vol. 69).

97. The effects of the process just described are easy to follow. The inflamed tissue becomes red, swollen, and hot: we have the inflammatory flush, and the inflammatory exudation or infiltration. The pain felt is referable to pressure, tension, or chemical irritation, acting on the sensory nerves in the tissue. It is plain, too, that the function of the part must be injuriously affected: the accumulation of exuded matter and the imperfect and disordered nutrition of the part are enough to account for that. The vascular disturbance is beyond doubt the most important and most characteristic factor in the entire process of inflammation. The other tissue-changes involved are not to be overlooked or undervalued; but it is the disturbances in the circulation which give inflammation its special character, and determine its course. The question as to the essential nature of inflammation is thus almost reduced to the question of the causation of these vascular disturbances.

The slowing of the blood-current, the dilatation of the vessels, the peripheral disposition of the white blood-cells, the migration of these from capillaries and veins, and the migration of the red cells from the capillaries, are all of them referable to a molecular **alteration in the vessel-walls** (SAMUEL). Mere paralytic dilatation does not give rise to slowing of the current, or to peripheral disposition of the white cells: mere slowing of the current is not followed by extravasation of the cellular elements of the blood. Increased activity of the neighbouring cells will not explain exudation, for white and red blood-cells will escape from the vessels into a tissue whose cells are already dead. COHNHEIM has shown that if the circulation through a vessel is interrupted for a certain time (in frogs, from 36 to 60 hours), the vessel-wall undergoes such changes that, when the blood is again allowed to circulate, an exudation makes its appearance just as in inflammation.

The alterations in the vessel which take place in inflammation cannot be histologically demonstrated. We infer them from the fact that the vessel-wall becomes more permeable. We must suppose that the elements composing the vessel-wall are in some way loosened: the cementing substance which unites the endothelial cells seems partially to give way. ARNOLD'S researches make it likely that the cells transude chiefly at places where the intercellular cement is abundant. The slowing of the blood-current itself may probably be due to endothelial changes, in virtue of which the frictional adhesion between blood and vessel-wall is increased (LISTER, RYNECK, COHNHEIM).

It may be accepted as an established fact that in inflammation the vessel-wall is affected (SAMUEL, *Virch. Arch.* vol. 43, and COHNHEIM, *loc. cit.*). But it is still questioned by some whether the affection is of the nature of a chemical alteration, or a mere widening of pre-existing intercellular apertures. ARNOLD, who has worked much at the subject, formerly thought that small openings (*stigmata*) normally existed between the endothelial cells, and that these enlarged in inflammation into wider *stomata*. He based this theory mainly upon injection-experiments, which seemed to show that the vessel-wall was permeable, even to blood-cells. COHNHEIM all along opposed the theory, and ARNOLD has now given it up. At the spots where *stigmata* were said to be we find nothing but little masses of cementing substance. COHNHEIM argued against the existence of openings, from the fact that the exudation has not the same composition as liquor sanguinis. The fact that inflammatory exudation is richer in albumen and in cells, and so coagulates more readily, than the liquid which transudes in simple engorgement, speaks for a change in the permeability of the vessel-wall. This has indeed been demonstrated by injection-experiments (WINIWARTER, *Wien. acad. Sitzungsber.* LVIII; ARNOLD, *loc. cit.*). COHNHEIM, like HERING (*Wien. acad. Sitzungsber.* LVII), regards the escape of the elements of the blood as due to a process of filtration. He thinks the altered quantity and quality of the transudation (in inflammation as compared with health) are referable simply to an alteration of the vessel-wall, that is to say, to an alteration of the filter. THOMA maintains (*Virch. Arch.* vol. 74), on the strength of certain experiments, that the white blood-cells never escape from the vessels unless they retain the power of independent movement. He would thus regard their migration as in some degree due to an active effort on their part. When the white blood-cells are deprived of the power of movement by irrigating the mesentery with 1·5 per cent. salt-solution, the migration at once ceases.

On the causes of the slowing and stasis of the blood-current see LISTER, *Phil. Trans.* 1858; RYNECK, *Rollet's Untersuch. Graz* 1870; COHNHEIM, *Op. cit.* 1873; GLAX and KLEMENSIEWICZ, *Wien. acad. Sitzungsber.* LXXXIV.

The increased temperature of an inflamed surface is due merely to the increased circulation of blood through the part; the loss of heat not keeping pace with the gain. COHNHEIM found by experiment that, in the same time, nearly twice as much blood flowed through the inflamed paw of a dog as through the non-inflamed one. This is quite enough to account for the rise of temperature.

98. The causes of the alteration in the vessels are thus the causes of the inflammation. In other words, the alteration in the vessels is the direct or indirect consequence of the injury which excited the inflammation. Or still more accurately—any injurious agency which is capable of altering the blood-vessels in a particular way is capable of producing inflammation. It is clear then that the number of agencies capable of exciting inflammation is indefinitely great: they are beyond enumeration or separate discussion. All we can say is that mechanical, thermal, and chemical agencies (and especially the latter) may act so as to alter the vessels and produce inflammation.

The exciting cause of inflammation may operate in one of three ways. It is in the first place conceivable that the injurious agent (noxa) may primarily attack the vessels. This will be the case when it is brought to them in the blood itself. The surrounding tissue suffers only by a secondary effect. In the next place, there are cases in which the exciting injury affects both tissue and vessels at the same time. In a third instance, the tissue alone is injured: the alteration in the vessel-wall is secondary to alterations in the surrounding tissue. Of course these cases are not always completely independent. In the same case textural lesions and vascular lesions may intercombine in various ways at different times.

To produce inflammation an injury must be of a certain severity, and yet must not be too severe. Thus a slight wound of the corneal epithelium does not excite inflammation: the defect is simply filled up by regenerative proliferation. On the other hand, a powerful caustic applied to the skin produces at the cauterised spot not inflammation, but necrosis. Inflammation is indeed excited; but only in parts beyond the cauterised region. In these the caustic has not acted fully, so as to kill the vessels: it has merely altered or damaged them by chemical action. This example shows that there are no noxae which can be described specifically as exciters of inflammation. Between the injury which is too slight to affect the vessels, and that which affects them too severely or kills them outright, there is an endless number of intermediate degrees.

The **repair of the damaged vessel-wall** is brought about by the *vis medicatrix* of the blood itself. If, when the injurious influence has ceased, the blood brings to the injured vessel the materials required for restoring it to its normal state, a *restitutio ad integrum* is effected. The inflammatory disturbance of the circulation thereupon comes to an end, and with it the exudation; and the process of healing is begun.

99. **The textural changes.** Inflammatory change in the vessels must of necessity be associated with tissue-change, antecedent, concomitant, or subsequent. An injury from without which excites change in the vessel must always in the first instance affect a certain number of tissue-cells. By what is said in Arts. 78—80 we see that all such an injury can do is to set up disorganising and degenerative changes in the cells. If the injury be slight, the cells may recover: if it be graver, a certain number of them will perish. Multiplication is never induced by excitation of the cells from without.

When the injurious agent affects the vessels primarily, being brought to them by the blood, there are two events possible. If the noxa be very powerful, it will attack (or even kill) not only the vessel-wall, but the surrounding tissue also. If it is of trifling intensity, and its operation is thus confined to the vessel-wall, the surrounding tissue escapes in the first instance. It will be affected secondarily only when the injury to the vessel-wall is great enough to lead to inflammatory disturbance of the circulation, and so to disordered nutrition of the tissue.

Experiment and post-mortem observation have alike shown that in severe inflammation a certain number of cells invariably perish. The so-called 'inflammatory stimulus' does not induce multiplication, but only degeneration and death, in the cells of the tissue. The slighter the inflammatory stimulus the less is the injury to the tissue. The degenerative and destructive effects of the exciting injury are least in the mildest forms of inflammation.

COHNHEIM'S discovery of the migration of white blood-cells suggested a possible source of the extraneous cells found in all inflamed tissues, and in particular a possible source of pus. But the question has often been raised whether all these extraneous cells (round-cells or leucocytes) are derived from the blood. Before the discovery of migration, it was assumed that these leucocytes were the product of the multiplication of tissue-cells, excited to proliferate by the 'inflammatory stimulus.' But it was quickly seen that there were well-founded objections to this hypothesis. COHNHEIM himself (*Virch. Arch.* vol. 40) had shown, and that before he made his discovery, that it was impossible to suppose that all pus-corpuscles arose from fixed cells: and that even the migratory connective-tissue cells of VON RECKLINGHAUSEN were inadequate to produce the enormous multitudes of cells found in pus. Numerous investigations made since then have shown that pus-corpuscles are derived solely from the blood, and that cells of the lymphoid type (such as pus-corpuscles) are never produced from fixed tissue-cells (COHNHEIM, *Neue Unters. üb. d. Entzünd.* Berlin 1873, *Virch. Arch.* vol. 61; KEY and WALLIS, *Virch. Arch.* vol. 55; EBERTH, *Unters. a. d. path. Inst. in Zürich* Parts 2 and 3). As has been stated in the text, the tissue-cells either show signs of degeneration or perish outright, and in this condition mingle with the exudations.

This doctrine has not been without its opponents. Among the chief are BÖTTCHER (*Virch. Arch.* vols. 58, 62) and STRICKER, with some of his pupils (*Studien aus d. Inst. für exper. Path. in Wien* 1870; various essays in the *Wien. med. Jahrb.* 1871—1880; *Vorles. üb. allg. Path.* Vienna 1877—1879; *Internat. Encyclop. of Surgery* vol. 1). BÖTTCHER'S objections have been completely answered by the painstaking experiments of the observers above cited. STRICKER'S observations are admirably described by BURDON SANDER-

SON in *Holmes's System of Surgery* vol. 5. Recent researches have not tended to confirm the results on which STRICKER'S objections are based. Experimental researches on the origin of pus-corpuscles have generally been made on the cornea: as this has no blood-vessels it offers a favourable opportunity for discerning the parts played by the blood and by the tissue-cells respectively.

100. The forms of necrosis and degeneration which may accompany inflammation are very various: they vary with the nature of the exciting cause, and with the intensity of the inflammation; with the character and extent of the vascular disturbance, and with the nature of the tissue. Any one of the forms of degeneration enumerated in Arts. 32—71 may occur. There is no rule determining in what cases any particular form shall appear. It deserves however to be specially mentioned, that a very common issue is the disintegration, solution, and liquefaction of the entire tissue—of its cells as well as its basis-substance. This is the case, for example, in all suppurations, to a greater or less extent. Another common occurrence is the coagulation of the exuded liquid, and also of the disorganised or necrosed tissue-cells. Fatty degeneration is not infrequently a secondary result of the vascular disturbance.

101. **Varieties of inflammation.** Inflammation is a process which may affect any tissue possessing vessels, or in connexion with vessels. In other words, it may affect any tissue in the body, except a few epidermoid structures. Its seat may vary greatly. It may lie within the parenchyma of an organ, or be confined to its surface: that is to say, we may have **parenchymatous** inflammation, or **superficial** inflammation. The former affects the interior parts of solid organs, like the glands, muscles, or brain. The latter form occurs on the exterior of the body, in mucous membranes, and in the lining membranes of the great serous cavities. In the former the exuded liquid saturates the tissues, and is spoken of as an **infiltration**. In the latter it is deposited on the surface, and is spoken of as an **effusion**, or an **exudation** in a narrowed sense of the term. Parenchymatous inflammations are still further subdivided. Glands, muscles, and nerves possess a fibrous framework in addition to their specific elements. Inflammation of the former must be distinguished from that of the latter: we have thus **interstitial** inflammation, as distinguished from parenchymatous inflammation in a narrowed sense of the latter term. There is really no essential difference between the two. The only value of the distinction is—that it allows us to indicate briefly the seat of inflammation in certain organs, whose fibrous framework is well defined from the specific parenchyma. Thus interstitial inflammation of the liver implies that the chief inflammatory changes are to be found in the interlobular fibrous tissue, the liver-cells being relatively less affected. If it is mainly the lobules which are affected, the inflammation is described as parenchymatous. Mistakes are often made by referring

simple degenerative changes in the liver-cells to parenchymatous inflammation.

In speaking of the parenchymatous inflammation of a particular organ, it is customary to make use of a term compounded of the Latin or Greek name of the organ and the affix **-itis**. Thus hepatitis, nephritis, encephalitis, oöphoritis, refer respectively to the liver, kidney, brain, and ovary. In some cases old specific names are used instead, as pneumonia (for pulmonitis), an inflammation of the substance of the lung.

Histologists often indicate that an organ has undergone inflammation by saying merely that it is infiltrated with small cells or leucocytes. This accumulation of cells is in reality the feature by which the fact of antecedent inflammation is most readily recognised.

102. The histological characters of inflammation depend on the one hand upon the nature of the exudation, on the other hand upon the changes in the tissue. Both factors have been utilised in classifying the forms of inflammation, according as one or the other happens to be the more prominent.

With respect to **varieties** in the nature **of the exudation**, the following types are distinguished.

(1) **Serous** and **fibrino-serous** exudation. When the inflammatory alteration in the vessels is not very marked, the exuded fluid may be relatively poor in cells, and in its constitution may resemble the transudation from vessels that are merely engorged. It is however distinguishable from the latter by its greater percentage of albumen and of white blood-cells, and by its greater coagulability. Where it collects in quantity, therefore, it looks more or less turbid, and contains flakes and threads of coagulated fibrin. Collections of this fluid in serous cavities are described as fibrino-serous effusions. When it infiltrates the parenchyma of an inflamed solid organ, it gives rise to **inflammatory oedema**. When it is effused on the surface of the skin or of a mucous membrane, it is spoken of as **serous catarrh**.

(2) **Fibrinous** or **croupous** exudation. When the exudation contains fibrinogenic and fibrinoplastic elements in abundance, it undergoes coagulation throughout. As explained in Art. 35, the fibrinogenic substance is contained in the exuded liquid, the blood-cells yielding the fibrinoplastin. The presence of a certain percentage of leucocytes in the exudation favours coagulation. The term fibrinous exudation is especially applied to effusions into the various body-cavities. The coagulated masses form toughish, yellowish white, adherent films or coverings over the affected organs. When tissues are infiltrated, or mucous membranes covered over, with the coagulated exudation, the term croupous is generally applied to it.

The croupous **false-membranes** formed on mucous surfaces

appear as yellowish white deposits, consisting chiefly of granular fibrinous trabeculae (Fig. 23 *c*) and filaments, interspersed with pus-corpuscles in varying amount.

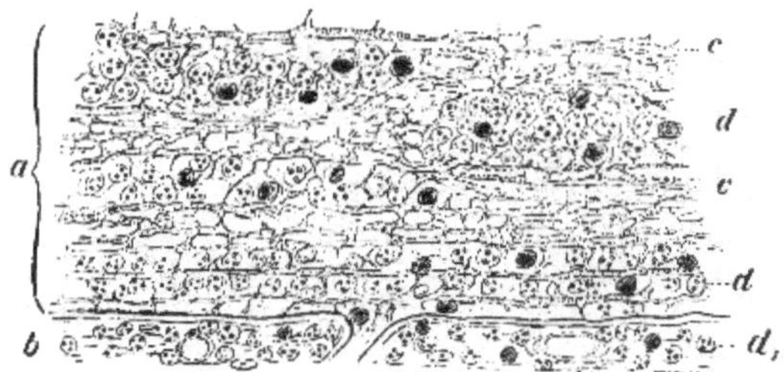

FIG. 23. SECTION OF A CROUPOUS MEMBRANE FROM THE TRACHEA. (× 250)

a false membrane
b surface layer of the mucous membrane infiltrated with leucocytes (d_1)
c fibrin
d pus-corpuscles

In other cases, the false membrane is chiefly made up of hyaline flakes and lumps (Fig. 24 *b*).

(3) **Purulent** or **fibrino-purulent** exudation. When the migration of white blood-cells from the vessels is very extensive, and coagulation does not immediately ensue, the exudation assumes a whitish milky or creamy appearance. It consists simply of a liquid plasma and small leucocytes containing from one to three nuclei, and is called '**matter**' or **pus**. It is commonly the consequence of bacterial infection. The bacteria seem to act so as to hinder coagulation. When the purulent liquid contains in addition white flakes of fibrin infiltrated with pus-cells, the exudation is described as fibrino-purulent. It takes this form chiefly in inflammations of the serous membranes. When purulent infiltration leads to liquefaction and dissolution of the tissues, so that a pus-containing cavity is formed, we have what is called an **abscess**. If the loss of tissue is superficial, and a morbid surface is formed which secretes pus, we have an **ulcer**. Secretion of pus from the skin, mucous membrane, or synovial membrane, constitutes **purulent catarrh**. An infiltration, partly purulent and partly serous, is described as **purulent oedema**.

(4) **Haemorrhagic** exudation. Blood may be mingled with serous, fibrinous, or purulent exudations, and is readily distinguished by its colouring them red. Such mixed exudations are called haemorrhagic.

(5) **Putrid** exudation. When from the presence of septic bacteria the exudation undergoes putrefaction, it is described as foul, putrid, or sanious.

103. We may likewise distinguish certain types of inflammation, according to the way in which the inflamed tissue is affected.

(1) **Desquamative catarrh.** In this form of inflammation, which affects the skin and mucous membranes, the epithelial cells are shed in large numbers and mingle with the secretion. It is also described as epithelial catarrh. Mucous catarrh is a variety of this, distinguished by free mucus-secretion from the surface epithelium, or mucous glands.

(2) **Necrotic inflammation.** This term is applied to cases in which an inflamed tissue dies over an extent that is perceptible with the naked eye. The form of necrosis may vary: it may be simple necrosis, gangrene, mummification, caseation, or coagulation (Arts. 32—42).

A special interest attaches to inflammatory coagulative necrosis or **diphtheritic inflammation** (Art. 38). In this form, the tissue which has been killed by the injury causing inflammation, or by the inflammation itself, coagulates into large flakes and reticulated masses. This happens, for example, in diphtheritic inflammation of the uvula, where the epithelium and infiltrated subepithelial

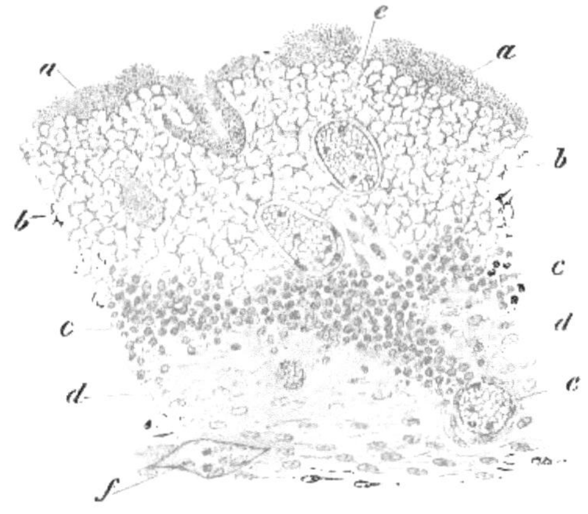

FIG. 24. SECTION OF UVULA FROM A CASE OF DIPHTHERIA.

(*The epithelium has been shed: aniline-brown staining:* × 100)

a micrococci
b sub-mucous tissue changed into amorphous flakes
c infiltrated leucocytes
d fibrinous exudation
e blood-vessels
f lymphatic vessel containing cells and fibrin

tissue are transformed into a coarse mesh-work interspersed with amorphous lumps and flakes (Fig. 24 *b*). The granulating tissue of a wound may in like manner become necrosed, and solidify into diphtheritic denucleated flaky masses.

Necrotic inflammation is of course always grave. It implies severe injury to the tissue, as well as serious alteration in the vessel-walls.

CHAPTER XXII.

LATER STAGES OF INFLAMMATION. RECOVERY. REGENERATION. GRANULATION. CICATRISATION.

104. Inflammation ceases to advance so soon as the blood circulating through the vessels restores their walls to a healthy state. When this happens **recovery** at once begins.

After a slight inflammation, *i.e.* one in which the vessel-walls are but slightly damaged, and the exudation trifling, the tissue affected may recover in a remarkably short time. So soon as the vessels perform their functions normally the exudation ceases to be formed; what is already effused forthwith undergoes **re-absorption** by the lymphatics or by the blood-vessels themselves. Simple serous exudations are those most readily absorbed, but corpuscular elements in moderate amount present no great difficulty. If any of the constituent cells of the tissue have been injured in the course of the affection, they may now recover. Their normal nutrition becomes possible as the circulation re-adjusts itself. In a short time nothing remains to show that inflammation has existed. The affected part becomes perfectly normal again.

If the inflammation has been more intense and the amount of exudation greater, and if in addition tissue-elements have been actually destroyed over a small extent, the process of recovery is somewhat different. When the circulation becomes normal the exudation is re-absorbed as before. Liquid and cells are alike taken up by the lymphatics and blood-vessels. Even coagulated exudations are gradually removed after undergoing liquefaction. The necrosed tissues, like the more solid masses of exudation, are ultimately disintegrated and liquefied, and then removed by absorption. If they lie on the surface they may be directly cast off (Arts. 112—115). If the loss of tissue be not too great, and the remaining parts are healthy and vigorous, **regeneration** or repair is effected by multiplication of the tissue-cells. Epithelium produces epithelium, muscle-cells form fresh contractile substance, periosteum generates new bone, &c. (Arts. 84—89). By and by the

10—2

lost tissue is replaced by new tissue after its kind. It may sometimes even happen that the amount of new tissue produced is in excess of what is needed, and hyperplasia succeeds inflammation. This will happen when the excessive nutrition of the tissue, which usually follows upon inflammation, is kept up for a considerable time.

The magnitude of the defect which can be filled up in this way, and the fitness of the new tissue to replace the old, are matters depending on the regenerative power of the affected structures. As we know, this differs greatly in different tissues (Arts. 84—89). The lining epithelia are able to cover over large denudations of surface, and, as in catarrhal desquamation, may be reproduced again and again. But it would seem that brain-tissue has no power to form a single fresh ganglion-cell.

For the efficient causes which call forth regenerative or hyperplastic proliferation, we refer the reader to Arts. 78—82. Here we have only to remind him once more that it is not the agency or noxa which excited the inflammation which now excites the cells to multiply, by some kind of direct stimulus. Multiplication is completely independent of the original cause of the inflammation. It is simply the result of changes in the vital conditions or environment of the cells; and these changes are the result of the inflammatory process itself.

105. If the inflammation continues for a time and is not too intense, and if the circulation is not too seriously interfered with, so that a good blood-supply is continuously kept up, we have all that is needed for the production of **inflammatory tissue**. The cells which build up the new tissue are the migrated white blood-cells or leucocytes: the new tissue which they form is described as **granulation-tissue** and **cicatricial tissue**. The most important factor in this plastic process is the formation of new blood-vessels. These alone make it possible to keep the young formative tissue supplied with adequate nutriment.

The factors which cause the inflammatory process to take on a formative or constructive character are not always the same. We must in general assume that some cause is acting which keeps up the morbid alteration in the vessel-walls, and so gives the inflammation in some degree a chronic character. In open wounds the inflammation is kept up by contact with the air, with the floating matters suspended in it, with the dressings, with the secretions from the surface. This continues till the skin, growing over from the margins of the wound, at length protects the vascular tissue from further irritation. In subcutaneous necroses following on acute exudative inflammation, the dead tissues or dead exudations are enough to maintain a certain irritation in their neighbourhood, especially as they undergo certain chemical changes before they are finally absorbed. In other cases, the original cause of injury persists and continues to excite ever fresh inflammation: or a new injury may affect a part in which inflammation is declining or overpast, and kindle it afresh. Which of all these possibilities applies to a given case is often hard to determine. Very frequently several such factors are in action, either at the same time, or at different stages of the process.

Plastic inflammation is, moreover, always associated with some form of degeneration. In parenchymatous organs, for instance, the growth of new fibrous tissue involves the atrophy or destruction of the proper and specific elements. Intrinsic sources of irritation of this kind are thus seldom wanting, and they maintain the inflammatory process, even when the original exciting cause has ceased to act.

106. The new tissue produced as a result of inflammation often fulfils the purpose of replacing tissue that has been lost. This application of the process is apparent in the healing of wounds. In an open skin-wound, for instance, there is formed first of all a delicate greyish-red vascular formative layer, the so-called **granulating surface**. This in a way unites the borders of the wound. After a time it becomes covered over with skin, and is transformed into fibrous tissue. The breach is thus filled up, the separated parts united, and a scar is formed. The **scar** or **cicatrix** is thus the result of an inflammatory plastic process. Scar-tissue is formed in other organs in the same way, and with the same result of replacing a loss of substance.

In many cases, however, the production of new tissue by inflammation does not serve so useful a purpose. It often takes the form of a useless or injurious hyperplasia. This happens, for example, when after inflammation the corium of the skin thickens, or the papillae become enlarged; or when the fibrous tissue of the kidney or the liver is morbidly increased, giving rise to disturbances in the nutrition of the organ. Even the formation of adhesions and adhesive membranes connecting the organs of the great serous cavities is often accompanied by impairment and hindrance of their functions.

107. As we have just stated (Art. 105), inflammatory tissues are developed from extravasated leucocytes, in cases where the circulation has not been very seriously interfered with. This last ensures that the exuded corpuscles are speedily irrigated with a sufficient but not too abundant stream of plasma. These conditions are perfectly fulfilled in the aseptic healing of an ordinary wound.

If an open wound be observed twenty-four hours after it is inflicted, the bottom and edges will be found to be intensely red and somewhat swollen. The elements of the tissue are still quite distinguishable, though the tissue seems turgid, and here and there small necrosed shreds are visible. On the second day, the tissues have a more gelatinous appearance, the outlines of the tissue-elements (cells and fibres) are blurred, and the colour is a greyish red. A reddish yellow liquid lies on the surface. After the second day little red nodules or granules begin to appear over the entire wound. These increase rapidly in size and number, and become at length confluent. After two or three days there is thus formed a continuous red granular layer—the granulating surface. It is covered with a more or less abundant secretion, which changes to a greyish gelatinous film, and afterwards becomes more yellowish and creamy in consistence. This film is composed of an albuminous coagulable exudation and numerous leucocytes, some of them with one nucleus, but most of them with two or three small rounded ones. These are **pus-corpuscles**. They are not capable of further development, but are rather to be looked upon as cells in process of decay. The multiplication of the nuclei is evidence, not of subdivision, but of disintegration.

The whole of the new tissue formed is derived from this delicate red formative or embryonic tissue, the granulation-tissue. From this the cicatricial tissue is developed.

It seems beyond doubt that the multiple nuclei of pus-cells (Fig. 25 a_1) are simply the result of disintegration. Nothing has been observed to indicate that the division of the nucleus is followed by a division of the cell, and nothing is known of their further development. Besides, it is noted that the combined size of the multiple nuclei is not greater than that of the single nucleus. This shows that the partial nuclei have not the power, like true daughter-nuclei, of growing by assimilation of substance from the protoplasm of the cell (KÜSS, *De la vascularité et de l'inflammation* Paris 1846; PAGET, *Surg. Path.* Lect. 10).

108. The naked-eye appearances in the healing wound are referable, partly to the accumulation of white blood-cells, partly to dilatation and distention of the vessels, and partly to the formation of new vessels. This latter takes place by means of off-shoots from the capillaries, as described in Art. 86. No other mode of vascularisation has been certainly made out.

The development of granulations and cicatricial tissue takes place in the following way.

The injury sets up inflammation, which leads to an infiltration of cells at the borders of the wound. Large numbers of migrated cells (with a certain quantity of fluid) are thus accumulated. Meanwhile parts of the existing tissue disintegrate by softening and liquefaction. A soft texture is in this way produced which is made up almost entirely of young round-cells, with very little intercellular substance. Some of these cells, chiefly those containing several fragmentary nuclei (Fig. 25 a_1), cease thereupon to live, and form true pus-corpuscles. They are either thrown off with the secretions from the wound, or are absorbed, or dissolved *in situ* and utilised to feed the more vigorous living cells. On the other hand another set of (uninuclear) cells (a) begin to grow. Their protoplasm increases in amount and becomes more markedly granular (Fig. 25 b). At the same time the cloudy finely-granular rounded nucleus becomes clearer, oval, and vesicular (*b*). The nuclear juice and nuclear substance become distinct, so that it becomes possible to discern clearly a nuclear membrane, nucleoli, and nuclear granules

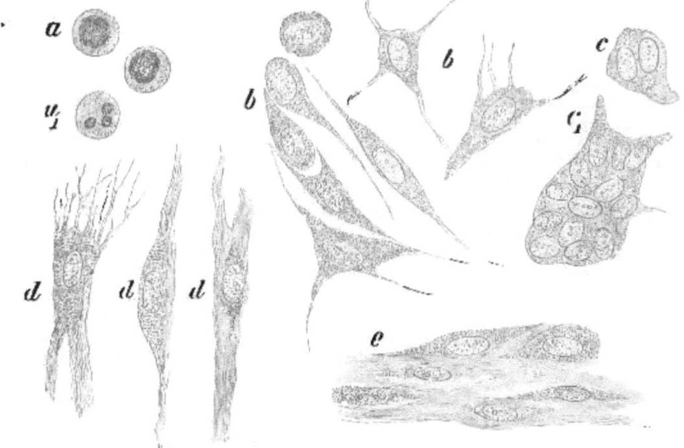

FIG. 25. GRANULATION-CELLS IN VARIOUS STAGES.

(*Picrocarmine staining*: × 500)

a uninuclear, a_1 multinuclear migrated white blood-corpuscles
b various forms of uninuclear formative cells
c binuclear, c_1 multinuclear formative cell
d formative cells developing into connective tissue
e developed connective tissue

and filaments. This differentiation of the elements of the nucleus gives the cell an altogether different aspect and habit. It resembles an epithelial cell, or as it is phrased—it becomes **epithelioid**.

The transformation of leucocytes into epithelioid cells is accompanied by cohesion of the protoplasm of separate cells. A growing cell may appropriate the substance of others which are decaying; or two equal cells may coalesce to form a single one.

The epithelioid cells are the formative cells of the granulation-tissue: they alone have the power of producing new connective tissue. They are best described as **fibroblasts**. They are usually uninuclear, and their numbers increase partly by successive transformations of round-cells, partly by subdivision. Very probably the division of their nuclei is of the karyokinetic type. If the protoplasm does not subdivide for some time after the nucleus has divided, binuclear (*c*) cells are formed; and even in some instances large multinuclear cells, the so-called **giant-cells** (c_1). In healthy granulations giant-cells are produced but sparingly.

ZIEGLER has endeavoured to prove experimentally that the migrated white blood-cells are capable of further development, and are the primary source of cicatricial tissue (*Exper. Untersuch. üb. d. Herkunft d. Tuberkelele-*

mente Würzburg 1875, and *Untersuch. üb. path. Bindegewebs- und Gefässneubildung* Würzburg 1876). He made a small disc-shaped chamber by fastening together two thin cover-glasses a slight distance apart. This was inserted under the skin of a dog and left for a certain length of time. When it was removed its contents could be examined microscopically. The thin interspace was found to be filled with cells, which either perished and broke up or underwent further development. In a single layer of cells obtained in this way, there were always some undergoing progressive change, and they could be observed with great ease. Thus not merely at the borders, but over the whole field, cells were found in all stages of development from the lymphoid to the epithelioid and giant-cell type. The actual formation of tissue from them could be followed. When large cells are formed, a certain number of the round-cells in their neighbourhood disappear. It is as if their protoplasm were appropriated by the larger growing cell. This is less surprising, as we know that migratory cells frequently pick up molecular matters (such as cinnabar) which they find in their way. The only difference is that the protoplasm is assimilated and utilised for growth; the cinnabar of course is not.

The various stages of nucleus-division cannot as yet be described in detail: only some of them have been observed. So far as is known, they correspond with the scheme of Arts. 74 and 75. Now and then a radial arrangement of the granules of the protoplasm is observed near the poles of the nucleus.

ZIEGLER's results have been called in question by various observers (EWETZKY, WEISS, BÖTTCHER, BAUMGARTEN, and others). These observers maintain that the migrated cells have no power of further development, and attribute the formation of new tissue to the multiplication of the fixed tissue-cells, especially in the case of the epithelia. Their experimental methods have been so different from ZIEGLER's, and their criticisms rest so much more on their own special theories of inflammation than on the facts adduced, that it is difficult to find a common basis for the discussion of them. Those who have used similar methods have in the main arrived at similar results. SENFTLEBEN (*Virch. Arch.* vols. 72 and 77) introduced fragments of dead lung or artery-wall into the peritoneal cavity of an animal. TILLMANNS (*Virch. Arch.* vol. 78) used bits of hardened organs with artificial cavities in them. HAMILTON (*Sponge-grafting, Edin. Med. Journ.* 1881) introduced bits of sponge. All of these have found that the cells which migrate into the receptacles thus artificially provided undergo further development. HEIDENHAIN had already discovered large cells in round bits of elder-pith, which he had inserted into the abdominal cavity of guinea-pigs (*Ueber d. Verfettung fremder Körper in der Bauchhöhle* Breslau 1872). SCHEDE (*Arch. f. klin. Chir.* XV), AUFRECHT (*Virch. Arch.* vol. 44), BIZZOZERO (*Annali universi di medicina* 1868), and others had already observed facts which were in favour of the notion that development does take place in migrated cells.

109. The newly-formed fibroblasts are rounded cells (Fig. 25 *b*). They soon change their form however by sending out processes and becoming elongated. In this way cells are produced which are club-shaped, spindle-shaped, or branched (*b*); and these cohere and coalesce in various ways. Meantime the larger formative cells are multiplied till at length they outnumber the small round-cells. Here and there they become tightly packed together. This is especially noticed in the deeper layers of the granulation-tissue. When their number has reached a certain point, fibrous tissue begins to be produced by the formation of a fibrillated intercellular substance. This latter arises in part directly from the cell-protoplasm, and in part from a homogeneous ground-substance derived from the fibroblasts. In the first case, from the ends and lateral

borders of the formative cells (*d*) there grow out fine fibrillae, which unite with those of the neighbouring cells. The direction and extent of the fibrous strands thus produced are independent of the original form and disposition of the formative cells. The run of the fibres is generally in the same direction for considerable lengths. When the fibrillae have reached a certain degree of definiteness and strength the process of fibrillation ceases, and the remaining cells with their nuclei remain as fixed connective-tissue cells (*e*). They lie along the surface of the fibrous bundles. The process is thus completed: granulation-tissue has become **cicatricial tissue**.

The formation of **new vessels** starts as soon as the first formative cells are developed. It proceeds rapidly, and even in a day or two multitudes of vascular loops are already produced. They bring the granulations the nutriment they need, and supply cells to fill the vacancies occasioned by absorption of the first leucocytes. The only part taken by the epithelioid cells in vascularisation is—that they serve to strengthen the thin-walled new capillaries, by disposing themselves along the outer surface of the vessels. It is possible that fibroblasts may now and then take part in the formation of new vessels. This they may do by attaching themselves to the budding off-shoots, and thus assuming the form of buds themselves. By excavation of their contents they are then converted into permeable channels.

Giant-cells, when they are present, seem to play no special part in the transformation of the granulations. They form fibrous tissue in the same manner as the other fibroblasts.

ZIEGLER has observed the process of scar-formation from granulation-tissue, both in ordinary granulations and by the cover-glass method. The latter yields preparations which are better than any sections, inasmuch as all the cells and cell-structures remain *in situ:* there is no possibility of disintegration or disturbance of the natural relations. TILLMANNS' (*loc. cit.*) observations agree with ZIEGLER'S.

The assertion is often made (BILLROTH'S *Surgical Pathology*, RINDFLEISCH'S *Pathological Histology*) that granulation-tissue passes into spindle-celled tissue. This is only partially the case. Spindle-cells are formed often enough, but the cells are just as often of many diverse shapes.

The granulations, when they are first formed, are nourished by the plasma which escapes from the existing vessels. THIERSCH has shown that the spaces in which this circulates among the granulations may be injected from the blood-vessels. This mode of nutrition is however inadequate for the complete formation of the embryonic tissue; new vessels are therefore required.

ZIEGLER (*loc. cit.*) and BRODOWSKI (*Virch. Arch.* vol. 63) have described a special relation of the giant-cells to the process of vascularisation, but this is no longer maintained.

110. The constructive processes taking place in the wound are completed when the cicatricial fibrous tissue is formed. The subsequent changes are limited to a certain amount of shrinking or contraction in the new tissue, and the suppression of some of the new blood-vessels. The scar, which from its vascularity is at first decidedly redder than its surroundings, begins to pale; and at

length becomes paler and whiter than its surroundings. A depression frequently results from the shrinking of the cicatricial tissue. The smaller the wound the smaller and less marked is the scar.

This form of healing, in which the wound is closed by means of its own granulations, is called healing by **second intention**. Healing by **first intention** occurs when two wounded surfaces come into contact and grow together without the intervention of visible granulations. In principle the process is the same as in the first case. An inflammatory infiltration is produced, and in this new vessels and new fibrous tissue are developed. The difference is merely quantitative. In skin-wounds, for example, the exudation and granulations are so insignificant in amount that they are imperceptible; they are very quickly bridged and covered over by regenerative multiplication of the epidermal cells.

The chronic inflammatory processes leading to fibrous hyperplasia follow in general the same course as when new tissue is being formed. In different organs however there are special peculiarities to be noted. They will be treated of in considering the special pathology of the several organs.

111. While cicatricial tissue is forming in an organ by means of granulations, it usually happens that the **fixed tissue-cells** also begin to multiply by subdivision. The extent to which this multiplication goes on, and the share it contributes to the final result, are by no means constant. But they are by no means negligible, especially in long-continued inflammations. Hence the different importance assigned to such cell-multiplication by different observers. Some ascribe all formation of new tissue to it, denying the existence of the inflammatory process above described. Others allow it small significance, or ignore it altogether. The truth is probably this—that accompanying the inflammatory constructive process, there is always some regenerative proliferation in the tissue, and that this is in inverse relation to the severity of the inflammation. Epithelium is a tissue which cannot be reproduced by means of granulations; it can be reproduced only by regenerative proliferation. Other specially differentiated tissues, such as muscles, nerves, bones, vessels, are in the same case. These, if replaced at all, must be replaced by regeneration starting in pre-existing homologous tissues. Cicatricial tissue pure and simple is therefore devoid of all such specialised structures, with the one exception of vessels.

If we were to define granulation-tissue according to its apparent purpose we might say—that it is a structure fashioned out of the cellular material gathered by the blood from the system in general, and utilised to make good a defect which the fixed tissue-cells of the injured region are unable to repair. This final purpose, unfortunately for teleology, only appears in the process by which wounds are repaired. It is not apparent in the fibrous hyperplasias of glandular organs, or in the formation of adhesions and false membranes; but the mechanism is the same.

CHAPTER XXIII.

IMPERFECT RE-ABSORPTION. FOREIGN SUBSTANCES.

112. The **re-absorption** of inflammatory exudations is not always so complete as we have hitherto assumed (Art. 104). Though it is true that in most cases even exudations containing numerous corpuscular elements are sooner or later absorbed, still there are limitations to this; or it may be that circumstances arise which directly check or hinder the process. If re-absorption (or briefly resorption) does not ensue, further changes take place in the exudation, whether it be an effusion into a cavity or an infiltration of a tissue. The commonest result is condensation, depending on loss of water and caseation. In purulent effusions, for example, the pus-cells undergo fatty changes (Fig. 26 *d*, 'GLUGE'S

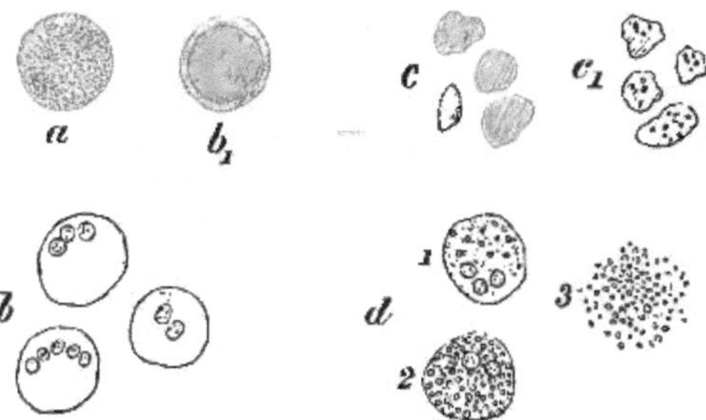

FIG. 26. PUS-CELLS BECOMING FATTY AND SHRINKING (× 400)

a pus-cell in solution of common salt
b pus-cell treated with acetic acid b_1 so-called granulation-cell
c shrunken pus-cells c_1 shrunken and fatty pus-cell
d pus-cells that have become fatty and broken up (GLUGE'S corpuscles)

corpuscles'). They then shrink and break up, so that presently all that is left is a mass of small irregular lumps (c and c_1), and granular detritus (d_3). The watery parts of the exudation being more or less absorbed, these products of disintegration form a creamy or cheesy pulp. Fibrinous effusions may also be transformed into a mass of cheesy detritus. These not infrequently become calcified as time goes on.

Condensed effusions of this kind may long resist resorption. It often happens that they cannot be removed in this way at all. Infiltrated tissues which have necrosed may in like manner resist resorption, and so persist for an indefinite time. Dead bone and fascia especially, which are hard to liquefy or disintegrate, may long be retained. But softer tissues may likewise become incapable of resorption, when necrosis has resulted in their caseation or mummification.

113. Tissues which have been killed by the original injury or by the subsequent inflammation, and inflammatory exudations, are no longer parts of the organism. They are **foreign substances**, and they act as such. In other words, they set up and maintain inflammation in their neighbourhood. They act like foreign bodies thrust forcibly into the tissues from without. Necroses other than inflammatory, such as those resulting from ischaemia, and haemorrhagic effusions or extravasated blood which has become necrosed, all act in the same way as foreign substances. To the tissue affected by them it matters nothing whether they once belonged to the organism or not. It is of more importance to consider the physico-chemical nature of the foreign substance. This it is which determines the intensity, the extent, the general character of the inflammation induced.

The great importance of the inflammations excited by such dead or foreign substances makes it absolutely essential to have a clear conception of their nature. And we must in especial discover the characteristics of the inflammation set up when the foreign substances are of corpuscular size. Stated generally, we may put it—that in such a case we have in addition to the ordinary phenomena of inflammation other processes whose object is the removal of the foreign substance. The peculiarities of special cases depend on the physico-chemical nature of the substance.

Foreign substances may be divided into two groups:—those which have but a slight effect or none in altering the surrounding tissue, and those which act destructively and excite violent inflammation. Among the first group are some substances easily absorbed, and others which are absorbed with difficulty.

114. The easily-absorbed substances include liquids and small solid matters which have no intense chemical action on the surrounding tissue. Of this latter kind are, for example, cinnabar, which is rubbed into the skin in tatooing; the dust of coal, lime, or iron, which is inhaled and passes from the alveoli into the lung-tissue; and lastly fatty and disintegrated exudations, softened and disintegrated tissues, and such like.

The effects produced in the organism by small corpuscular bodies of the above kinds are not serious. Perceptible inflammatory changes are brought about only when large quantities of them are present together: their effects are thus integrated as it were.

Most of the pulverulent or corpuscular matters referred to are removed from the tissue containing them by resorption. If they lie within a liquid exudation (as do fatty pus-cells or free oil-globules) they may be taken up along with it into the lymphatics, and so carried off. A large number of them would still however remain, if another means were not at hand for disposing of them. The additional resource is brought into play by the mild inflammation which the foreign substance excites. The agents are the white blood-cells which thereupon migrate from the blood-vessels.

These migratory cells appropriate the foreign substances lying in the tissue (Fig. 27 h h_1 h_2 h_3). They let their protoplasm flow

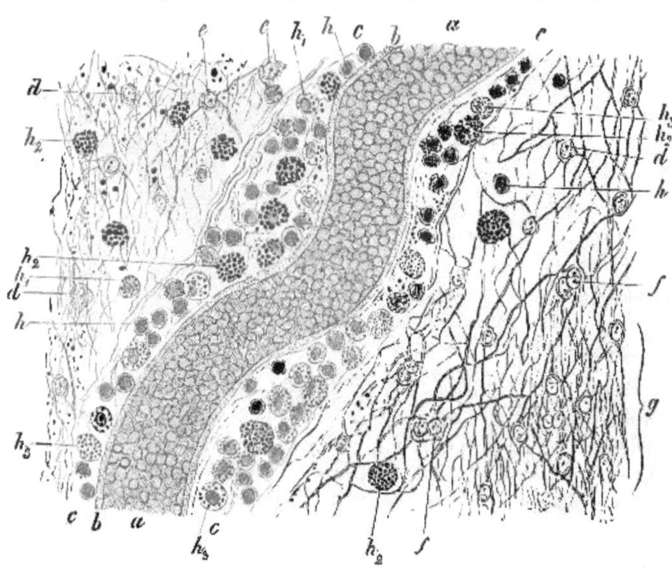

FIG. 27. SECTION THROUGH A DEGENERATING PATCH FROM THE BRAIN.

(*Osmium preparation:* × 200)

a blood-vessel filled with blood
b tunica media
c adventitia with its lymph-sheath
d unaltered neuroglia-cells
e fatty neuroglia-cells
f binuclear neuroglia-cells
g sclerosed tissue
h round-cells
h_1 round-cells containing single oil-globules
h_2 fat-granule carriers
h_3 pigment-granule cells, some containing blood-cells

round them, and so take them up into their interior. By frequent repetition of this process granule-carrying cells are produced. According to their contents, these have been variously described as fat-granule carriers (h_2), blood-cell carriers (h_3), pigment-granule cells (Fig. 28 *c*), dust-cells, cinnabar-carrying spherules, &c. In cerebral degenerations, we constantly find cells containing granules and minute drops (Fig. 27 h_1 h_2): these are migratory cells, which have taken up some of the products of disintegration of the brain-substance.

The carrier-cells ultimately reach the lymphatics. Thus in the brain they accumulate in the lymph-spaces surrounding the adventitia of the arteries (Fig. 27 *c*). Hence they are carried on by the lymph-current, and at length reach the lymphatic glands. Here they are retained for a time, and ultimately filtered away—at least in part. In Fig. 28 is represented a lymphatic gland infiltrated

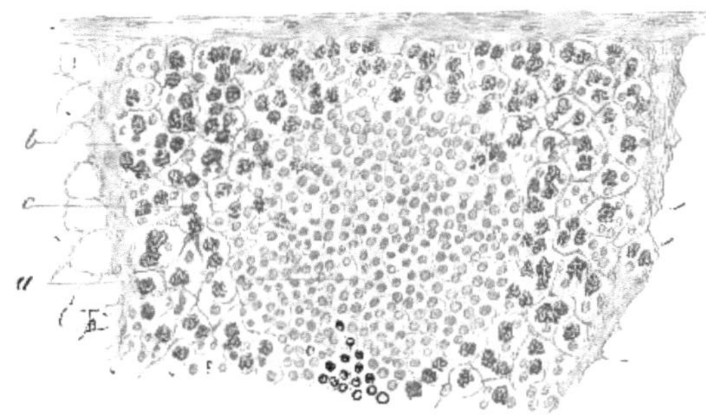

FIG. 28. SECTION OF A LYMPHATIC GLAND WHOSE SINUSES AND ALVEOLI CONTAIN PIGMENT-GRANULE CELLS. (*Carmine staining*: × 80)

a follicle *b* trabeculae *c* pigment-granule cells

with pigment-carrying cells; these were derived from an extensive haemorrhage which had undergone resorption. The pigment-carriers for the most part remain within the lymph sinuses: only a few have penetrated the follicles. The greater portion of the foreign substance absorbed usually remains in the lymphatic gland: but it may happen that a part filters through it and reaches the next gland, or ultimately the blood-vessels. A considerable quantity of corpuscular foreign matter can in this way be removed. Often however the resorption is inadequate, and a portion of the substance remains *in loco*.

Foreign substances may be deposited along the walls of the lymphatics as well as in the glands. The granules inclosed in the carrier-cells are set free as the cells decay. Hence it often happens that lymphatics, which have conveyed away quantities of pigmented substance, show traces of pigmentation all along their course. This happens likewise in the corresponding glands. The deposits may even excite the respective tissues to inflammatory hyperplasia.

The above process is, of course, only carried out in its entirety when the foreign substances are insoluble and indestructible. Soluble and destructible matters like chalk, fat, myeline, are sooner or later dissolved or attacked; the agency of the cells, of oxygen, or of non-organised ferments completes their destruction.

References :—VIRCHOW's *Cellular Pathology*; PONFICK, *Virch. Arch.* vol. 48; RINDFLEISCH, *Exper. üb. d. Histol. des Blutes* 1863; ORTH, *Virch. Arch.* vol. 56; BIZZOZERO, *Med. Jahrb.* 1872.

115. The process of resorption and the associated inflammation are somewhat different in character when the foreign substance forms a compact mass, offering more or less resistance to removal. Such are, for example, ligatures, drainage-tubes, ivory pegs, leaden pellets, necrosed bone, compact haemorrhagic patches, haematomata and infarcts, thrombi, coagulated or condensed exudations, necrotic cheesy masses, &c.

All of these excite in the surrounding tissue a certain amount of inflammation, though its intensity is very various. If the foreign body is quite insoluble in the juices, as glass is, and if the introduction of it is unaccompanied by any injury to the tissues among which it lies (*e. g.* in the abdominal cavity), then the effect may be almost nothing. Bodies which are soluble, and undergo chemical changes in the tissues, usually irritate them much more, and the inflammatory processes excited are generally intense. This is also true of bodies (like bullets) which produce laceration as they penetrate the tissue.

The first stage is the formation of a zone of inflammatory infiltration around the foreign body. This is followed by the development of granulation-tissue, and at length of fibrous tissue. If the foreign body is not meanwhile absorbed, it thus becomes encapsuled. Only insoluble and compact bodies can remain quite unaltered, for resorption is as it were attempted, even though it be in vain. Bodies which are at all assailable are sure sooner or later to undergo changes. These ensue as follows:—the migratory leucocytes, transformed into uninuclear or multinuclear formative cells, attach themselves to the surface of the object. If this be made up of smaller parts, or if particles of necrosed tissue be mingled with it (such as decomposed blood in haemorrhagic patches), these are taken up by the cells and carried off in the manner set forth in Art. 114. If the body be compact and not to be broken up, the cells cling to its surface. If there be accessible cavities or clefts in it, they penetrate into these. If the cells be insufficiently nourished, they become fatty and die. If new vessels are formed to supply them, they develope as granulations. Very often indeed multinuclear or giant-cells are found in such circumstances. A dead piece of bone inserted under the skin of an animal, and examined a few weeks after, will be found interpenetrated with vascular granulations, and the trabeculae will be beset in many places with giant-cells. The whole process is very similar to that of physiological bone-resorption. By means of the clinging cells blood-clots, necrotic patches, inserted pieces of dead liver or lung, ligatures, &c. are absorbed amid the granulations. They are partly softened and dissolved, partly broken up and carried away.

This process is peculiarly modified when the foreign substance is firmly connected with the surrounding tissue; when it is in fact a necrosed fragment of the tissue itself, such as bone or kidney. In this case the first step is the separation of the living tissue from the dead. At the common boundary of the two an inflammatory zone is formed, which by the softening and resorption of the border-tissue leads to the loosening of dead from living. This zone is called the **zone of demarcation**: the loosened piece is a **sequestrum**. The sequestrum is by and by broken up and absorbed. If it lies on the surface it is thrown off as a **slough**: it leaves an **ulcer** behind it.

A further modification ensues when the foreign substance simply lies on the surface of an organ. This occurs, for example, in the fibrinous effusions which form on the surface of the pleura. The deposit is in this case invaded by granulations and cicatricial tissue from one side only. If it lies between two separate organs or lobes it may be invaded from both sides.

LANGHANS (*Virch. Arch.* vol. 49) was the first to describe minutely the processes by which the larger foreign bodies are absorbed. He pursued the subject experimentally by producing extravasations of blood in various animals. He thus discovered the giant-cells. HEIDENHAIN (In. Diss. Breslau 1872) also found them in pieces of elder-pith, which he had inserted in the abdominal cavity of animals. ZIEGLER always met with them on the surface of his cover-glasses (Art. 108). By introducing bits of boiled bone into the abdomen of animals, he found that granulations always penetrated to the interior, and that large **osteoclasts** or resorption-cells (with one or many nuclei) were developed in contact with the bone. SENFTLEBEN (*Virch. Arch.* vol. 77) and TILLMANNS (*Virch. Arch.* vol. 78) have gone further into the matter, and find that hardened aseptic animal tissues, such as bits of liver, kidney, or lung, are partly absorbed and partly adhere and heal in. Fresh tissues are absorbed faster than hardened tissues. HEGAR (*Klin. Vorträge* No. 109) and ROSENBERGER (*Langenbeck's Arch.* XXV) have shown that absorption is most speedy in the case of tissues taken quite fresh from a living organ, and introduced into the body. The inflammatory reaction is very slight, and ends with the process of resorption. The resorption of bone has excited special attention. KÖLLIKER (*Die normale Resorption des Knochengewebes* Leipzig 1873) and WEGNER (*Virch. Arch.* vol. 56) have studied it minutely. They as well as others have made out this process to be something quite peculiar. ZIEGLER (*Virch. Arch.* vol. 73) has sought to do away with the attempted isolation of the process, and to put bone-resorption on a level with other resorptions. He thinks it possible to view all processes of resorption from the same stand-point. In every case the process is carried out with the purpose of removing from the organism a substance which is foreign and useless to it. Giant-cells are very usually formed in such circumstances, and it is possible that they take up the soluble parts of a tissue when it undergoes liquefaction. But resorption is not confined to their agency: it goes on where they are absent. It remains a remarkable fact that they should so frequently be found on the surface of solid objects. It is perhaps conceivable that the contact of the cell with a foreign body hinders in some way the process of cell-division, without affecting the subdivision of the nucleus.

It has long been known that foreign bodies may 'heal into' a tissue. Details of the histological process will be found in the memoirs quoted above. HALLWACHS has lately published some observations on the subject (*Langenbeck's Arch.* XXIV).

116. Many foreign substances, and especially certain altered organic products, have a far more baneful effect on the surrounding tissues than any we have yet considered. Such, in a high degree, is dead tissue which from contamination with septic matters has passed into a state of putrid decomposition.

In the course of this decomposition various chemical compounds are formed which act harmfully on the tissue (Art. 42), and set up in it progressive destructive changes, and violent haemorrhagic or purulent inflammation. Under the action of the pus-cells, which form in great quantity, and of the septic ferments, the necrosed tissue becomes dissolved. If it is connected with living tissue, a suppurative zone of demarcation is formed and sets it free: the result is a cavity filled with pus—an **abscess**. The process often continues, the infiltration and dissolution of tissue go on, and the abscess grows larger and larger.

If decomposing matter from the abscess reach the blood-vessels or lymphatics, and is so conveyed to other regions, it may lead to putrid decomposition and purulent inflammation at the spots where it lodges. In this way **metastatic abscesses** are formed.

If the inflamed region be near a free surface and at length breaks through it, we have a **suppurating ulcer** formed.

Should death not result from this destructive suppuration or purulent necrosis, the injury done may be repaired by the formation of granulation-tissue at the boundary of the living tissue and the dead. In the course of time the pus secreted may be absorbed, or solidified and encapsuled.

CHAPTER XXIV.

THE INFECTIVE GRANULOMATA.

General characters.

117. The granulative formations we are about to discuss are all distinguished by similar characters. Their development usually stops short at the fibroblast stage, and having reached it (or even before that) the constructive process gives place to retrogressive changes. Cicatricial development being arrested, the granulation-tissue persists for a time unmodified, and often developes to a considerable amount. For this reason VIRCHOW described the formations as **granulative growths** or **granulomata**. All of these growths have furthermore the clinical character of **infectiveness**. Hence they have been termed infective growths by KLEBS and COHNHEIM, and specific inflammations by RINDFLEISCH.

Their infective character may be recognised by various signs. Thus they are all locally **invasive**; *i.e.* the granulation-tissue spreads centrifugally from a centre into the surrounding structures. At the same time the central (or oldest) part of the new formation usually dies and disintegrates. In many cases the lymphatic system becomes affected, so that secondary granulative foci are formed in it. From the lymphatics the process is at times transferred to the blood; or it may invade the blood-vessels directly. The final result is the spread of the disorder to various organs, or throughout the system.

In most of the granulomatous disorders we may have not merely a diffusion of the disease throughout the individual organism, but also a transference of it from one individual to another: the affection is **inoculable**. If one person be inoculated with the inflammatory products derived from another, he acquires a disease whose course is exactly similar to that of the original one, and which yields identical inflammatory products. This latter character of infectiveness is that by which it is most readily recognised.

To this group of infective granulomata belong the neoplastic formations found in tuberculosis, syphilis, leprosy, lupus, glanders, and actinomycosis. All these affections are due to the invasion of the body by a virus or poison derived from the outer world, or from the body of another individual. This virus may probably be produced by vegetable parasites. In leprosy (ARMAUER HANSEN, NEISSER), tuberculosis (KOCH), and syphilis (KLEBS) bacteria have been found, and in actinomycosis a special fungus. These are declared to be the originating causes of the respective diseases. Our ideas as to the nature and character of these affections are as yet mainly based upon their clinical course; but we have also derived something from inoculation-experiments. Tuberculosis and syphilis are thus known to be communicable from one person to another; tuberculosis is also communicable from man to lower animals.

It was VIRCHOW who invented the term 'granulative growth' or 'granuloma' for these formations, which he was the first to define accurately (*Die krankhaften Geschwülste* II). He set it down as characteristic of them—that they usually fail to develope beyond the stage of granulation-tissue; that this is unstable in character; and that the regular issue is in ulceration. He laid stress on their near alliance to the products of inflammatory processes. KLEBS (*Prager Vierteljahrsschr.* vol. 126) called such growths 'infective growths or tumours,' and the name has been adopted by COHNHEIM. Neither description is exactly adequate. VIRCHOW'S takes no account of their infective character: KLEBS' bears no reference to their structure. As it is by no means certain that there are no other new formations of infective origin, some apter designation seems called for. Even RINDFLEISCH'S term 'specific inflammation' is too indefinite, for it might perfectly well apply to a number of other processes, such as those of pyaemia, erysipelas, variola, &c. In this book the term 'infective granuloma' will be used: this serves to keep in view both the structure and the clinical character of the morbid formations in question.

Tubercle and Tuberculosis.

118. The structure characteristic of tuberculosis is the **tubercle**, or tuberculous nodule. The notion of tuberculosis is thus primarily an anatomical one—tuberculosis is a tubercular (*i.e.* nodular) disease.

Of course it does not follow conversely—that every nodular growth found in the organism implies tuberculosis: the special nodule of tuberculosis, the tubercle *par excellence*, is a structure of definite and special constitution. VIRCHOW (*Die krankhaften Geschwülste* II, 636) describes a freshly-formed tubercle as—a small grey translucent nodule, not exceeding a millet-seed in size, mainly composed of cells, and developed from connective tissue. The cellular elements (he adds) are essentially similar to those of lymphatic glands: they are round cells of various sizes, some of them like white blood-cells, some larger, some smaller. Their nuclei are homogeneous and bright, small and spherical or large and oval, vesicular, and transparent; they contain nucleolar corpuscles. The larger cells often contain two nuclei, and frequently more—to the number of twelve or over. Between the cells are found fibrous filaments arranged in a network, and sometimes vessels also. The latter are never new-formed: they existed before the tubercle was developed, and lie within the tubercle only because the tubercle has grown around them. The nodules occur either singly or in numbers; or they may be grouped in confluent masses. In the latter case, the internodular tissue does not remain unchanged: it seems made up of imperfect granulation-tissue, or inflammatory fibrous hyperplasia takes place. The appearance is then rather that of a mass of compact uniformly diseased tissue, than of normal tissue containing nodular deposits.

When the nodule becomes older, the centre of it is invariably found to be caseated. It is then yellowish-white and opaque. Under the microscope it appears as a granular friable mass, while the periphery still shows its cellular constitution. The aggregations of cells may stretch out in various directions through the tissue, as if the nodule threw out pseudopodia.

The nodular groups undergo caseation like the single nodules. The internodular granulation-tissue also becomes cheesy, so that at length large and continuous caseous patches are formed. It is much rarer to find the nodules undergoing fibrous transformation. **Caseation** is characteristic of the later stages of the tuberculous nodule.

The term tubercle (*tuberculum*) was formerly applied to all varieties of nodular growth. BAILLIE (1794) and BAYLE (1810) were the first to direct attention to the grey miliary nodules which we now call tubercles. BAYLE however applied the term to other growths in the lung. LAENNEC applied it mainly to the cheesy masses found in phthisical lungs. Larger caseous foci and caseous lobular infiltrations were also described as tuberculous. The caseous nodes and masses were simply **'tubercles,'** the diffused infiltration was **'tuberculous infiltration,'** the grey nodules (or true granulative tubercles) were **'miliary tubercles.'** Cheesy change was thus made the main characteristic of tuberculosis; caseation was spoken of as 'tuberculisation.' In opposition to this view, VIRCHOW maintained that caseous masses might arise in many different ways, and hence had very various significance in different cases. He laid it down that the anatomical basis of tuberculosis is the cellular tubercle (VIRCHOW, *loc. cit.*; WALDENBURG, *Die Tuberculose* Berlin 1869; GRANCHER, *L'Union méd.* 1881).

119. We may define a tubercle, then, as a non-vascular cellular nodule, which does not grow beyond a certain size, and at a certain stage of its development becomes caseous. This definition includes all that we can say, in general terms, of tubercle from the histological point of view. The histological researches of the last fifteen years (by LANGHANS, SCHÜPPEL, KÖSTER, RINDFLEISCH, COHNHEIM, ZIEGLER, KLEIN, SANDERSON and others) have added only this—that the tubercle possesses in many cases a special structure, and that certain cell-forms frequently occur in it and give it a characteristic appearance. The central part of the tubercle usually contains **giant-cells** (Fig. 29 *a*). These possess numerous nuclei, which are not uncommonly arranged round the periphery, or gathered together at one pole of the cell. The uninuclear cells

are partly lymphoid, partly larger and like swollen epithelial or endothelial cells—these are called **epithelioid** (Fig. 29 *b*). Giant-cells and epithelioid cells are marked by their coarsely granular

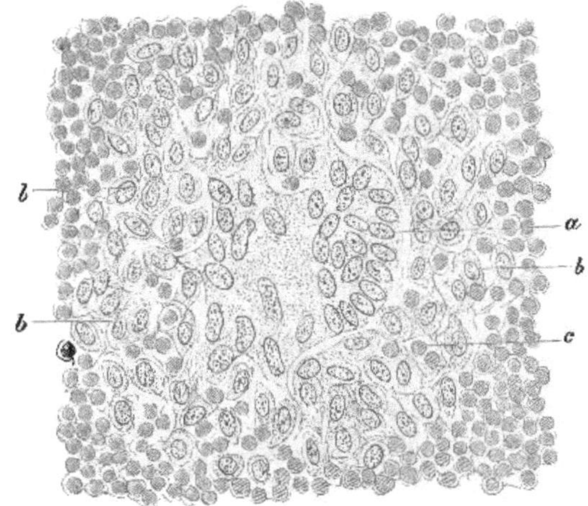

FIG. 29. TUBERCLE FROM A FUNGATING GRANULOMA IN BONE.
(*Aniline-brown staining:* × 250)
a giant-cell *b* epithelioid cells *c* lymphoid cells

protoplasm, and large vesicular oval nuclei with clear nuclear juice and nucleoli. The round or lymphoid cells (*c*) are finely granular, with a small round nucleus in which the nuclear juice and nuclear substance are not clearly distinguished.

These cells lie in a stroma which in many cases exhibits a reticular arrangement.

120. The epithelioid cells and giant-cells have been thought by some to be characteristic of tuberculosis. Many writers have thus come to speak of specific tubercle-cells, and have based the diagnosis of tuberculosis merely on the presence of these larger varieties of cells. This is certainly unjustifiable. Such cells, indeed, are common enough in tuberculous affections, but they are by no means exclusively confined to them.

All inflammatory tissue-formation is preceded by a stage in which large cells are developed. It is very easy to generate experimentally in such formations all the various elements found in tubercle, and especially the giant-cells. The constituent cells of tubercle are precisely equivalent to the corresponding cells of granulation-tissue. All the evidence points to the conclusion that tubercles arise in the same way as granulations. The chief materials are derived from the migrated white blood-cells; and the endothelial cells and fixed connective-tissue cells supply only a minor part.

So far as the cell-forms are concerned, the only difference between tubercle and granulation is—that in tubercle the larger cells are often found in relatively greater numbers.

The characteristic features of tubercle, therefore, do not lie in the forms of its cellular elements. As has been already said, the characteristic features are these,—that the cells form a definite nodule, which does not exceed a certain size, contains no new-formed vessels, and in consequence at a certain stage of its development ceases to progress; that the nodule thereupon undergoes retrogressive changes, and becomes fatty, necrotic, and caseous.

If this proposition be duly considered, it will be seen that the diagnosis of tubercle cannot be made to depend on anatomical structure and constitution alone. A cellular nodule made up of round-cells only without a single giant-cell, or a nodule whose general texture is fibrous, may perfectly well be characterised as a tubercle, if its life-history corresponds with what we have set down. As an actual fact, in perfectly typical cases of tuberculosis we may find such nodules close by others that contain giant-cells. We may explain the occurrence of the former, by supposing in the one case that the aggregated round-cells have prematurely ceased to develope or have not yet had time to reach their full development; in the other case the fibroblastic stage (that of epithelioid cells and giant-cells) has been exceptionally transcended, and that of fibrous-tissue formation has been reached. The physiological analogue of the last is of course the transformation of granulations into cicatricial tissue.

According to the recent investigations of KOCH (Art. 127) the definition of tubercle just given must be amended. By tubercle we are it seems in future to understand—a cellular nodule containing within it the specific tuberculous virus, the **Bacillus tuberculosis** of KOCH.

The general doctrine of tuberculosis must be altered in many points in consequence of KOCH's discovery. The text has been allowed to remain as representing the hitherto accepted doctrine, and as containing what is probably the truth, though not the whole truth.

LANGHANS was the first to examine carefully the giant-cells (*Virch. Arch.* vol. 42) and to describe their forms. SCHÜPPEL (*Untersuch. üb. d. Lymphdrüsentuberculose* Tübingen 1871) maintained that they were always present in tuberculosis, and based the diagnosis of the affection upon them. KÖSTER (*Virch. Arch.* vol. 48), BUHL (*Die Lungenentzündung* Munich 1872), and RINDFLEISCH (*Pathological Histology* I, 136 and *Ziemssen's Cyclopaedia* vol. V), have also insisted on their importance in diagnosis. The latter has even declared that any large-celled infiltration of a tissue is to be regarded as tuberculous or scrofulous in character. In opposition to this view HERING (*Stud. über Tuberculose* Berlin 1873) has disputed the specific significance of giant-cells and epithelioid cells, and has demonstrated that they are often absent in undoubted tubercles. The second constituent of the tubercle, the fibrous reticulum, has been investigated by SCHÜPPEL (*loc. cit.*), WAGNER (*Das tuberkelähnliche Lymphadenom* Leipzig 1871), KLEIN (*Report of Med. Officer of Privy Council* 1874). CORNIL and RANVIER (*Man. of Path. Histology* vol. I. 1882) maintain that the reticulum is produced *post mortem* by the action of hardening reagents on the intercellular substance. For further references to the history of the question the student may consult TREVES (*Scrofula and*

Tubercle London 1882), HAMILTON (*Practitioner* 1879—1881), KLEIN (*Practitioner* 1881), BURDON SANDERSON (*Practitioner* 1882), GEE (Article *Tuberculosis*, *Quain's Dict. of Medicine* 1882).

ZIEGLER (*Ueber die Herkunft der Tuberkelelemente* Würzburg 1875, and *Ueber path. Bindegewebsneubildung* 1876) has sought to show that neither giant-cells nor epithelioid cells are exclusively confined to tubercle, but are to be found in all granulations. Between the latter and tubercle the only difference is—that in healthy granulations the multinuclear cells occur but sparingly, while in tubercle they are in great numbers and highly developed. In tubercle the formative material is abundantly provided and fibroblasts produced, but they are not utilised for further development into fibrous tissue.

The giant-cells of granulation-tissue are to be distinguished from those which arise from epithelial cells. When tubercles form in epithelial ducts, such as those of the liver or testis, the affected epithelial cells seem to coalesce and form structures much resembling the giant-cells of granulations (cf. KLEIN, *Lymphatic System* part II London 1875). They have properly nothing to do with the formation of the granulomatous tubercle. They are accidental consequences of the locality in which the tubercle is developed. To draw conclusions from them (as do GAULE, *Virch. Arch.* vol. 49, and LÜBIMOW, *Virch. Arch.* vol. 75) with regard to the genesis of all tuberculous giant-cells is not permissible.

121. **Diffusion of tubercle.** When a tuberculous organ is examined we do not usually find the tubercles in their earlier stages; they have already undergone certain advanced changes. Parenchymatous organs contain caseous nodulated patches or foci, which are either firm and compact in texture or are already softened and broken down towards the centre. In surface-tissues, ulcerations are produced by this softening process, and their edges and base are caseous. The caseated tissue passes at its boundaries

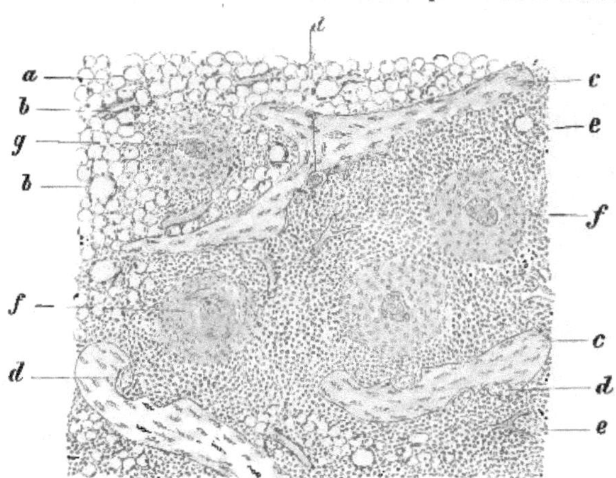

FIG. 30. FUNGATING GRANULOMA WITH TUBERCLES FROM THE CALCANEUM.
(*Haematoxylin staining*: × 60)

a medullary tissue containing fat
b blood-vessels
c bone trabeculae
d osteoclasts (Art. 115)
e granulation-tissue
f tubercles in the granulation-tissue, some containing giant-cells
g isolated tubercle

into a zone of grey or greyish-red translucent tissue, reminding one exactly of granulation-tissue. This grey or greyish-red tissue is found in other parts of the affected organ in the form of larger or smaller patches: these often quite visibly contain small grey or yellowish-white and opaque nodules.

Lastly, the affected organ also contains small grey nodules lying in apparently unaltered tissue; and sometimes surrounded by a hyperaemic zone, sometimes not.

The grey or greyish-red translucent tissue, whether it surrounds the caseous focus, or forms the base of an ulcer (Fig. 31 *h* and h_1), or occurs in isolated patches, is nothing else but tissue infiltrated with cells; it is granulation-tissue. The grey and the yellow nodules are fresh or **'crude'** tubercles generally containing giant-cells (Fig. 30 *f*), and old already caseated tubercles (Fig. 31 i_1), respectively. The grey and yellow isolated or aggregated nodules in the neighbourhood of the larger patches are of the same character (Fig. 30 *g* and Fig. 31 *i* and i_1).

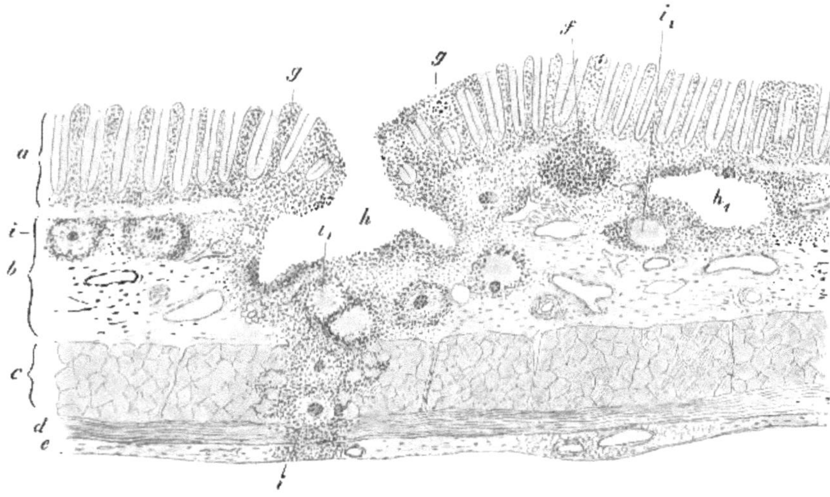

FIG. 31. SUBEPITHELIAL TUBERCULOUS GRANULATIONS AND DISCRETE TUBERCLES IN THE WALL OF THE LARGE INTESTINE. (*Bismark-brown staining:* × 30)

a *mucosa*
b *submucosa*
c *muscularis interna*
d *muscularis externa*
e *serosa*
f solitary gland
g *mucosa* infiltrated with cells
h tuberculous ulcer
h_1 focus of softening or tuberculous abscess
i 'crude' or fresh tubercle
i_1 caseous tubercle

From these observations we may gather—that tubercles sometimes occur aggregated or grouped within a tissue which is already infiltrated with cells; and that the affection spreads by the formation of fresh nodules in the neighbourhood of the old. In other cases granulation-tissue and fibrous tissue may develope between and around the aggregated tubercles. The process may thus begin with an eruption of tubercles, or with a more diffused inflammatory infiltration. These propositions practically include all that is important concerning the diffusion of tubercle in the tissues.

It is not usually difficult to recognise tubercles in the substance of tuberculous granulation-tissue. The giant-cells and epithelioid cells seen in microscopical sections do not take colour nearly so well as the small round-cells which form the main component of the tissue. Three zones are usually distinguishable in a tubercle. In the centre lies the core of aggregated giant-cells of a dark or dull colour. Then comes the zone of faintly-stained epithelioid cells, and finally at the periphery the zone of deeply-stained round-cells; these last are usually deeper in tint than the granulation-cells around them. When the middle of the tubercle has already become caseous, giant-cells are generally to be made out here and there over it.

It is not always correct to say that tuberculous patches take their rise from single nodules. The formation of nodules may be preceded by a diffused infiltration, or even the development of granulation-tissue; the nodules only making their appearance as secondary growths.

122. The eruption of fresh tubercles in the neighbourhood of an existing tuberculous focus is usually followed sooner or later by the appearance of nodules in the lymphatic system. The nearest lymphatics are of course the first to be affected: they receive their lymph from the region primarily affected. Thus in tuberculous ulceration of the mucous and submucous coats of the intestine, first the lymphatics of the muscular coats (Fig. 31 *c d*) are infected, and then those of the serous coat. In this way strings of tubercles may be formed along the course of the vessels.

From the nearer lymphatics the eruption may pass in succession to others, and at length approach the thoracic duct. More frequently the affection is not uniformly diffused in this way, but attacks certain parts of the lymphatic system rather than others, especially those through which the lymph is as it were filtered, namely the lymphatic glands.

It is in the glands that the tuberculous eruption is most intense. Generally the process makes a kind of halt at these gland-stations: but it sooner or later finds opportunity to spread onwards, and at length reaches the main trunks and the thoracic duct itself.

Wherever the tuberculous process has become established, it is distinguished by the development of tubercles, and this in the lymphatic vessels as well as the glands (Fig. 32).

A more or less intense inflammation of the surrounding tissue is always associated with the tubercular eruption: it is manifested by hyperaemia with infiltration and swelling. If the process last for a certain time, it not infrequently happens that young connective tissue is developed at the seat of the eruption. The usual fate of the tuberculous growth is caseous necrosis and disintegration. It rarely issues in the formation of fibrous tissue, and still more rarely in complete resorption of the tubercle.

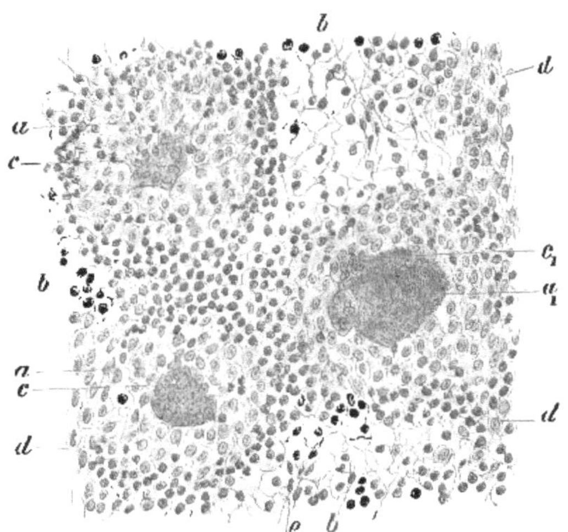

FIG. 32. TUBERCULOSIS OF A LYMPHATIC GLAND.
(*Haematoxylin staining:* ×150)

a large-celled tubercle with giant-cell (*c*)
a_1 tubercle with central caseation and giant-cells (c_1)
d epithelioid cells lying outside the tubercles in the adenoid reticulum (*b*) of the gland
e lymphoid cells

123. The virus which engenders tubercle may be carried out of the lymphatic system into the blood, either from a tuberculous focus in a gland or a tuberculous ulcer in the thoracic duct. It may thus be conveyed to distant organs. This will also happen when the virus passes directly from a tuberculous focus into an artery or vein. The result is an eruption of new tubercles either local or general.

When the infection of the blood results in a general eruption of tubercles throughout all the organs or in most of them, the affection is called **acute miliary tuberculosis**. The various organs are beset more or less densely with minute (miliary) grey or translucent nodules, or here and there with yellowish-white opaque nodules with cheesy centres. This is the case whether the affection extend to several organs or to one, or even to a single arterial territory within an organ.

All these nodules are made up of cells. In their earliest stages they are nothing but little heaps of small round-cells (Fig. 33 *b*), unquestionably derived from the blood. Many foci maintain this character until they are mature: all the cells do is to multiply. In other cases giant-cells and epithelioid cells (Fig. 32 *a*) are developed. In these cases as in the others the nodule ultimately becomes caseous. Very seldom does fibrous transformation or resorption occur.

Diffused and wide-spread inflammatory disturbance of the circulation is very often associated with the eruption of the nodules.

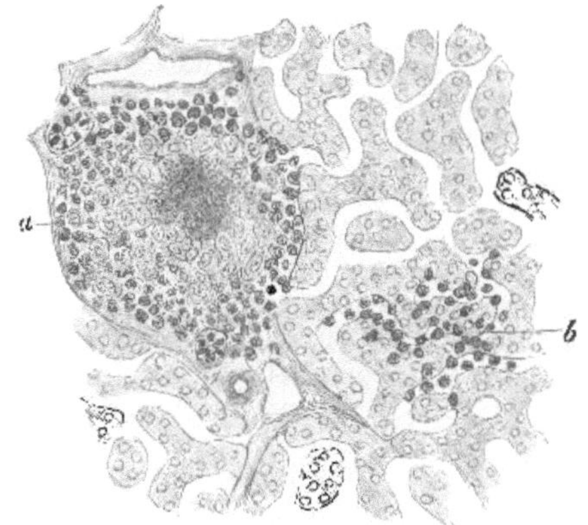

FIG. 33. MILIARY TUBERCULOSIS OF THE LIVER. (*Carmine staining*)
a mature tubercle in the portal sheath
b tubercle beginning to develope in a liver-cell

This is especially the case in the pia mater, the serous membranes, and in the lungs, where the process is often accompanied by copious and diffuse exudation. In the liver, kidney, thyroid gland, &c. on the other hand, the changes elsewhere than in the immediate neighbourhood of the nodules are usually but slight.

ZIEGLER has investigated the development of miliary tubercles occurring in very diverse structures, and maintains that their basis is always a collection of white blood-cells which have migrated from the veins and capillaries. These indeed often form the entire mass of the tubercle. In other cases the endothelia contribute something. When the nodule has reached a certain size it becomes difficult to make out certainly the behaviour of the fixed cells of the tissues. He has not been able to confirm the often-made assertion that miliary tubercle is specially apt to develope round the smaller arteries.

The direct penetration of the tuberculous virus into the blood-vessels may be the result of tuberculous change in their walls. If a considerable number of sections of phthisical lung be examined, there will here and there be found vessels whose walls are the seat of tubercles. If these penetrate the intima, they may then break into the blood-channel directly. WEIGERT has shown that large venous trunks may be invaded in this way.

There are two reasons for the fact that all organs are not simultaneously and equally attacked when the blood is infected with the tuberculous virus. One is that the virus, though it is circulating in the blood, may not reach all the organs alike. The other is that all the organs are not equally predisposed to infection. The skin, for instance, seems to enjoy almost perfect immunity.

General miliary tuberculosis is not an inevitable result of tuberculosis occurring in an organ. The rule rather is that the tuberculous process does not extend beyond the boundaries of the organ primarily affected, and the lymphatic glands pertaining to it. What most commonly leads to general infection of the blood is the disintegration of caseous tuberculous glands.

124. Tubercle may be disseminated in other ways, and independently of the lymphatics and blood-vessels. Consider, for example, the mode in which it spreads on the surface of mucous membranes. It is easy to verify that solitary nodules, as well as tuberculous patches and ulcers of larger size developed in mucous membrane, do not long remain isolated, but soon give rise to new foci. These are situated not merely in the immediate neighbourhood of the first, but often at a considerable distance from them. They may even appear unconnected with the first lesions; while it is certain that they are not at least in every case propagated through the lymphatics. In pulmonary tuberculosis, for instance, which has already passed into the ulcerative stage, it is not at all uncommon for the mucous membrane of the air-tubes to become affected. This is especially apt to occur in the larynx, epiglottis, and at times in the pharynx: and the affection often extends to the lower segments of the large and small intestines. When the kidneys become tuberculous, and contain caseous ulcerations, the ureters, bladder, seminal vesicles, and prostate may become consecutively diseased. In other cases the process commences in the latter organs and extends upwards.

From such instances it becomes plain that the infective virus may actually be transported along the surface of the mucous membrane. It attacks the spots at which it is allowed to linger, and penetrates the mucous tissue. It there sets up the specific inflammation manifested by the development of nodules, which disintegrate and produce ulcerations.

Tubercle is in like manner disseminated on the surface of the serous membranes lining the great body-cavities. In their case it is obvious that the transport of the virus is favoured by the normal movements and displacements of the contained organs.

It must be remembered, in connexion with this question, that all mucous membranes are not equally susceptible with regard to the tuberculous virus. The mucous membrane of the mouth, pharynx, and oesophagus is far less susceptible than that of the larynx and trachea. The stomach duodenum, and bile-ducts, as also the urethra, are very rarely attacked. This is explicable now that we know that the virus is a special micro-organism (Art. 127): for the secretions of the stomach, duodenum, and common bile-duct are prejudicial to the development of bacteria. The oesophagus and urethra have this advantage—that they are continually being swept clean, as it were. In the small and in the large intestine, where the process of absorption goes on most actively, the ingesta and with them any tuberculous sputa which may happen to have been swallowed, may lie a long time in contact with the mucous membrane. In the neighbourhood of the larynx, the bronchial secretion continually accumulates before it is coughed out, and the virus has thus abundant opportunity of attacking its mucous membrane. The bladder, in like manner, contains the accumulating secretion of the kidneys, while the urethra is only 'flushed' with it from time to time. In addition to these factors, however, we must not leave out of account the possibility of special predisposition in the various structures and tissues.

125. **The clinical significance of tubercle.** The processes just described (Arts. 118—124) are comprehended under the term

tuberculosis. Tuberculosis, so defined, is distinguished by two chief characters. The one is anatomical, namely the development of specific nodules: the other is clinical, namely the consecutive invasion of one or more parts of an organ or of the entire system.

As a disease, tuberculosis is distinguished by its progressively destructive tendency. It not only destroys gradually the organ first attacked, but it seizes by various routes upon other organs, or spreads throughout the organism.

In addition to this clinical characteristic of progressive invasion, we have the anatomical characteristic—the tubercle. Tuberculosis is anatomically an inflammatory process; but its course does not correspond with that of other inflammations. It is sharply distinguished from them by the development of nodules both in its original seat and in the parts that are secondarily attacked: and these nodules have a definite type and structure—they are cellular and non-vascular.

There is still another characteristic, but we owe our knowledge of it not so much to observation at the bed-side or at the post-mortem table, as to direct experiment. VILLEMIN and KLEBS were the first to show—what many investigators (such as WALDENBURG, COHNHEIM, ORTH, BOLLINGER, SIMON, WILSON FOX, KLEIN, and BURDON SANDERSON) have since verified—that tuberculosis is transmissible to animals. In other words, when animals are inoculated with matter from fresh or caseous tuberculous foci, they are forthwith attacked by a disease which, judging from its clinical course and anatomical products, is identical with human tuberculosis.

This character determines the genus of tuberculosis in the classification of human diseases. It is an infective disease.

The proposition that tuberculosis is anatomically an inflammatory process is disputed by many pathologists. There has always been a strong inclination to reckon tubercle among the true tumour-formations, like cancer. Such a view will hardly be maintained now. The genesis of tubercle, its cellular constitution, its whole life-history, are all in favour of its kindred with the inflammatory new-formations: they offer no fair grounds for comparing it with the tumours. We may add—that the possibility of generating tubercles by inoculation with caseous or necrotic tuberculous matter is a strong argument for regarding tubercle not as a tumour but as a product of inflammation.

The fact of the transmissibility of tuberculosis to animals is now placed beyond doubt. It is true that the experiment does not always succeed; for though some animals are very susceptible, such as rabbits, guinea-pigs, and ruminants generally, others like dogs enjoy a certain degree of immunity. This only proves, not that tuberculosis is not infective, but that the tuberculous virus is not a universal poison, capable of attacking each and every organism. This is likewise the explanation of the fact that physicians have observed comparatively few cases of quite indubitable transmission of the disease from man to man. Among human beings there are predispositions: tuberculosis does not attack all with equal readiness. Nor must we forget in criticising the clinical data—that it is scarcely possible to discern the exact time at which tuberculosis sets in. The clinical manifestations may not appear till long after the first infection, when it is impossible to make out anything that throws light on the origin of the disease (BUDD, *Lancet* 2, 1867; WEBER, *Clin. Soc. Trans.* 1874; RINDFLEISCH, *Virch. Arch.* vol. 85; BURNEY YEO, *Contagiousness of Pulm. Consumption* London 1882).

A short but very comprehensive summary of the evidence for the transmissibility of tuberculosis from man to man, and from man to lower animals, is given by KLEIN (*Practitioner* Aug. 1881). The student who desires to know the 'state of the case' for the specific nature of tuberculosis immediately before KOCH's discovery cannot do better than to consult this article.

Inoculation-experiments have been made in various ways. The tuberculous matter has been inserted under the skin, into the peritoneal cavity, into the eye, and into the joints: it has been mixed with the food: it has been pulverised and conveyed to the lungs with the respired air.

References:—VILLEMIN, *Gazette hebd.* 50, 1865; *Comp. rend.* 61, 1866; *Etudes sur la tuberculose* 1868: LEBERT, *Bullet. de l'acad.* XXXII; *Gaz. méd. de Paris*, 25—29, 1867: LEBERT and WYSS, *Virch. Arch.* vols. 40 and 41: ROUSTAN, *L'inoculabilité de la Phthisie* Paris 1867: FELTZ, *Gaz. méd. de Strasbourg* 1867: WILSON FOX, *The artificial production of Tubercle* London 1868: CHAUVEAU, *Gaz. méd. de Lyon* 1868: LANGHANS, *Die Uebertr. der Tuberculose auf Kaninchen* 1868: WALDENBURG, *Die Tuberculose* Berlin 1869: VIRCHOW and HIRSCH, *Virch. Jahresber.* 1868—1870 (containing full and very useful references to previous research): *Trans. Path. Soc.* 1873 (an instructive discussion of current views): KLEBS, *Virch. Arch.* vols. 44, 49; *Arch. f. exp. Path.* I; *Naturforscher-versammlung in München* 1877: COHNHEIM and FRAENKEL, *Virch. Arch.* vol. 45; *Die Tuberculose vom Standpunkte der Infectionslehre* Leipzig 1880: KLEIN, *Lymphatic System* II London 1875: TAPPEINER, LIPPL, SCHWENINGER, *Naturf.-versamm.* 1877: TAPPEINER, *Virch. Arch.* vol. 74: ORTH, *Virch. Arch.* vol. 76: BOLLINGER, *Arch. f. exp. Path.* I: H. MARTIN, *Recherches sur le tubercule* Paris 1879; *Arch. de Physiologie* 1881; *Revue de méd.* April 1882: SANDERSON, *Report to Med. Off. of Privy Council* 1868—9 (republished in *Practitioner* Sept.—Dec. 1882; a critical summary of preceding researches is given in the latter of these reports): KIENER and others, *L'Union méd.* 1881.

126. Two important questions remain unanswered. Tuberculosis is an infective disease: and it bears the anatomical character of a destructive nodular inflammation. It is important for diagnostic purposes to know something more. Does the tuberculous inflammatory process manifest itself by the formation of nodules only? Conversely, are all varieties of cellular nodules, exhibiting the general structure of tubercles, to be regarded as evidence of tuberculosis? The second question is—What is the nature of the tuberculous virus? In answer to the former question, clinical observation and experiments on animals have shown that all nodular eruptions are not tuberculous. Thus when small irritating foreign bodies are introduced into the body of an animal, it sometimes happens that a nodular affection is produced which anatomically simulates tuberculosis. Yet these nodules have in reality no kindred with true tubercles. The exciting cause is essentially different (Art. 127) from that which engenders true tuberculosis; while neither the life-history of the nodules, nor the course of the process as a whole, corresponds with what is observed in human tuberculosis.

Moreover, there occur in man certain nodular inflammations whose clinical course is radically different from that of tuberculosis, though the nodules in some degree resemble tubercles. The best known instance is lupus of the skin (Art. 132). In this affection perfectly typical tubercles are frequently formed; but they never induce tuberculosis in other organs, or general tuberculosis. In the peritoneum, again, there are now and then found tuberculoid nodules; but they have probably nothing whatever to do with tuberculosis as a disease.

While the domain of tubercular eruptions is on one hand somewhat wider than that of tuberculosis, on the other hand the domain of tuberculosis goes beyond that of tubercular eruptions. In other words, there may be tuberculosis without isolated tubercles. It not infrequently happens that in the course of tuberculous disease inflammatory patches are formed, consisting of diffuse continuous granulations in which no tubercles can be detected. These patches must nevertheless be acknowledged to be tuberculous: the clinical course of the process, and the life-history of the new inflammatory tissue, indicate this; while tubercles may actually be developed in later stages of the same affection. In such cases it may be hard to determine whether the process is really tuberculous; especially in organs like the lungs where the usual inflammatory changes are at all times apt to make the recognition of tubercle a difficult matter. Experimental inoculation, or the detection of the specific virus (Art. 127), can alone settle the question. As regards the latter test we may expect that the near future will bring us much additional information. It is fortunate that these ambiguous cases are not very numerous. Although therefore the anatomical notion of tubercle and the clinical notion of tuberculosis do not precisely correspond throughout their full extension, they do correspond in the vast majority of cases. It is a rule almost without exception—that tuberculosis is distinguished microscopically and on the post-mortem table by the presence of tubercles.

Much confusion has arisen in the discussions on tuberculosis from the assumption that the production of a nodular or tubercular eruption in an animal is necessarily the same as the production of tuberculosis. The result of the assumption has been, that observers have fancied they have induced tuberculosis in animals by the introduction of all sorts of foreign bodies. The diagnosis is not to be based on the presence of nodules simply: the life-history of the nodules and the general course of the whole process are also of essential importance (H. MARTIN, *Arch. de Phys.* 1881).

127. We are now able to give a definite answer to the second question raised in the last article—What is the nature of the tuberculous virus?

At the meeting of the Berlin Physiological Society held on the 24th of March 1882, Dr R. KOCH communicated some results of his researches on tuberculosis, which constituted a distinct advance in our knowledge of its aetiology.

He announced that the tuberculous virus is a special bacillus (**Bacillus tuberculosis**, Art. 206). Its length is about a third of the diameter of a red blood-cell, and its breadth one-fifth to one-sixth of its length. Individual bacilli contain clear bright spores. The bacilli are chiefly found in fresh tubercles, more sparingly in older ones. Some of them lie within the cells and especially within the giant-cells, others lie outside. They are generally single and scattered; at times they are found in prettily grouped clusters. By treatment with methylene-blue and vesuvin, they take up a different tint from that of the surrounding tissues. The tissues stained in the first instance with methylene-blue have their colour discharged by vesuvin, while the tubercle-bacilli retain it.

EHRLICH, GIBBES and others (*Brit. Med. Journ.* Oct. 14, 1882) have devised simpler and speedier methods than KOCH's for staining and so detecting the bacilli. These methods are readily applicable to the clinical examination of phthisical sputa.

KOCH has shown that the bacilli may be cultivated in the serum of ox-blood. The bacilli so bred may then be introduced into the bodies of various animals, such as rabbits, rats, and dogs, and tuberculosis is thereupon induced; in other words, they are attacked by a disease characterised by a progressive formation of cellular nodules. The nodules always contain the characteristic bacilli. In guinea-pigs the first appearance of disease is manifested ten days after inoculation.

It may therefore be accepted as an established fact that tuberculosis is an infective disease, induced by the presence of a specific bacillus.

In the light of this knowledge, the various theories which have been advanced with regard to the causation of tuberculosis become in some respects irrelevant. It will be matter for further experimental investigation to determine the vital properties of the tubercle-bacillus. Among other points, it will have to be settled whether the bacillus can develope only within the bodies of men and other mammals, or whether it may not pass through some stage of its existence outside the body: in other words, whether the disease is strictly contagious, *i.e.* transmissible directly from one subject to another; or whether it is due to something of the nature of a miasma—a poison which may develope outside the body. According to KOCH, the bacillus can only be bred between the temperatures of 30°C and 41°C (86°F—105·8°F). If this be so, it is hard to see how it can multiply outside the body. With regard to the transmission of tuberculosis from animals to man, it is to be noted that KOCH has found the specific bacillus in the nodular growths which occur in the 'pearly disease' or 'grapes' of cattle (*Perlsucht* or bovine tuberculosis).

Clinical experience would seem to indicate that the tubercle-bacillus is no ordinary bacterium, such as may enter and affect any organism without distinction. It would seem rather as if infection occurred only where a definite predisposition exists, or where a considerable quantity of the virus is introduced. This predisposition may be local as well as general. The local predisposition may perhaps depend mainly on antecedent inflammatory change. A general predisposition is attributed to **scrofulous** subjects especially. These are persons whose tissues exhibit a certain frailty or susceptibility to injury, that makes them particularly liable to chronic inflammatory disorders. It is however not at all uncommon for the term 'scrofulous' to be applied to individuals actually affected with tuberculosis, as well as to those who are only predisposed to it.

We may imagine the course of the infection to be this—the bacilli settle in a tissue accessible from without, pass thence into the deeper structures, and ultimately into the blood: or, without any primary local settlement, they may be taken up by the circulating juices directly, and carried to various parts; wherever they settle they begin to develope, and so set up inflammation and the formation of cellular nodules.

KOCH has found the bacillus not only in general miliary tuberculosis but in caseous pneumonia, caseous bronchitis, intestinal and glandular tuberculosis, 'pearly disease,' spontaneous and inoculated tuberculosis in various animals, and in the so-called scrofulous hyperplasia of lymphatic glands. All these affections are thus to be included under the head of tuberculosis: they are all the result of the same bacterial infection. Tuberculosis from this point of view is an infective disease not always manifested by the formation of tubercles. It may even appear as a purely local affection, and yet be unaccompanied by tubercles.

It is of special interest to note that KOCH has detected the bacillus in the sputa of phthisical patients. As the bacillus produces spores within the body, it is very likely that the virus exists and diffuses itself outside the body mainly in the form of spores.

KOCH finds that the bacilli grow very slowly, and after inoculation proceed to develope and multiply only when they reach a spot where they are not subject to much mechanical disturbance or displacement. From this we may understand how it happens that many persons, though again and again exposed to the invasion of tubercle-bacilli, yet remain uninfected. It is moreover conceivable that individuals, in whose tissues inflammatory changes have already occurred, are those who are most disposed to tuberculous infection.

At the time when KOCH was bringing his researches to an end, BAUMGARTEN (*Centralblatt f. d. med. Wiss.* 15, 1881) succeeded in detecting bacilli in tubercle by treating microscopic sections with dilute solution of caustic potash. He did not however go on to cultivate and inoculate the bacilli. AUFRECHT had already described bacilli which he had found in tubercle (*Path. Mitth.* Magdeburg 1881); but his demonstration was likewise defective. He did not show that the bacilli were peculiar and specific as regards tuberculosis.

It has been a much-debated question whether or not human tuberculosis is identical with the bovine 'pearly disease.' Anatomically the pearly disease is a progressively advancing affection in which nodes and nodules are formed. These may be single or agglomerated into masses as big as a potato. They are chiefly found in the serous membranes, as also in the lymphatic glands, lungs, and liver. In the serous membranes, the nodular masses are often pedunculated and pendulous. Caseation is not very common; calcification much more so. The nodules are essentially cellular in structure, often contain giant-cells (VIRCHOW, *Virch. Arch.* vol. 14), look very like tubercles, and may lie together in great numbers in the midst of a cellular stroma.

A. C. GERLACH (*Jahresb. d. k. Thierarzneischule in Hannover* 1869) fed and inoculated rabbits and goats with matter from such nodules, and on the strength of his experiments maintains that the pearly disease is transmissible to other animals and is identical with human tuberculosis. SCHÜPPEL (*Virch. Arch.* vol. 56), and CREIGHTON (*Bovine Tuberculosis in Man* London 1881), from microscopic comparison of tubercles and the pearly nodules, declare that they are identical. ORTH (*Virch. Arch.* vol. 76) arrived at the same conviction through experiments in which the animal was fed with the infective matter; as did also BOLLINGER and KLEBS (*Arch. f. exp. Path.* 1), CHAUVEAU (*Jahrb. der ges. Med.* 1872), and BAUMGARTEN (*Berl. klin. Woch.* 49, 1880). On the other hand COLIN (*Compt. rend.* 1876), GÜNTHER, HARMS, and MÜLLER (*Jahrb. der ges. Med.* 1873–74) obtained only negative results. VIRCHOW (*Berl. klin. Woch.* 1880 and *Virch. Arch.* vol. 83) also made experiments by the method of feeding, but his results were ambiguous. He thinks that so far as experiments have hitherto gone the transmissibility of the pearly disease to other animals (by feeding them with diseased milk or meat) is not yet certainly established.

KOCH's observation of the specific bacillus in the pearly nodules seems to remove all doubt of their identity with tubercles. How far the bovine disease may be transmitted to man is not yet made out. The transmission is at any rate possible, and that by various channels.

Syphilis.

128. **Syphilis** is an infective disease, originating in a fixed contagium. It starts at a wounded or abraded spot, gives rise there to certain local tissue-changes, and thence spreads through the entire system. The poison of syphilis occurs in the human organism only; it is nowhere reproduced but within the human organism; and it is conveyed to other individuals only by direct transference. When transplanted into a new organism, it excites inflammatory processes of the most diverse intensity and extent—from simple localised and transitory hyperaemia to the formation of enormous exudations, or granulomatous growths, or extensive fibrous hyperplasias. If a child be procreated while the infection lasts, the disease may be transmitted to it from the mother's side as well as from the father's.

The primary inflammatory focus is formed at the seat of infection as an **indurated chancre** or 'hard sore.' It is an ulcer with an hardened bacon-like or gristly base and margin. It generally begins as an excoriation, *i.e.* a slight and superficial loss of substance, and over this a vesicle or pustule is formed. In other cases it is developed from a node formed (for example) in the scar of a former ulcer; this then breaks, giving rise to the characteristic ulcer with its hardened gristly base. In other cases again the ulcer is first formed, and the induration follows later on.

The node or induration which forms the **primary lesion** of syphilis appears under the microscope at first as a dense infiltration of the connective tissue with small cells (Fig. 34 *a*). The process may not advance beyond this: but in many cases the infiltrating cells proceed to develope further. From the small round-cells larger formative cells (Fig. 34 *b*), and not infrequently giant-cells (*c*), are formed. The development does not advance beyond this point: the greater part of the affected tissue breaks down and ulcerates, or is re-absorbed. Some part of the cells go to form a cicatrix.

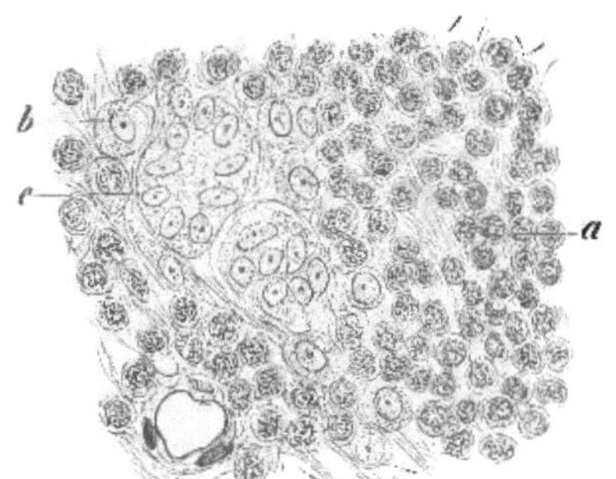

FIG. 34. SECTION OF A SYPHILITIC HARD SORE.
(*Alum-carmine preparation*; × 350)
a infiltration with round-cells *b* large uninuclear, *c* multinuclear, formative cells

Nothing certain is known concerning the nature of the syphilitic virus. KLEBS (*Arch. f. exp. Path.* x) regards the disease as a parasitic bacterial affection. Our histological knowledge of syphilitic growths is mainly due to VIRCHOW (*Krank. Geschwülste* II), E. WAGNER (*Arch. d. Heilk.* IV, 1863), AUSPITZ and UNNA (*Vierteljahrsschr. f. Derm. und Syph.* IV, 1877). See also BÄUMLER, *Ziemssen's Cyclopaedia* vol. III; VAN OORDT, *Des tumeurs gommeuses* In. Diss. Paris 1859; CORNIL and RANVIER, *Man. of Path. Hist.* vol. I.

129. After a certain time the 'initial sclerosis' or hard sore is followed by inflammations of the lymphatic glands, skin, and mucous membrane. These are the '**secondary symptoms**.' Still later appear syphilitic inflammations of the viscera and bones. These are the '**tertiary symptoms**.' The various inflammations are for the most part similar to other, non-syphilitic, inflammations. Certain special granulomatous formations are also developed which are called syphilomata (WAGNER) or gummata, and condylomata.

The syphilitic **condyloma** (*condyloma latum* or **mucous patch**) is a raised level patch on the skin or mucous membrane, due to inflammatory change in the epidermis and corium, or in the epithelium. The upper layers of the corium, and especially the papillae, swell up greatly owing to infiltrations of cells and liquid exudations. The cutis appears as a loose sodden gelatinous tissue infiltrated with cells (Fig. 35 *i* and *k*). There is no true granulation-tissue as a rule, for no organisation of the cellular material takes place, and no new vessels are formed. In condylomata of the mucous membranes, the tissue may take on something of the look of granulations owing to abundant cell-production. The epithelium is usually swollen (Fig. 35 *e f g*) and infiltrated with cellular and liquid exudations.

The syphilitic **gumma** in its earlier stages is histologically very similar to the condyloma. The gumma is a circumscribed patch of morbid tissue, not unlike granulation-tissue. It occurs chiefly in the periosteum, muscles, brain-substance, and membranes, as well

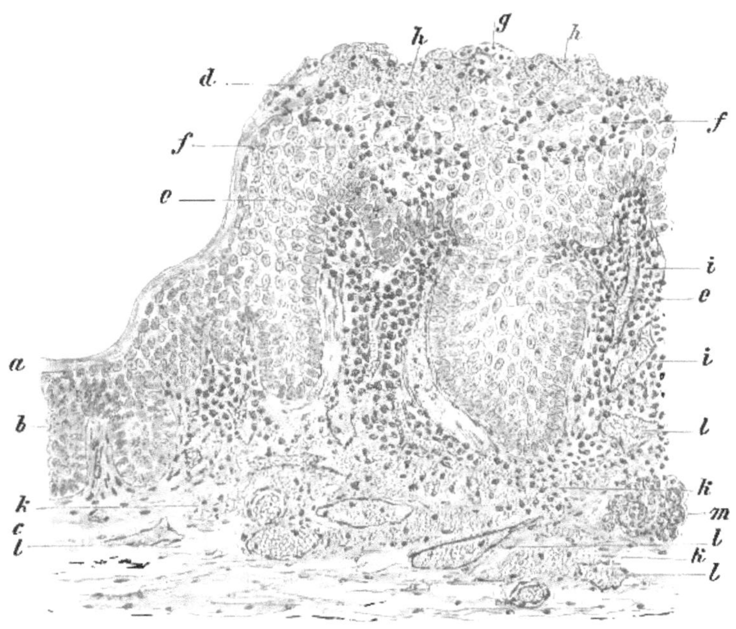

FIG. 35. *CONDYLOMA LATUM ANI* OR 'MUCOUS PATCH.'

(*Aniline-brown staining* : × 100)

a horny layer *b* rete Malpighii
c corium
d loosened horny layer infiltrated with leucocytes
e rete Malpighii swollen and (*f*) infiltrated with cells
g degenerate epithelial cells containing leucocytes
h granular coagula
i papilla swollen and infiltrated with cells and exuded liquid
k corium infiltrated with cells, exuded liquid, and coagula
l lymphatic distended with coagula
m sweat-gland

as in the parenchymatous organs of the abdomen, such as the liver, spleen, and testis. The relative proportion of cells in the gumma varies with its site. Varieties which are poor in cells, such as are found at times in bone, are soft and gummy in texture. On section they have a gelatinous look, the liquid constituents exceeding the cellular in quantity. The older surrounding tissue undergoes in part a mucoid change. Varieties rich in cells, met with chiefly in the pia mater and arachnoid, and the spleen, form nodes or patches which are translucent, grey or whitish or greyish red in colour, and rounded (spleen) or irregular (brain-membranes) in shape. They have in fact the exact appearance of granulations.

In the affected organs or tissues there are usually found, in addition to the gummata, more diffused and extensive inflammatory changes.

130. These syphilitic granulomatous growths are generally of a very perishable or unstable nature. Frequently there is no proper granulation-tissue developed: that is to say, no vessels are formed and no further development of the extravasated leucocytes takes place. The leucocytes usually perish by fatty degeneration. Small infiltrated patches may often disappear by re-absorption. In other cases, as in the bones, suppuration or fatty necrosis and ulceration is the issue. In larger patches abounding in cells, caseous nodes are not infrequently formed: they may be either rounded and spherical, or irregular in shape. If the caseous process is still in a comparatively early stage, these patches are found surrounded by highly cellular granulations. After a time these latter pass into dense fibrous tissue (Fig. 36), and contract into a narrow zone surrounding the caseous patch. Lastly, this zone may be further transformed into connective tissue of a more ordinary type. Caseous nodes, thus imbedded in an irregular puckered capsule of scar-tissue, are found most commonly in the liver and testis.

It is these scar-surrounded caseous nodes which are chiefly referred to when **gummatous nodes** are spoken of. They have of course ceased to be strictly gummatous, for they contain merely the caseous detritus of the original cellular gumma. The caseous change often involves not merely the cellular new-formation, but also the normal tissue of the affected organ. The node comes thus to contain more than the necrotic remains of the true gumma; it includes all or most of the proper or specific tissue affected and destroyed by the original infiltration.

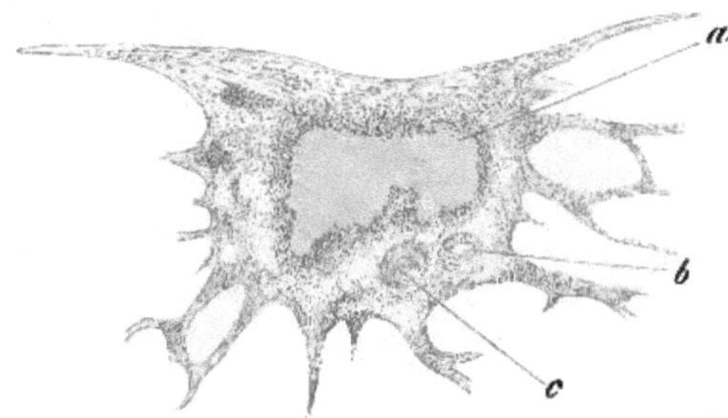

FIG. 36. GUMMA OF THE LIVER UNDERGOING CASEATION. (× 25)

a gumma enclosed in an irregular capsule of scar-tissue
b artery with thickened wall *c* obliterated portal vein

This common issue of syphilitic inflammation in disintegration and necrosis seems to depend chiefly on the nature of the virus which produces the disease. It is not however impossible that another factor may lie in the aptness of the vessels and especially the arteries to be attacked by the specific inflammation. Wherever granulations are formed or hyperplasia set up in consequence of syphilitic inflammation, the vessel walls and chiefly the intima are observed to thicken. The lumen is thus narrowed, and often entirely occluded (Fig. 36 *b* and *c* and Art. 297).

On syphilitic disease of the arteries see GREENFIELD &c., *Trans. Path. Soc.* vol. 28; HEUBNER, *Die luetische Erkrankung der Gehirnarterien* Leipzig 1874; LANCEREAUX, *Gaz. des Hôp.* 21, 1876.

Leprosy.

131. **Leprosy**, lepra or *elephantiasis graecorum*, is a disease distinguished anatomically by the formation of nodes and tubers in the tissues. These when cutaneous are usually seated on the surfaces exposed to the air—the face, hands, and feet. They may at times occur elsewhere. The subcutaneous tissues, nerves, mucous membranes, and viscera may also be affected. The nodes may reach the size of a walnut.

When a node is about to form in the skin, there appears first a red spot, which becomes bluish and then brown: the underlying tissue becomes meanwhile thickened and indurated. The swelling then increases, and the patch becomes gradually transformed to a firm red protuberance, which later on becomes softer and paler.

The basis of the node is made up of cellular granulation-tissue, lying immediately beneath the epidermis. It is spread in a uniform layer, or sends down cellular processes into the deeper structures. In colour it is greyish-white and somewhat translucent. The cells are of various sizes according to their stage of development. When the nodes break down, leprous ulcers are formed, though these are more commonly the result of external injury. Fatty metamorphosis of the cells and resolution of the tumour thereby are not unknown, but the process is very slow. The nodes of the mucous membrane are more apt to ulcerate than those of the skin: this occurs, for example, inside the nose, and in the conjunctiva, mouth, and larynx.

Leprous growths in the nerve-sheaths may lead to disturbance of the nerve-functions: we may thus have local amyotrophy and anaesthesia, as in *Lepra anaesthetica*. Visceral leprosy is rare.

ARMAUER HANSEN and NEISSER have discovered that leprosy depends on the presence of a specific bacillus (**Bacillus leprae**) in the affected tissue. The bacillus is found in all leprous foci (NEISSER), generally enclosed in the larger cells. The hereditariness of leprosy has not been proved. It is but slightly contagious; yet in certain regions it is endemic. It is nowadays rare in Europe: Norway and Sweden, Finland, and the Baltic provinces of Russia, are the regions where it is most prevalent. It occurs (but more rarely) in special districts of Greece and Italy. It is prevalent in Central and South America, and in Southern Africa and Asia.

VIRCHOW's *Onkologie* (vol. II) contains a full account of leprosy, from which the above details are chiefly drawn. THOMA (*Virch. Arch.* vol. 57) gives a description of the histological characters of the disease agreeing in essence with VIRCHOW's. NEISSER's discovery of the *Bacillus leprae* was announced in the *Breslau. ärzt. Zeitschrift*, 20 and 21, 1879: ARMAUER HANSEN's in *Virch. Arch.* vol. 79. See also NEISSER, *Virch. Arch.* vol. 84. The bacilli have been found in the nodes of the skin, oral epithelium, and larynx—as well as in diseased foci in the nerves, cartilages, testes, lymphatic glands, liver, and spleen. NEISSER has inoculated rabbits and dogs with leprous matter, and so produced inflammatory nodes corresponding with those of human leprosy. He supposes that the bacilli enter the system as spores, and develope wherever they find a suitable nidus, especially in the lymphatic glands. Thence they invade the entire body.

KÖBNER (*Virch. Arch.* vol. 88) found the bacilli in the blood. His attempts to transmit the disease to monkeys did not succeed. He is thus inclined to question NEISSER's demonstration of its transmissibility.

In *Lepra anaesthetica* the skin is usually smooth and shining. This form has therefore been distinguished as *L. laevis* or *glabra*. White or brown stains appear on the skin at times, probably at the site of a former infiltration. This variety is described as *Lepra maculosa;* the patches as *morphoeae nigrae* or *albae* (not to be confounded with the skin-disease Morphoea).

Lupus.

132. **Lupus** (or '*noli me tangere*') is an affection of the skin and contiguous mucous membranes. The surface becomes red, and this is followed by the formation of large or small nodules (Fig. 37 *d*) with more diffused swellings. Granulation-tissue is formed in the corium and subcutaneous connective tissue.

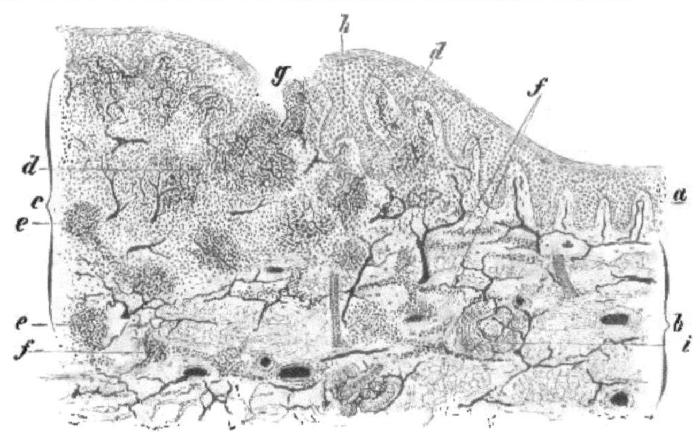

FIG. 37. SECTION OF SKIN THROUGH A LUPUS-PATCH.

a normal epidermis
b normal corium with sweat-gland (*i*)
c focus of lupus-tissue
d vascular nodule surrounded by diffuse cellular infiltration
e non-vascular nodule
f strings of cells
g lupous ulcer
h proliferating epithelium

The granulations are generally vascular, the cells small, spherical, and lymphoid: but at times numerous epithelioid cells and giant-cells may also be found. In the latter case, nodules may also develope having the exact appearance of tubercles. Surrounding the true granulomatous focus there are found nests and strings of cells following the course of the lymphatics (Fig. 37 *e f*). When the subepithelial granulations have reached a certain degree of development, they begin to break down and ulcerate (Fig. 37 *g*). It seldom happens that ulceration is averted by re-absorption or cicatrisation.

The exciting cause of lupus is unknown. The general course of the process, and especially its progressive character, seem to indicate that it is due to some virus capable of reproduction.

SCHÜLLER (*Centralb. f. Chir.* 49, 1881) has found certain micrococci in lupus-tissue, which he holds to be the cause of the affection. His observations are not however enough to establish the fact with certainty.

Glanders.

133. **Glanders** (or *Equinia*) is a contagious disease of the horse, communicable to man by direct transmission. Glanders and **farcy** are manifestations of one and the same infective disease: the first affects chiefly the nasal mucous membranes, the second the skin.

The initial lesion in the horse is usually situated in the nasal mucous membrane. The submaxillary gland is then affected: and then, by metastasis, various other organs. The first effect of the infection is to give rise either to wide-spread cellular infiltration of the mucous membrane, or to subepithelial nodules from the size of a millet-seed to that of a pea, and not unlike those of lupus.

In chronic farcy larger nodes and nodules form in the skin, and sometimes link themselves into vermiform cords ('corded veins').

The epithelial nodules are very unstable in structure. The cellular elements of which they are built up maintain throughout the characters of lymphoid cells or pus-corpuscles. Owing to fatty change, disintegration, softening, or suppuration in the nodules, ulcerations are soon formed which have a yellowish infiltrated base. These grow by progressive nodular (or simply diffused) infiltration of their borders, followed by gradual disintegration. In this way contiguous ulcers may become confluent. In horses that have died of glanders, the mucous membrane of the nasal septum is beset with large irregular excavated ulcers with eroded edges and greyish or yellowish bases. In addition to these, there are other minute lenticular ulcerations, and grey or yellow nodular patches on the point of breaking down. The whole process is near akin to that of suppurative inflammation. The ulcers may heal up by the formation of irregular puckered cicatrices.

The cervical glands are always inflamed and swollen. Among

the viscera the lungs are the most liable to be affected. They contain either nodes with caseous detritus in the centre and a greyish cellular periphery; or on the other hand lobular pneumonic patches of a light grey or blood-stained colour, or opaque and yellow from fatty and caseous change. At times the alimentary mucous membrane contains nodes of various sizes, composed either of light grey cellular tissue, or of opaque yellowish-white caseous or suppurative matters. In farcy, which is usually chronic, the nodes ('buttons' or 'buds') formed in the skin and muscles are made up of small-celled granulation-tissue, which later on undergoes retrogressive change, and becomes caseous or breaks down.

In man, as in the horse, infection with glanders-poison is followed by the formation of nodes and nodules, especially in the nasal cavities and frontal sinuses, and in the larynx and trachea. At the same time vesicular and pustular eruptions appear on the skin, followed by phlegmonous abscesses in the skin and muscles. The viscera are also affected in like manner. The development of the granulation-tissue is generally very imperfect: the inflammation tends rather to take on a suppurative character. In chronic farcy large nodes ('farcy buds') are formed in the skin and muscles. When these break down they give rise to indolent and obstinate ulcerations.

For a fuller description of equine glanders and farcy see YOUATT, *On the Horse* London 1859; FLEMING, *Man. of Veterin. Sanitary Science* vol. I London 1875: on the human affection see POLAND, *Holmes's System of Surgery* vol. I.

The nature of the glanders-poison is unknown. See VILLEMIN (*Études sur la tuberculose* Paris 1868), BOLLINGER (*Ziemssen's Cyclopaedia* vol. III), and PÜTZ (*Die Seuchen und Herdekrankheiten* Stuttgart 1882).

Actinomycosis.

134. **Actinomycosis** is a progressive inflammatory affection, set up by a certain fungus, the *Actinomyces*. It results in the formation of granulations and fibrous tissue, and in suppuration. It attacks human beings, cattle, and swine; and may be communicated to cattle by inoculation.

The disorder was first recognised and described in man by ISRAEL (1877), and in cattle by BOLLINGER (1877).

The parasite which causes the disorder is a peculiar fungus. It first appears as a tufted rosette of radiating pyriform or club-shaped structures: these are either simple or divided by dissepiments, and are of considerable bulk. They are possibly the conidia (Art. 213). The fungus on reaching its full development appears as a peculiar gland-like body, with the outward form of a mulberry. It is produced by the aggregation of the club-shaped conidia: these spring in all directions from the filaments of a matted tuft which we may provisionally call the mycelium, and are thus crowded into a compact mass. The true botanical position of the fungus is as yet undetermined.

When the actinomyces settles in a tissue, it at once sets up inflammation in its neighbourhood. While the spore is developing its mycelium and its bunch ('gland' or 'core') of conidia, a nodular inflammatory focus is formed around it, which in its structure exactly resembles a tuberculous nodule. Recent nodules consist chiefly of round-cells: in less recent ones the zone in contact with the fungus-core contains epithelioid cells and giant-cells. The core is yellowish in tint, and in later stages of the process it often becomes calcified.

When the nodules increase greatly in number and become confluent, the internodular inflammation also extending, large areas of inflammatory swelling are formed. In many cases, and especially in cattle, scar-like bands of fibrous tissue may be formed in the spaces between the nodules. The nodules themselves usually break down and suppurate. If the tendency to further development be strong enough, we may have, instead of suppuration, large nodular patches of new tissue formed. These may grow for weeks or months and finally become as large as the fist, or larger. The tumour is made up partly of coarse fibrous tissue, partly of granulations, with the intermediate stages. It always contains small pus-cavities and other excavations, in which the fungus-cores are found as small white or yellow greasy-like masses lying among the purulent detritus.

If on the other hand the tendency to disintegration and suppuration prove the stronger, we have formed large sacculated cavities with branching intercommunicating fistulae. The walls of these are lined with granulations and hyperplastic fibrous tissue, containing here and there colonies of the fungus.

135. In the case of cattle the disorder attacks chiefly the lower jaw; then the upper jaw, tongue, pharynx, larynx, oesophagus, stomach, and intestinal wall. The skin, the lungs, and the subcutaneous and intermuscular connective tissue, are also liable to invasion. In these sites it generally gives rise to nodular tumours of various sizes, such as we have described. Till the true nature of the disease was made out, these were described by a multitude of names such as osteo-sarcoma, bone-canker, bone-tubercle, fibroplastic degeneration, woody-tongue, lingual tuberculosis, lymphoma, fibroma, spina ventosa, tubercular stomatitis, etc. In the cases observed in the human subject, the disease has chiefly attacked the soft parts of the neck, the thorax near the spine, the mediastinal tissue, and the lungs. In one case the infective matter had entered the blood, and gave rise to metastatic foci in the viscera (PONFICK).

The inflammatory growths seldom reach any great size in man: they are apt rather to break down early. In the cases referred to, cavities and fistulae were formed, some of them subcutaneous and some extending deeper. Among their purulent contents were found the fungus-cores. Where the process invaded the bone, it led to destructive caries; this was notably the case with regard to the vertebrae. In all the affected regions the destruction of tissue was very considerable.

As regards the genesis of the disease, it seems very probable that the mouth is the starting-point of the infection. ISRAEL, JOHNE, and PONFICK affirm that in healthy individuals the specific fungus is now and then found lying in the follicular crypts of the tonsils. It has also been discovered in concretions from the lacrimal duct, and in hollow teeth. The observations of the above authors, with those of BOLLINGER, make it probable that infection often follows upon wounds of the oral cavity (*e.g.* those left after the extraction of teeth). ISRAEL believes that the spores or fungi may be inhaled, and so give rise to the disease in the lungs.

Clinically speaking, the disease is chiefly marked by its chronic course and local malignancy. Metastasis is not common.

ISRAEL'S researches were published in *Virch. Arch.* vols. 76, 78: BOLLINGER'S in the *Centralb. f. med. Wiss.* 27, 1877. Since then the affection has more than once been observed in man. JOHNE and PONFICK have been the chief writers on the human affection. JOHNE demonstrated the inoculability of the disease in animals (*Deutsch. Zeitsch. f. Thiermed.* VII, 1881). PONFICK has quite recently published a monograph (*Die Actinomycose des Menschen* Berlin 1882), in which the published observations on the disease are brought together; light is thrown on its aetiology by new observations and experiments; and the significance of the various morbid processes is explained. GANNET gives a useful summary in *Bost. med. surg. Journ.* Aug. 31, 1882.

PFLUG has described a case of actinomycosis in a cow, which took the form of miliary nodules disseminated through the lungs (*Cent. f. med. Wiss.* 14, 1882); HINK (*ibid.* 46, 1882) gives another case, in which the nodular affection was confined to a part of one lung.

SECTION VI.

TUMOURS.

CHAPTER XXV.

GENERAL CONSIDERATIONS.

136. In Arts. 79—92 under the heading of Hyperplasia and Regeneration we discussed a series of progressive or formative disturbances of nutrition. Some of these were the result of normal development carried to an excessive degree. Others seemed due to the resumption or intensification of processes of growth which had been interrupted or enfeebled. These processes led to the formation of new tissue, which either resembled exactly the matrix-tissue from which it arose, or at least was composed of the same elements.

Another mode of tissue-formation was discussed in the last section, under Inflammation. This process, as we saw, gave rise only to a single form of new tissue: it resulted in the development of granulations and fibrous tissue from them.

The mode of tissue-formation which leads to the development of a **tumour**, neoplasm, or new growth in the restricted sense of the term, is not comparable either with hyperplastic proliferation or with inflammation. It differs from the former in this, that the new tissue is not similar to the matrix-tissue but specifically different from it. A true tumour or neoplasm proper is always composed of tissue differing in type from that out of which it grows. It is distinguished from inflammatory tissue by the great variety of forms it may assume, and by the mode of its genesis.

The diversity existing between the neoplasm and the matrix is manifested in two ways. First, the new-formed tissue appears as a more or less sharply bounded and defined mass. Secondly, its texture and structure differ from those of its matrix, and generally to such an extent that the difference is recognisable with the unaided eye; it is of course still more plainly marked under the microscope. These two marks are generally enough to determine the diagnosis of tumour, though not invariably. In a whole series of new-formations, it is difficult or even impossible to distinguish anatomically between hyperplastic or inflammatory tissue and true neoplasm. The distinction must in such cases be based on the life-history of the tissue in question.

It should be noted—by way of distinction between inflammatory tissue and a neoplasm—that the latter does not originate in extravasated blood-cells, so far at least as its essential elements are concerned. As distinguished from hyperplasia, the genesis of a neoplasm is not dependent on exaggerated function or increased activity in the affected organ: moreover it does not retrogress, but continues to grow on without reaching any particular or typical termination.

The term tumour or neoplasm has been very differently interpreted by different writers. VIRCHOW, for example, includes all hyperplasias and inflammatory or granulomatous formations among the tumours; while COHNHEIM definitely excludes them. Others take up a middle position. This difference of view is closely connected with the different theories held concerning the aetiology of tumours (Arts. 177—181). We think with COHNHEIM that it is better to narrow the meaning of the term tumour so as to exclude hyperplasias and the infective granulomatous growths.

References :—VIRCHOW (*Die krankhaften Geschwülste*); LÜCKE (*Handb. d. Chir. v. Pitha u. Billroth* vol. II); R. MEIER (*Lehrb. d. allg. Path.* 1871); COHNHEIM (*Allg. Path.*); PAGET (*Surgical Path.*).

137. Tumours have been distinguished by various names according to their external form. **Nodular** tumours are made up of circumscribed nodes or nodules, single or grouped. Nodules of the size of a millet-seed are called miliary; smaller ones subminiliary. If the neoplasm is imperfectly marked off from its matrix, and extends into it by continuous or disconnected outgrowths, it is called **infiltrating**. The terms nodular and infiltrating are not however antithetical. A tumour may have nodes and nodules, and yet infiltrate the tissue in which it lies. This latter depends on the mode of growth. If the tumour increase interstitially ('central' or 'expansive' growth), it merely compresses and thrusts away the surrounding tissue, but does not infiltrate it. If it grows at the periphery by including ever fresh portions of the matrix-tissue ('appositional' or 'excentric' growth), it will give rise to the appearance of infiltration.

A tumour seated on any of the surfaces of the body, and protruding so as to form a segment of a spheroid, is said to be **tuberous**. If the base be smaller than the body of the tumour, it is **fungous**. If stalked, it is **polypous** or pedunculated. If it consist of several small and close-set protuberances, like the papillae of the skin, rising from a common stalk or base, the tumour is called warty, verrucose, papillomatous, or briefly a **papilloma**. If the papillae are very long and branched, it is described as a dendritic or ramifying growth.

138. The texture and structure of tumours are very various. A large group consist of tissues resembling some of the adult or embryonic connective tissues; they are thus made up solely of

mesoblastic elements. Such are distinguished as **histioid** tumours, or more simply as **connective-tissue** tumours. Some of them are firm and of the texture of fibrous tissue, cartilage, or bone. Others are soft and contain adipose tissue, mucous tissue, or embryonic or indifferent tissue. Very soft varieties, resembling brain on section and yielding a white creamy juice on being scraped, are described as encephaloid or medullary. Not uncommonly a tumour may have a different texture in different parts of it; it is then spoken of as a mixed tumour. It arises when two distinct tissue-forms are simultaneously developed, or when a single tissue has undergone partial transformation into another.

A second group of tumours are more complex in structure. They consist not only of mesoblastic elements, but of epiblastic and hypoblastic elements in addition; in other words they contain elements derived from epithelial cells. They are therefore described as **epithelial** tumours, in contradistinction to the connective-tissue group. Inasmuch as they exhibit a certain similarity of structure with various organs of the body, they have also been called **organoid** tumours. Their structure may often be recognised with the naked eye. On section the general appearance is that of a dense basis-substance, built up of reticulated bands and trabeculae, and containing within its meshes a substance of different colour and softer consistence. The latter often takes the form of a milky or creamy juice. Medullary forms are also met with in this group.

A tumour resembling its matrix-tissue in texture VIRCHOW calls **homoeoplastic**: one which differs widely is **heteroplastic**. The latter term implies—that in normal circumstances tissue like that of the tumour never occurs at all at the spot in question; or at any rate not at the particular stage of development reached at the time in question. A tumour may thus be heteroplastic as regards its site (heterotopic), or as regards its date (heterochronic). By excluding the mere hyperplasias from the category of tumours, we are bound in strictness to regard all tumours as heteroplastic: they never are of exactly the same structure as the matrix-tissue. A division of tumours into homologous and heterologous growths has been proposed. Homologous growths are such as resemble some normal tissue of the body: heterologous growths such as resemble no mature normal tissue. Unless a homologous growth is heterotopic it is not distinguishable from a hyperplasia. A growth which is strictly heterologous must be heteroplastic.

139. Every tumour is developed from pre-existing tissue-cells by proliferation: in some tumours new blood-vessels are also formed. The processes of cell-division and of vascularisation are identical with those described in Arts. 74 and 86. Nuclear subdivision is indirect: new vessels are formed by off-shoots from existing ones.

Tumours usually develope from small beginnings. It is rarely that their site of origin extends over an entire organ. From this it follows—that they do not usually lead to an enlargement of the organ as a whole, but rather tend to form definite nodes or protuberances. Some grow with great rapidity; others slowly and intermittently. There is no limit to their growth; they often reach enormous dimensions. They may cease to grow at all for years together, and then suddenly begin again.

Neoplastic or tumour tissue is very liable to retrogressive changes; this is especially true of quickly-growing cellular tumours. All the retrogressive changes which affect normal tissues are observed in tumours—fatty degeneration, mucoid degeneration, necrosis, caseation, disintegration, softening, liquefaction, gangrene, infarction, calcification, pigmentation (as in melanoma), &c. Inflammations are also very common in tumours.

Any of these processes may lead to partial destruction of a tumour. Cavities or ulcers are often formed in consequence of softening, and the new tissue may thus be disintegrated and destroyed—slowly or rapidly as the case may be. It is unfortunate that this process does not usually bring about the removal and eradication of the tumour, especially in the so-called malignant forms. The centre may break down, but the periphery continues steadily to advance. It may even happen that the peripheral advance is accelerated by the inflammatory disintegration of the central parts.

It is highly probable that, during the development of a neoplasm, the walls of the blood-vessels are somehow damaged or impaired. In support of this it may be mentioned—that in the neighbourhood of tumours we always find aggregations of small extravasated leucocytes. The manner in which this impairment of the vessel-walls is brought about remains unknown.

140. Most tumours are solitary. In other words there is originally but a single primary tumour. It is less frequent to find two tumours growing in an organ simultaneously, or in quick succession. In the latter case we must suppose that appropriate conditions arise at the same time at the different sites. Now and again it happens that several tumours, all of different structure, appear simultaneously in the same person.

From such multiple primary neoplasms we must of course distinguish what are called metastatic formations. **Metastasis** in this case implies a secondary neoplastic eruption, resulting from the transmission of elements of the original or parent tumour to a remote part of the body, and the development of a daughter-tumour from these germinal elements.

The germ or other virus given off by the parent tumour is conveyed to other regions through the lymphatics, or through the blood-vessels. According to the channel of transport, we find metastatic affections in the lymphatic vessels and glands which receive the infected lymph; or in remote organs irrigated by the infected blood, either directly or after passing through the heart. Thus in cancerous disease of the intestine we find secondary nodules developed in the liver, through the medium of the portal system: from the liver some germs may even find their way into the lungs. The germinal elements usually reach the blood by the direct penetration of the tumour-tissue into the lumen of a blood-vessel.

The development of the daughter-tumour starts unquestionably from these transported germs. This is probable *a priori* from the fact—that the metastatic or secondary tumour has always the same structure as the primary. The germs are, furthermore, essentially composed of cells in a condition of vital activity. The share taken by the matrix-tissue in which the germs are deposited is not always the same. In all cases it must furnish the necessary nutriment and blood-vessels, for without these no new growth is possible. But it very often furnishes other elements, and especially connective tissue. Proliferation is set up around the transplanted germs, and tissue is thereby formed; while migratory leucocytes generally contribute something to the whole. The secondary tumours developed may vary greatly in number. They are usually marked off definitely from the surrounding tissue; it is very uncommon for metastases of the kind to take the form of diffuse infiltration. This happens (if at all) in the case of bone, which may be transformed into tumour-tissue by secondary change affecting almost the entire skeleton.

Metastases are not invariably produced by all tumours: many of these never extend beyond the limits of their primary seat. The clinical character of **benignancy** or innocency is generally correlated with this property of tumours: **malignancy** is a character of the metastatic varieties. Other marks of malignancy are—the tendency to infiltrate and so destroy the surrounding tissue; and the tendency to recur after apparent extirpation.

Malignancy, or the tendency of a tumour to invade the neighbouring tissue and to produce metastatic tumours, is usually regarded as an inherent property of the tumour. COHNHEIM has recently expressed a different opinion (*Allg. Path.* I). He tries to explain malignancy by assuming that the physiological resistances to invasion are somehow diminished. Germs transplanted into fresh tissue are sure, he thinks, to perish in consequence of the normal chemical or metabolic changes which go on in the tissue. They can only develope when these metabolic changes cease to be normal. His main ground for this view is derived from an experiment made by himself and MAAS (*Virch. Arch.* vol. 70). They introduced pieces of living periosteum into the pulmonary vessels, and found that they grew for a time, but were ultimately absorbed and disappeared. The diminished resisting power of the tissues may be either congenital or acquired. The latter is especially the case in advanced age.

ZIEGLER is unable fully to agree with this view. Though the condition of the tissue has undoubtedly a great influence on the development of a germ transplanted into it, yet this alone cannot determine the malignity of the parent tumour. It surely depends on the structure and texture of the tumour whether its germs can be carried off at all, and transported by the stream of lymph or blood. And the faculty of developing in proper circumstances must be inherent in the germs themselves. ZAHN (*Sur le sort des tissus emplantés dans l'organisme* Geneva 1878) found that foetal tissues continued to grow for a time, when introduced into the body of an animal. LEOPOLD has quite recently confirmed this observation (*Virch. Arch.* vol. 85). Pieces of living tissue, taken from embryo rabbits and transplanted into other rabbits, are in part absorbed, and in part continue to grow. The latter is especially true of embryonic cartilage.

141. The formation of a tumour is always more or less fraught with injury to the affected organ, and in many cases to the entire system. The least harmful tumours are those which grow slowly and by expansion, so that they merely compress the surrounding tissue. If this is expansible or yielding like the skin, the resulting changes may be trifling. But it is not rare for the compressed tissue to become atrophied or absorbed. If the neoplasm be an infiltrating one, the surrounding tissue suffers much more seriously. It either perishes outright, or begins to proliferate and so contributes materials to the general growth. This is especially the fate of tissues which have specific functions; the specific elements die, while the fibrous or connective framework persists and becomes hyperplastic.

A tumour requires to be fed if it is to grow: hence the organ in which it is placed and the system generally are deprived of a certain proportion of nutriment to supply the tumour. If growth is slow the deprivation is unimportant, but it may become grave in the case of rapidly increasing tumours.

The seat of the tumour is of serious import. It need hardly be said, for instance, that a tumour growing in the brain or spinal cord has an altogether different significance, so far as life is concerned, from that of one developed in the skin. So also a tumour in the oesophagus obstructing the passage of food, or one in the stomach interfering with digestion, will lead to more serious results than one, say, in the bone of the finger. In the one case the function of an essential organ is impaired by the presence of the tumour, in the other the effects are merely local.

Metastatic or secondary formations have always an unfavourable significance. As the neoplastic foci become more numerous, so also do the organs exposed to the risk of injury by pressure, invasion, or abstraction of nutriment.

Disintegrative changes and ulcerations connected with tumours are specially destructive. There is nearly always an active secretion and loss of substance from the surface of such ulcers, and the body is reduced by the constant drain. Moreover it is not uncommon for putrefactive changes to be set up in the products of disintegration, and then the risk of blood-poisoning by absorption of septic matters becomes considerable.

Tumours may thus impair the function of essential organs, or give rise to a serious drain of matter from the body, or bring about a kind of blood-poisoning through the absorption of deleterious products of decay; in any or all of these ways the general nutrition may be profoundly disturbed, and the patient fall into grave ill-health. This is spoken of as the **cachexia** of tumour. It may become so profound that the patient dies of exhaustion.

CHAPTER XXVI.

TUMOURS DEVELOPED IN MESOBLASTIC TISSUES. CONNECTIVE-TISSUE TUMOURS.

a. Fibroma.

142. A **fibroma** is a tumour made up of fibrous tissue. It usually takes the form of a sharply defined node or lump, and occupies a part only of the organ in which it is seated. More rarely the organ (as *e.g.* the ovary) becomes transformed throughout into a fibrous mass. Fibromata occurring on epithelial or mucous surfaces often take a papillomatous form.

The fibroma is of very varying consistence, according to the texture of its component tissue. It is often very firm and tough, grating under the knife, and having a glistening gristly look on section (desmoid fibroma). In other instances it may be soft and flabby, with a greyish translucent section. Other specimens will be found in which the scattered fibrous bands are dense and white and glistening, but the general structure is loose and incompact; so that the tumour as a whole is rendered limp and flabby. All varieties of intermediate forms occur between the firm and the soft, and even within the same tumour different parts may be of different consistence. The firm varieties are seen under the microscope to be made up chiefly of large coarse fibrous bundles, interspersed more or less thickly with cells whose protoplasm is scanty.

The softer fibromata, with their translucent greyish section, are usually richer in cells. By teasing out a fragment it is easy to isolate numbers of slender spindle-shaped or caudate cells. The intervening substance is more scanty, the fibrils less coarse and gathered into smaller bundles. Stained sections of such fibromata appear as if they were full of nuclei (Fig. 38).

In loose-textured fibromata a clear juice is contained between the fibrous bundles, which are crossed and plaited and interwoven in all directions.

The fibroma is developed from proliferous connective-tissue cells. Accordingly spots are often to be found in it where cells

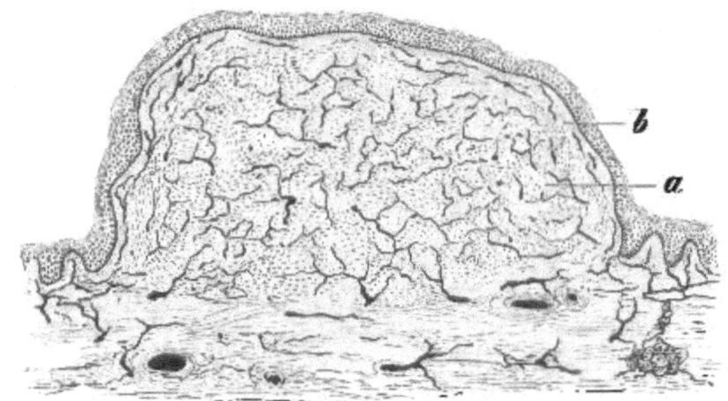

FIG. 38. FIBROMA MOLLUSCUM OF THE SKIN.
(Injected preparation stained with haematoxylin: × 25)
a fibroma *b* papilla thinned out by distension

are more abundant than in the tumour generally: in such spots we find not only the slender spindle-shaped kind, but also round and oval cells, and even stellate cells. The transformation of the proliferated cellular tissue into fibrous tissue is effected by the same steps as in fibrous hyperplasia (Art. 85).

Fibromata may occur in very various tissues; in any structure indeed which contains any form of connective tissue. Thus they are found in the skin, nerves, ovary, periosteum, fasciae, uterus, and less often in the mamma, alimentary canal, &c. Their appearance is always manifestly different from that of the matrix in which they are seated (Fig. 38).

Fibromata do not give rise to metastatic or secondary tumours, though they are often enough multiple, especially in the skin, nerves, and uterus. Within the same tumour we may often make out several centres of growth: the fibroma is in fact composed of several nodes separated by ordinary fibrous tissue. Such tumours can only do injury in virtue of their size or of their site.

Now and then fibromata undergo degenerative changes. They may become fatty, or may soften and break down, so that cavities form within them. They may give way at the surface and so ulcerate; sometimes they become partially calcified, as in the case of uterine 'fibroids.' They may be highly vascular, or the reverse (Fig. 38).

In rare cases the blood-vessels become wide and dilated, so that the tissue is pierced with capacious channels and cavities containing blood. In other instances the lymphatics are similarly dilated.

It is not always easy to distinguish between true fibroma and fibrous hyperplasia. In general the fibroma is characterised by the difference between its texture and that of the surrounding tissue, from which moreover it is for the most part sharply defined. These characters are usually wanting in hyperplasias, such for instance as those consequent on chronic inflammation. Now and then however we meet with inflammatory hyperplasias which are circumscribed—such as venereal warts in the skin, and the nodes developed in the lungs around inhaled dust-particles. As in the last instance, their texture may be different from that of the matrix. It is the life-history and mode of genesis to which we must appeal in such cases. Inflammatory hyperplasias, being mere products of inflammation, cannot properly be reckoned among the true tumours.

b. *Myxoma.*

143. When the ground-substance of a fibroma swells up by the imbibition of fluid, it becomes gradually more and more translucent and may even become transparent. The tumour at length resembles a mass of jelly. A swollen fibrous tumour of this kind is best described as an oedematous fibroma. The texture of many oedematous fibromata much resembles that of the umbilical cord in nearly mature foetuses; where the cells and fibrils are more or less thrust asunder and interpenetrated by a transparent juice (Wharton's jelly).

Adipose tissue, whether neoplastic (Art. 144) or normal, may similarly become transformed into a gelatinous mass. The fat disappears from the cells, and a dense saline liquid collects between them. They ultimately assume a ramified or stellate form.

No sharp line can be drawn between jelly-like oedematous fibromata and lipomata, and true **myxoma**. Many writers do not hesitate to include the former class among the myxomata. It is

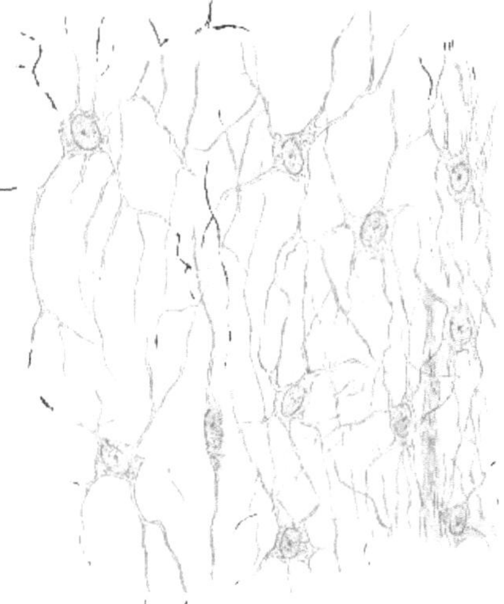

FIG. 39. CELLS FROM A PERIOSTEAL MYXOMA OF THE THIGH. (*Gold staining:* ×400)

perhaps more correct to reserve the name for tumours in which we have not only a swollen and semi-liquid condition of the interfibrillar substance (a substance normally containing mucin), but also an actual solution of the fibrillae and replacement of them by dense saline juice. Such a tissue is highly translucent, almost transparent in fact. The cells it contains are generally much ramified, though some remain rounded (Fig. 39). They here and there undergo mucoid degeneration and so perish. Pure mucous tissue, such as we have just described, is never uniformly present throughout the tumour: there is no such thing as a perfectly pure myxoma. The bulk of the tumour is generally made up of oedematous connective tissue: some parts of it may even be coarsely fibrous. It is thus best described as **myxofibroma** or **myxolipoma** as the case may be.

Myxomata are most commonly found in the fibrous tissue of the periosteum, skin, fasciae, and muscular septa, as also in the subcutaneous and subserous fat, and in the marrow of bone. They are innocent and rarely give rise to metastases. On the other hand they may grow to an inordinate size, and may also be multiple.

KÖSTER (*Sitzungsb. d. niederrhein. Ges. f. Natur- und Heilk.* 17 Jan. 1881) and his pupil RUMLER (In. Diss. Bonn) have investigated the relation between myxoma and oedematous fibroma. KÖSTER regards swollen and saturated connective tissue as identical with mucous tissue. Myxomata arise merely from the swelling up (by imbibition) of the ground-substance of the various connective tissues.

c. *Lipoma.*

144. **Lipomata** are tumours composed of adipose tissue. They form soft or firm lobular masses, often of considerable size. Their structure is very much like that of the subcutaneous *panniculus adiposus;* it is made up of a series of fatty lobules bound together by fibrous septa of varying thickness. The lobules of the tumour are however rather larger than the normal ones.

If, as is not uncommon, we have mucous tissue associated with the adipose, the tumour is described as a **lipomyxoma:** if it contains abundant fibrous tissue it is a **lipofibroma.**

Lipomata generally arise from normal adipose tissue, though they may also be developed in connective tissues which normally contain no fat, such as the submucous coat of the intestine, and the dura mater. The larger lipomata not infrequently undergo either calcification, necrosis, gangrene, or putrid decomposition. They do not form metastases, though they are often multiple. The fat they contain is never completely absorbed, even when the patient becomes utterly emaciated.

d. *Glioma.*

145. **Gliomata** are tumours which develope from the neuroglia-cells of the central nervous system, and when mature are largely made up of neuroglia-cells. They are formed in the brain, and

more rarely in the spinal cord. They appear as tumours which are imperfectly marked off from the healthy brain- or cord-substance; the margin of the tumour gradually merges into the healthy tissue. They have thus the look rather of localised swellings than of tumours: but the difference in tint, and the blurring of the normal distinctions between the various elements of the brain-substance, serve to make good the diagnosis.

Their appearance varies. Some are light grey and translucent like the cortical substance, and fairly firm in consistence. Others are whiter, coarser, and firmer. Others again are greyish red or even dark red, in which case they are traversed by large and numerous blood-vessels. Vascular gliomata often enclose haemorrhagic patches. They are subject to fatty degeneration, caseation, softening, and disintegration.

A section of a mature glioma exhibits under the microscope a kind of felted texture, made up of excessively fine lustrous filaments (Fig. 40 *B*) interspersed with a multitude of slightly oval nuclei. The nuclei are surrounded by a scanty hardly-visible protoplasm. If however the preparation be examined when quite fresh, or after treatment with Müller's fluid, it is readily seen that the nuclei belong to cells which are furnished with numerous delicate ramifying processes going off in various directions (Fig. 40 *A*).

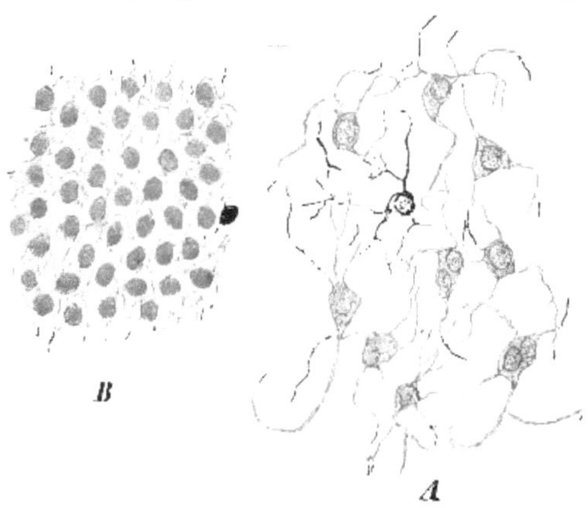

FIG. 40. GLIOMA FROM THE BRAIN.

A, cells isolated by teasing and stained with carmine. *B*, section of the same tumour hardened in Müller's fluid, mounted in Canada balsam, and stained with aniline brown: ×350.

These cells are very similar to neuroglia-cells, though they are often decidedly larger and coarser. Some of them may contain two, three, or more nuclei.

Researches on the development of glioma have shown that the neuroglia-cells are the parent cells of the tumour. The ganglion-cells take no part in the proliferous process. The proportion of cells in the tumour varies greatly: sometimes the cells form the bulk of it, and sometimes the fibrous framework.

The vessels are often highly developed, and may be sacculated or generally dilated.

Glioma is usually solitary, and as regards metastasis is innocent: it is only locally malignant.

Certain cellular tumours of the retina have been described as gliomatous: their elements resemble the cells of the granular layer. As they grow they invade on the one hand the orbital cavity behind the eye-ball, or on the other hand break through the cornea and sclerotic, passing forwards. They recur after apparent extirpation, and give rise to metastases. The cells of which they are made up are partly round and simple, and partly ramified. It seems questionable whether we are justified in calling these tumours gliomata. We are inclined to maintain that they are really sarcomata.

Glioma was first defined and named by VIRCHOW (*Die k. Geschwülste* II. ch. 18). KLEBS has recently propounded the theory (*Beiträge zur Geschwulstlehre* I, 1879) that the ganglion-cells play an active part in the formation of gliomata. ZIEGLER and CHRISTOPH examined a large number of gliomata both fresh and hardened, but failed altogether to find evidence for this view. The nuclei of the ganglion-cells seemed never to subdivide. In the instances where this at first sight appeared to occur, closer investigation showed that the suspected ganglion-cell had merely incorporated a neuroglia-cell.

e. *Chondroma.*

146. **Chondromata** (or enchondromata) are tumours which consist essentially of cartilage. The slight amount of fibrous tissue usually present in a chondroma is of altogether minor importance. It either serves to cover the surface of the tumour, or penetrates the interior carrying the nutrient blood-vessels.

Cartilaginous tumours are chiefly developed in regions which normally contain cartilage; that is to say, in the osseous system or in the cartilaginous parts of the respiratory system. They may occur however in tissues which are normally devoid of cartilage, such as the testis and parotid gland, and more rarely in other organs. They are of very various size: the smaller ones are generally globular, the larger are lobed or nodular. The several lobes are in the latter case separated by fibrous tissue. They are often multiple, especially in the skeletal structures of the hands and feet.

The tumour-tissue has usually the structure of hyaline cartilage, though sometimes yellow cartilage or fibro-cartilage largely replaces it. Even in hyaline chondromata, however, there are always patches in which the matrix-substance is beset with fibres. At the periphery the cartilage passes gradually into fibrous tissue, which forms a sort of perichondrium. The hyaline matrix often has a dusty or ground-glass appearance.

The number, size, shape, and grouping of the cartilage-cells vary much in different cases, and even within the same tumour. Many tumours abound in cells, in others they are sparse: in some the cells are large, in others small. They may be surrounded by capsules, or they may be naked; and crowded in groups within single capsules, or more uniformly scattered. Every variety of normal cartilage may occur also in chondromata. The form of the cells varies accordingly: they are usually spherical, but fusiform and stellate cells are not uncommon, especially in the neighbourhood of the fibrous septa which divide or surround the lobules of the tumour. So far as the development of the tissue is concerned, all that was said in Art. 87 applies also here. The matrix is derived either from pre-existing cartilage, or from marrow, periosteum, bone, or other connective tissue. Cartilaginous tumours which originate in cartilage have been called **ecchondroses** (*cf.* exostoses).

Chondromatous tissue is very apt to undergo retrogressive change. Some of the cells generally contain oil-globules. In large tumours the matrix-substance frequently undergoes mucoid softening and liquefaction, at points scattered here and there through it. This results in the formation of mucous tissue (Arts. 90—92); or in complete liquefaction of the matrix and destruction of the cells, and so in the formation of cysts containing liquid. In other cases the cartilage becomes calcified, or true bone is developed (Art. 165). Sarcomatous tissue may be produced when the cartilage-cells multiply rapidly.

Chondromata are generally speaking innocent, though metastases are occasionally met with.

In reference to cartilaginous growths, we must be careful to distinguish hyperplasia from true neoplasm. We must not set down all cartilaginous formations as chondromata, even when they are extensive. We often find considerable cartilaginous growths in connexion with bones (especially at the articular ends), which are quite certainly to be regarded as hyperplastic. It is the general course of the process which must decide in each case. The more completely a growth differs from its matrix, and developes as an independent tissue, the more certain we are that it is a real tumour.

VIRCHOW (*Monatsber. d. Acad. d. Wiss.* Berlin 1875) has made it probable that many osseous enchondromata originate in remnants of cartilage which have abnormally remained unossified. Such quiescent islands of cartilage certainly exist and are not at all uncommon; it may well happen that they suddenly resume the habit of growth and begin to proliferate. VIRCHOW suggests (by way of accounting for parotid enchondromata) that outlying bits of foetal cartilage may lodge in the rudimental parotid gland, which properly belong to the rudimental pinna of the ear. See PAGET, *Surg. Path.* Lect. 26; *Med. chir. Trans.* 1855; RANVIER, *Bull. Soc. Anat.* 1865; VIRCHOW and HIRSCH, *Virch. Jahresber.* 1869.

f. Osteoma.

147. The **osteomata** are tumours composed of osseous tissue. Their usual seat is in connexion with the bones, though they may occur elsewhere.

Osseous formations connected with the bones have received different names according to their site and disposition. **Hyperostosis** is diffused and extensive overgrowth in a bone. When the new-formed tissue is seated upon a definite spot in the old bone it is described as an **osteophyte**; or, if it be larger and more like a tumour, as an **exostosis**. Circumscribed bony growths in the interior of bones are called **enostoses**. Bony growths which are not rigidly connected with the bone are divided into—mobile periosteal exostoses, which are seated on the periosteum though separate from the bone; parosteal osteomata placed near to the bone, but not connected with it; independent osteomata remote from the bone and seated in tendon or muscle; and finally, the strictly **heteroplastic osteomata**, which may be seated in the lungs, brain-membranes, diaphragm, skin (rarely), parotid gland, &c.

Excrescences also occur in connexion with the teeth. If they consist of cement or *crusta petrosa*, they are called dental osteomata: if they consist of dentine they are odontomata. The latter originate in a hyperplasia of the pulp during the development of the tooth.

The texture of an osseous tumour may resemble that of ivory, as in eburnated osteoma; or it may be soft and spongy, as in spongy or cancellous osteoma; the former varieties are built up of dense and compact tissue with narrow nutrient canals, and similar to the cortical layer of the long bones. The latter are built of thin and delicate trabeculae enclosing large medullary spaces; they are allied in texture to cancellous bone.

The surface is sometimes uniform and smooth, so that the entire tumour is conical, spherical, or pyriform: sometimes it is irregular, rough, or tuberculated, without any definite figure. Ivory-like tumours are generally of the first kind: they occur most commonly as exostoses of the skull. Spongy exostoses are of the second kind, as are also the independent and heteroplastic osteomata.

The development of the osseous tissue in tumours follows the course described in Art. 88. It is effected partly by the agency of osteoblasts, partly by metaplasia of the existing tissue. The ground-substance is chiefly derived from the connective tissue of the periosteum and of the structures in which the tumour is bedded; as well as from cartilage and bone-marrow. When cartilage is first produced by periosteal proliferation, and then transformed into bone, the growth is described as a cartilaginous exostosis. When bone is directly produced, by suppression of the cartilaginous stage, we have a fibrous exostosis.

Many abnormal bony growths are not strictly speaking tumours, but rather hyperplasias resulting from excessive growth or inflammation. This is true not only of most hyperostoses, osteophytes, and exostoses, but also of some parostoses and independent osteomata. Of this nature are the bony growths produced in the adductors of the thigh by constant riding, and in the deltoid by the shouldering of the rifle in manual-exercise. In what way fibrous tissues which never produce bone normally are excited to produce it by long-continued irritation, is not easy to determine. We only know that the occurrence is not by any means impossible. The diagnosis between true and false osteoma is not always easy. If the new growth is unaccompanied by signs of irritation or of inflammatory change in its neighbourhood, it is probably a true osteoma.

References :—MÜLLER, *Zeitsch. f. wiss. Zool.* IX ; PAGET, *Surg. Path.* Lect. 27 ; VIRCHOW, *Die k. Geschwülste.*

g. Angioma.

148. **Angiomata** are tumours principally made up of blood-vessels. Some of these blood-vessels may be new-formed, others are pre-existing vessels more or less altered. The alteration is chiefly in the direction of dilatation, or thickening of the walls. Angiomata are not sharply marked off from the surrounding tissue. According to our definition of tumour, which makes the formation of new tissue an essential feature, we should exclude from the angiomata all vascular tumours which are produced merely by the dilatation or overgrowth of pre-existing vessels.

General usage has however sanctioned a certain relaxation of this strict rule ; inasmuch as simple vascular dilatations extending over a definite region, and so giving rise to a definite tumour-like swelling, are universally described as angiomata. According to its structure the angioma is spoken of as simple or cavernous Racemose aneurysms, and racemose varices, have also been included among vascular tumours ; and a fifth variety is furnished by lymphatic angioma or lymphangioma.

149. **Simple angioma** (telangiectasis or simple erectile tumour) is a structure made up of some normal basis-tissue, containing an abnormal number of distended and altered veins and capillaries.

Such formations are most frequently met with in the skin: they are usually congenital, and after birth merely increase in size. They are described as vascular **naevi**, and chiefly occur at places where foetal clefts have become closed (fissural angiomata). They can hardly be spoken of as tumours, for they do not raise the skin. A simple naevus merely looks like a level patch of a different tissue substituted for the normal skin. The colour is either bright red (*n. flammeus*, strawberry mark), or livid (*n. vinosus*, port-wine mark). It is not usually marked off very sharply from the normal tissue. Small circumscribed red specks are often found round the edges and in the neighbourhood of the chief patch. The red colour is due to the wide and distended blood-vessels, which are seated in the corium or subcutaneous fat. In the latter site they are often beset with minute sacculations. It is rare for such naevoid angiomata to be found elsewhere than in the skin ; but they occur now and then in glands like the mamma, in bone, and in the brain. They occur also, and more frequently, in the interior of morbid growths, such as gliomata and sarcomata.

When the vascular changes are more closely examined, by isolating the vessels or by making sections of the tumour, it is seen that they depend essentially on localised dilatations of new-formed or pre-existing capillaries (Fig. 41). The dilatations are fusiform, cylindrical, sacculated, or spherical; and these varieties of form

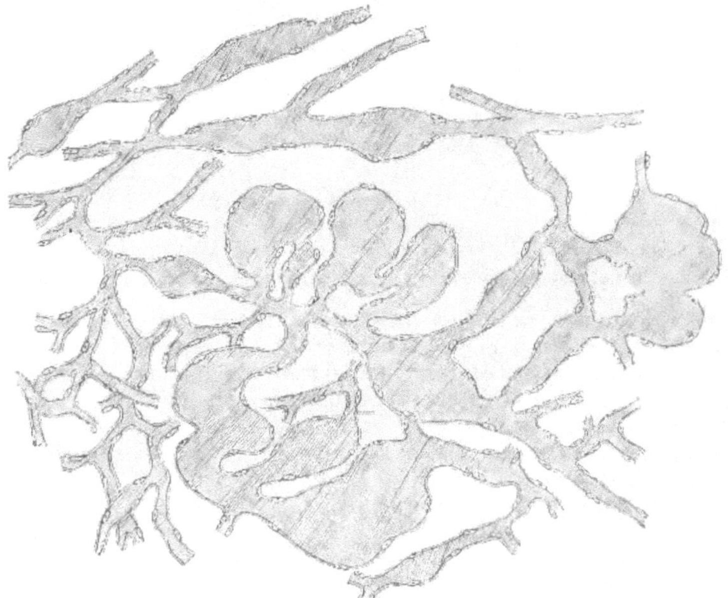

FIG. 41. DILATED CAPILLARIES FROM A SIMPLE ANGIOMA OF THE BRAIN.
(Isolated by removal of the basis-tissue: × 200)

are combined in all possible ways. In naevi the dilatations are even more exaggerated than those in the figure. They form wide cavities connected together by normal or but slightly dilated capillaries. The walls of the capillaries are not perceptibly thicker than the normal: they have thus the appearance of being rather thin than otherwise.

Another form of simple angioma, best described as the hypertrophic form, is made up of dilated capillaries whose walls are very considerably thickened. The dilatations are not usually so extreme as in the former varieties; but the number of vessels is so vast that on section they seem everywhere contiguous, the basis-tissue being as it were thrust out of sight (Fig. 42). The capillary-walls are abnormally thickened and beset with nuclei, resembling somewhat the walls of the arterioles. When the blood is abstracted and the lumen of the vessels diminished as much as possible, so that the nuclei are set radially, the section looks very like one through the glomerulus of a sweat-gland.

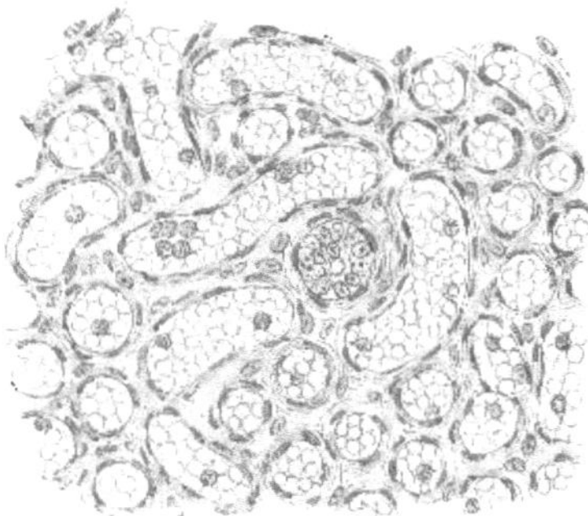

FIG. 42. SECTION OF A SIMPLE HYPERTROPHIC ANGIOMA OF THE SKIN. (× 200)
The duct of a sweat-gland has been cut across at the middle of the section.

This resemblance is further increased by the fact that the tumour is made up of a number of lobules or nodules separated by fibrous tissue, each composed of a convoluted knot of hypertrophied vessels. Moreover, as these angiomata occur in the skin, and chiefly in the deeper parts of the cutis and subcutaneous connective tissue, it sometimes happens that the section includes actual sudoriferous tubules (Fig. 42).

A third form of simple angioma is the venous or varicose tumour: it likewise occurs chiefly in the skin and subcutaneous tissues. In the forms already described the smaller veins are often dilated, but this feature is not marked in comparison with the capillary changes. In the venous angiomata the dilatation is almost entirely confined to the smaller veins, the anastomosing capillaries remaining almost unchanged. The venous dilatations or varices are cylindrical, ampullate, or saccular, with distinct and somewhat thickened walls. **Haemorrhoids** or piles are of this nature: they are tumours formed in the mucous membrane of the rectum near the anus, and consist mainly of hyperplastic submucous tissue, and of blood-containing saccules, derived from the small veins by morbid dilatation.

References:--ROKITANSKY, *Lehrb. d. path. Anat.* 1855; VIRCHOW, *Die krankhaften Geschwülste;* BILLROTH, *Arch. f. Chir.* XI; LÜCKE, *Chirurgie v. Pitha u. Billroth* II; MONOD, *Étude sur l'angiome simple* Paris 1873; PAGET, *Surg. Path.* Lect. 28 (containing further references).

150. The **cavernous angioma** is distinguished from the simple angioma by the fact that the tubular form of the vessels is more or less lost. In its fully developed form, the tumour is made up of a series of wide variously shaped cavities, separated

from each other merely by fibrous septa (Fig. 43). In section these cavities appear as sinuses of various size, separated by

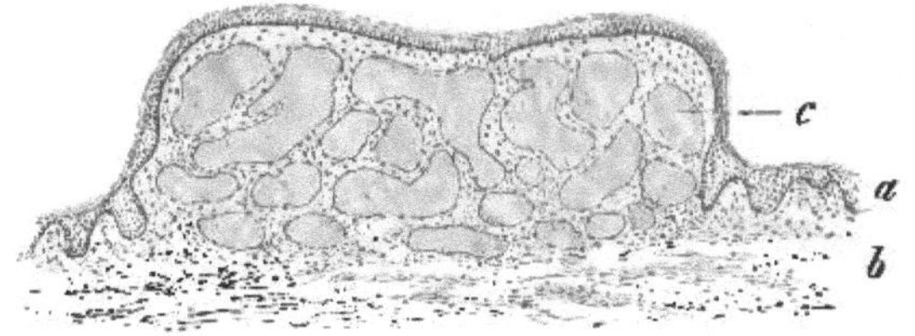

FIG. 43. CONGENITAL CAVERNOUS ANGIOMA OF THE SKIN.
(*Haematoxylin staining*: ×20)
a epidermis *b* corium *c* cavernous blood-spaces

a trabecular network of nucleated fibrous or spindle-celled tissue. The separation is not complete, as the spaces communicate with each other. The mass resembles greatly the corpus cavernosum of the penis, and is sometimes described as composed of 'erectile' tissue. The walls of the cavities are lined with endothelium.

These tumours are commonly seated in the skin, and may be congenital (Fig. 43). In other cases they are developed from simple angiomata by continued dilatation of the already dilated vessels. In the skin they form livid raised and sometimes uneven patches (*naevus prominens*). Among the viscera the liver is by far the commonest seat. Here they take the form of dark brown patches, not raised above the surface, and not compressing the liver-tissue, which indeed they simply replace. They are never congenital, but are developed in advanced age when the liver is tending towards atrophy. It is easy to make out in favourable specimens that the cavities have arisen from the varicose dilatation of individual capillaries within the lobules, the liver-cells disappearing simultaneously (Fig. 44). At first there

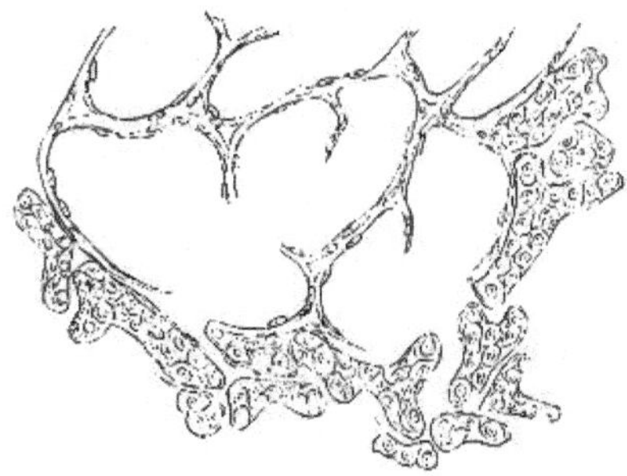

FIG. 44. SECTION FROM THE ADVANCING BORDER OF A VERY SMALL CAVERNOUS ANGIOMA OF THE LIVER. (×150)

is no proliferation from the vessel-walls. Then several capillaries coalesce by disappearance of the septa, and so form larger cavities. When the cavernous metamorphosis reaches the border of a lobule, the periportal fibrous tissue forms a capsule round the transformed vascular mass, which at first has no definite boundary. At this stage proliferation of the tissue not infrequently sets in (*cf.* RINDFLEISCH, *Path. Hist.* vol. I p. 163).

Angiomata are found, though very rarely, in the kidney, spleen, uterus, intestine, bladder, muscles, bones, &c.

The above account of the development of cavernous tumours in the liver is considerably at variance with that given by VIRCHOW (*Die k. Geschwülste*, III). VIRCHOW supposes that the first step is not a dilatation of the vessels, but the formation of new granulation-tissue. In this the vessels and vascular sinuses are formed. ZIEGLER is unable to find any traces of such a mode of genesis. He examined a liver which contained a multitude of angiomata varying from a scarcely perceptible speck to a tumour the size of a walnut. All stages of development were represented, from the dilatation of a single capillary up to the cavernous metamorphosis of an entire lobule. Yet in no instance was there any sign of proliferation at starting: atrophy and dilatation only were observed. PAYNE describes a remarkable case of a similar kind in the *Trans. Path. Soc.* 1869.

The term angioma nowadays embraces formations which are genetically very diverse. Some angiomata are congenital, and are therefore conditioned by some disturbance of development. Others arise from new-formed vessels. Others again are the result of a kind of degenerative change; vascular dilatation following on abnormal relaxation of the vessel-wall, or on atrophy of the intervascular parenchyma. Formations of this kind, produced merely by dilatation and cavernous degeneration, should be excluded from the category of true tumours.

151. **Aneurysm by anastomosis** (anastomotic or racemose aneurysm) is not properly a neoplasm; it is rather a morbid change affecting a vascular territory. The arteries of the territory become dilated and convoluted, while the intervening tissue atrophies. The pulsating growth feels to the finger like a knot of writhing worms. Many of these growths originate in congenital faults, especially those which occur in the scalp, and lead at times to erosion of the bone. Others are acquired, and follow upon mechanical injuries. The dilated arteries generally have thickened walls.

The racemose or **anastomotic varix** is analogous to the racemose aneurysm. It is a common affection of the veins in the leg, the labia pudendi, and the spermatic cord (varicocele).

Further details concerning aneurysm and varix will be found in the Special Pathological Anatomy under Vascular Affections.

152. **Lymphatic angioma** or lymphangioma is, in relation to the lymphatic system, what angioma (as hitherto considered) is to the haemic system. The essential character of the growth is dilatation of the lymphatic vessels, associated at times with hypertrophy of the vessel-wall and atrophy of the intervening tissue. We may distinguish the various forms into simple lymphangioma or lymphatic

telangiectasis, and cavernous lymphangioma; together with a third form, the cystoid lymphangioma. As in the foregoing cases, the magnitude and arrangement of the dilatations may vary greatly. In the extreme stages actual cysts may be formed. The cavities contain lymph, which is generally clear and limpid, though it is sometimes milky.

The growth may be congenital or acquired. Congenital lymphatic dilatations take various forms according to their seat, which may be the tongue (macroglossia), lips (macrocheilia), skin (lymphatic naevus), labia, &c. Lymphangiectasis of the skin is not rare as an acquired affection; it chiefly occurs in the thigh and thorax. Sometimes it gives rise to considerable tumours, which fluctuate on palpation. The section represented in Fig. 45 was taken from a tumour as large as the fist, which had formed in the subcutaneous fat of the thigh. The dilated and sacculated lymphatics have their walls more or less thickened, and they are generally embedded in the adipose tissue.

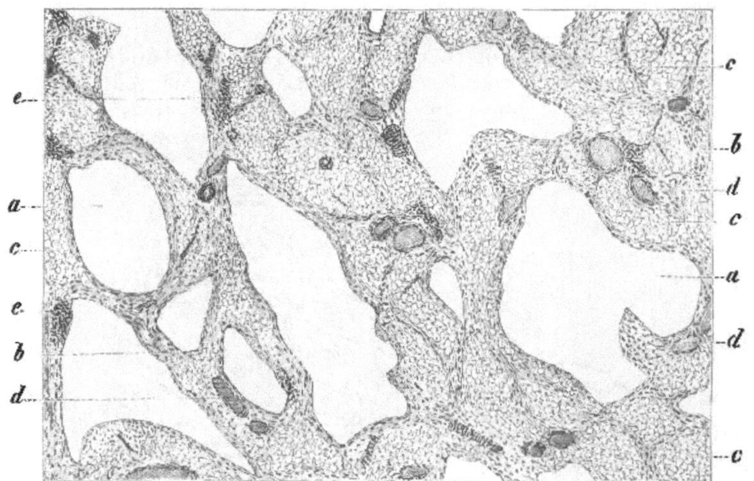

FIG. 45. SUBCUTANEOUS CAVERNOUS LYMPHANGIOMA.

(*Section mounted in Canada balsam, and stained with alum-carmine:* × 20)

a dilated lymphatics
b connective tissue
c adipose tissue
d larger blood-vessels
e groups of small cells or leucocytes

If the more superficial cavities of a cutaneous lymphangioma should rupture, a grave lymphorrhoea may ensue. The affection is often complicated with fibrous hyperplasia of the skin (as in elephantiasis lymphangiectodes), or of other organs.

References :—MAIER, *Lehrb. d. allg. path. Anat.*; VIRCHOW, *op. cit.*; ARNSTEIN, *Virch. Arch.* vol. 54; ANGER, *Tumeurs érectiles lymphatiques*, In.

Diss. Paris 1867; GJORGEWIC, *Arch. f. klin. Chir.* XII; REICHEL, *Virch. Arch.* vol. 46; WEGNER, *Langenbeck's Arch. f. klin. Chir.* XX; PINNER, *Centralb. f. Chir.* 12, 1880; POSPELOW, *Vierteljahrs. f. Derm. u. Syph.* 1879; HEBRA and KAPOSI, *Diseases of the Skin* (Syd. Soc.) vol. III; NIEDEN, *Virch. Arch.* vol. 90.

h. Myoma.

153. **Myoma** is a tumour consisting essentially of new-formed muscular fibres. It occurs only in certain parts of the body. If the fibres are non-striated the tumour is described as a leiomyoma, if striated as a rhabdomyoma.

Leiomyoma (or levicellular myoma) is of frequent occurrence in the uterus, less frequent in the muscular coats of the intestine. It takes the form of a spherical nodulated growth, not unlike a fibroma. The smooth muscular fibres form bundles (Fig. 46), which are plaited and interwoven. They are usually surrounded by abundant fibrous tissue, which binds the fibres and the bundles together. If the fibrous tissue form a considerable part of the bulk, the tumour is described as a **fibromyoma**. Most of the uterine 'fibroid' tumours are of this nature. The fibrous bands are white and lustrous, the muscular elements are pink, or reddish grey, or white. It is often by no means easy to distinguish the muscular elements from the purely fibrous. To make an exact

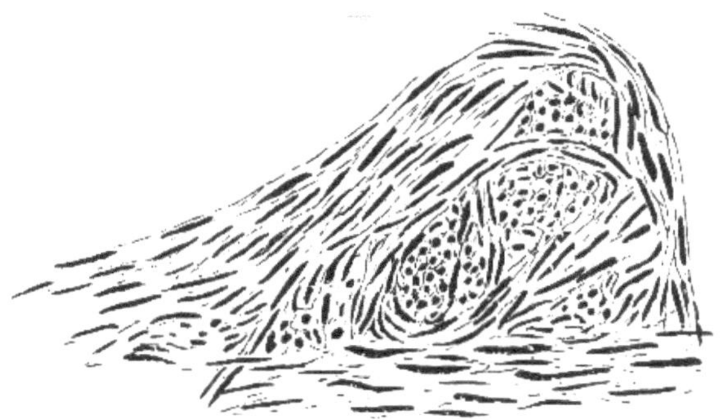

FIG. 46. SECTION THROUGH A LEIOMYOMA (*from PERLS*).
The nuclei are shown partly lengthwise, partly cut across.

determination, it is advisable to isolate the muscle-cells by teasing while the preparation is fresh. The isolation is easier if small fragments of the tumour have been steeped for twenty-four hours in a 20 per cent. solution of nitric acid, or for twenty to thirty minutes in a 34 per cent. solution of caustic potass. The nuclei of the muscle-cells are then easily recognised. Under the microscope the muscle-fibres are distinguished by their rod-like nuclei (Fig. 46) and by the regular structure of the tissue they form. In cross-section the muscle-spindle is seen as a small polygonal area enclosing the rounded section of the nucleus. Leiomyomata are invariably innocent; though they may cause danger by their tendency to bleed. They are liable to fatty change and to softening, which may lead to their disintegration or putrefaction, or to cystic excavations. Calcification is not infrequent.

On the nature of so-called uterine 'fibroids' see BRISTOWE, *Trans. Path. Soc.* 1853; OLDHAM, *Guy's Hosp. Rep.* (2nd series) vols. 2, 8; WILLIAMS, *Lancet* 1, 1880; COURTY, *Dis. of Uterus* London 1882 (contains full references).

Rhabdomyomata are very rare. They are hardly ever made up entirely of striated muscular fibres. In cellular sarcomatous tumours, chiefly of the kidney and testis, spindle-cells with more or less perfect striation are found associated with smooth muscle-fibres (**myosarcomata**). It is probable that such tumours (which are found only in children, and are of great size) are due to foetal deposits of muscular elements in the rudimental kidney and testis.

References to the literature of rhabdomyoma are given by HUBER and BOSTRÖM (*Arch. f. klin. Med.* XXIII). The name is due to ZENKER: VIRCHOW uses the term striocellular myoma. See also EBERTH, *Virch. Arch.* vol. 55; COHNHEIM, *Virch. Arch.* vol. 65; MARCHAND, *Virch. Arch.* vol. 73; KOCHER and LANGHANS, *Deut. Arch. f. Chir.* IX; BRODOWSKI, *Virch. Arch.* vol. 67.

i. Neuroma.

154. **Neuroma** is a term which in strictness should be applied only to tumours composed essentially of new-formed nerve-fibres. What we are accustomed to describe as neuroma is a growth occurring indeed in a nerve, but due to multiplication of the cells of its neurilemma and perineurium, not to the formation of new nerve fibres. It is generally a fusiform, oval, or cylindrical outgrowth, whose axis may coincide with that of the nerve, or deviate laterally. Such tumours are very often multiple, and may affect either single nerve-territories or the entire system. Neuromatous nodes may also occur in the central nervous organs: they may be as large as a hen's egg, or (rarely) larger. If the nodular changes affect an entire nerve-territory, a network of course bands and nodes may be formed. This form has received the name of plexiform neuroma (VERNEUIL). Sometimes painful nodular growths form at the ends of divided nerves, as in amputation-stumps. They are spoken of as amputational neuromata.

Almost all of these varieties are false neuromata: they are really fibromata and myxomata of the connective tissue of the nerve, unassociated with any multiplication of its nerve-fibres. The latter indeed are compressed and atrophied. This is true of the multiple varieties as well as of the amputational neuromata. The latter are in most cases due to inflammatory fibrous hyperplasia.

It is asserted however that, in some neuromatous tumours, a true new-formation of nerve-tissue may occur. Amputational neuromata have furnished examples of this, as well as the tumours

14—2

of various sizes which develope in the continuity of a nerve without any discoverable cause. These then would be instances of true neuroma.

Nerve-fibres are said to multiply by subdivision and by offshoots. According as the new-formed fibres are medullated or not, we have the varieties myeline neuroma and amyeline neuroma. Neuromata are entirely innocent: they never give rise to metastases. It has been shown that the multiple false neuromata are apt to be inherited, or at least to depend on some congenital fault. (See Special Pathological Anatomy of the Nerves.)

References :—VIRCHOW, *op. cit.* and *Gesammelte Abhand.*; SMITH, *On Neuroma*; PERLS, *Handb. d. allg. Path.*; VERNEUIL, *Arch. gén. de méd.* vol. 18 (5th series); CZERNY, *Arch. f. klin. Chir.* XVII; SOYKA, *Prager Vierteljahrs.* 35, 1877; PERLS, *Arch. f. Ophthalm.* XIX; P. BRUNS, *Virch. Arch.* vol. 50; VON RECKLINGHAUSEN, *Ueber d. multiplen Fibrome d. Haut* Berlin 1882.

j. Lymphoma and Lymphosarcoma.

155. **Lymphoma** is a comprehensive term, and includes formations which are not strictly tumours, but rather hyperplasias of the tissue proper to lymphatic glands—lymphadenoid (or briefly adenoid) tissue, as it is called. Lymphoma, as a neoplasm, would imply the development and deposit of new lymphadenoid tissue in the form of a tumour within a lymphatic gland, a follicle, or some other structure of the connective-tissue group. In what is usually called lymphoma, this does not happen. What does happen is—that the tissue of the lymphatic gland or follicle increases in size because the lymphoid cells it contains are multiplied, while the reticular tissue undergoes hyperplasia. The process is often inflammatory in character, and should then be classed with the inflammations: in other cases the lymphoid hyperplasia seems to begin idiopathically, *i.e.* without any cause hitherto discovered. It may often be doubtful whether the increased growth of a lymphatic gland should be regarded as neoplastic or as hyperplastic. Many cases of lymphoma, especially the leukaemic kinds, seem referable to hyperplasia. The lymphatic glands, lymphadenoid structures of the intestine, and lymphoid follicles of the spleen, all maintain their structure as they grow in size, or alter but slightly. Moreover the functions of the glands seem to be more actively performed. This does not seem to indicate that they are invaded by anything of the nature of a neoplasm.

In addition to the hyperplastic lymphomata, there is a true or heteroplastic tumour whose structure agrees with that of lymphadenoid tissue. As the term lymphoma has been perverted to describe the hyperplastic formations, we may do well to distinguish the genuine tumour as **lymphadenoma** or lymphosarcoma. This latter title corresponds with the fact—that the tumour agrees in its characters with the sarcomata. It will therefore be treated in connexion with them (Art. 158).

The relations of lymphoma and lymphadenoma to Hodgkin's disease and to leukaemia are discussed in the Special Pathological Anatomy.

Recent researches have shown that lymphadenoid tissue is in normal conditions widely distributed throughout the body. The overgrowth of some such normal deposit may simulate a heteroplastic formation.

k. Sarcoma.

156. The **sarcomata** are tumours constructed on the type of the connective tissues, in which however the cellular constituents predominate over the intercellular substance. In this respect they resemble the immature connective tissues; so that the comparison of sarcoma to embryonic formative tissue is perfectly apt.

Sarcoma originates invariably in a structure belonging to the connective-tissue group; *i.e.* in formed or unformed fibrous tissue, in cartilaginous, bony, mucous, lymphoid, neurogliar, or adipose tissue. The transformation of these into tumour-tissue is effected by the growth and multiplication of the constituent cells.

In favourable circumstances it is possible to follow up this mode of genesis histologically. At the advancing margin of a growing tumour we may find all kinds of transitional cell-forms, from the small cells of the normal connective tissue to the large cells of the tumour. Fig. 47 represents the advancing margin of a

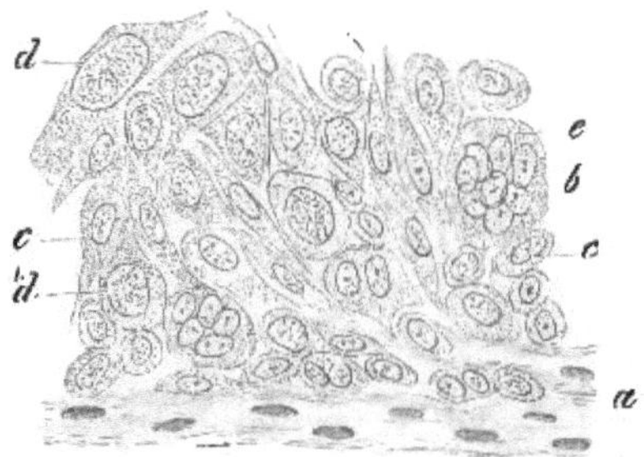

FIG. 47. SECTION THROUGH THE ADVANCING MARGIN OF A SMALL SARCOMATOUS NODULE FROM THE MAMMA. (× 300)

a fibrous tissue
b cells of the sarcomatous tissue
c smaller cells
d cells with hypertrophied nuclei
e multinuclear cells

small sarcomatous nodule from the mamma, and in it the various stages of development can be made out. Enlarged and swollen cells (*c*) lie beside the small cells of the fibrous tissue (*a*): others with enormous nuclei (*d*), or with several (*e*), are also noticeable. At the same time the number of the cells is vastly increased.

In bone and cartilage it is possible to demonstrate the subdivision and multiplication of the fixed cells even more clearly than in connective tissue. The multiplication sometimes occurs in the substance of non-vascular cartilage or bone away from the medullary spaces, and thus the part played by the individual cells within their cavities is very readily followed (ZIEGLER, *Virch. Arch.* vol. 73). In connective tissue it is less easy to exclude the possibility of cell-infiltration from neighbouring parts. VIRCHOW has thus shown that sarcoma-cells may arise by proliferous multiplication from connective-tissue cells of perfectly normal aspect. This is the process in a large number of cases; but it may vary to this extent—that the development begins in tissue which is already morbidly altered. Thus new-formed cartilage may pass into sarcoma by over-intense proliferous growth of the cartilage-cells, and disappearance of the matrix-substance.

It is of great interest to note that cells, which form part of what we might call congenital heteroplastic foci, may often serve as the starting point of a sarcoma. Congenital warts and pigment-spots are specially remarkable for this. The transformation into sarcomatous tissue is effected by the growth and multiplication of the nests of cells that are always found in such spots.

Summing up what we know of the development of sarcoma we may say—that sarcomatous tissue may arise either from connective tissues which up to then seem normal, or from tissues that are to be regarded as already morbid.

References on the genesis of Sarcoma:—VIRCHOW, *Die kr. Geschwülste* II; R. MAIER, *Allg. path. Anat.*; PERLS, *Allg. path. Anat.*; BIZZOZERO, *Med. Jahrb.* IV, 1878; BILLROTH, *Arch. f. klin. Chir.* XI; STEUDENER, *Virch. Arch.* vol. 59; SOKOLOW, *Virch. Arch.* vol. 57; CORNIL and RANVIER, *Man. Path. Hist.* vol. I.

157. The form and mode of growth of the cells varies much in different varieties of sarcoma. The intercellular substance is sometimes scanty, soft, and stringy: in other cases its texture approaches that of the mature normal tissue. The various varieties are distinguished according to the constitution of the ground-substance as well as of the cells, but chiefly of the cells. That constituent is taken as characteristic, which prevails in the tumour in question. Seeing that a sarcoma is continually in process of growth, it always contains some parts which are as yet immature, and merely represent an earlier stage of development of the tumour. In settling the classification of the tumour such parts are not taken into account.

The texture of the sarcoma, as made out by the unaided eye, varies much in the different forms. In its mature condition it is generally more or less sharply marked off from its surroundings. It may occur in any locality where connective tissues are found, but the frequency of its occurrence is different in different tissues. Thus it is much commoner in the skin, fasciae, intermuscular fibrous tissue, bone, periosteum, lymphatic glands, brain, and ovary—than in the liver, lungs, intestine, or uterus.

The amount of intercellular substance present chiefly determines the consistence and the tint. Forms which are soft, marrowy, and white or greyish-white on section, are rich in cells and poor in intercellular substance. Firm and coarse-grained forms are poorer in cells and abound more in fibrous intercellular tissue. The latter kinds pass without any break into the fibromata. Intermediate forms are described as **fibrosarcomata**. The cut surface of a sarcomatous tumour has a uniform look throughout; unless indeed it has undergone retrogressive changes, or the amount of blood in it varies from part to part. It looks evenly smooth, in medullary tumours milk-white, in firmer kinds clear greyish-white and translucent, or greyish-red or brown. The hard forms are white or yellowish-white, and lustrous on section.

The blood-vessels are variously developed: now and then they are exceptionally wide and numerous, or even irregularly dilated, as in telangiectatic sarcoma. Lymphatics have not been shown to exist in sarcomata.

Retrogressive changes are apt to happen, such as fatty change, mucoid change, liquefaction, caseation, disintegration, haemorrhage, putrefaction, ulceration, &c.

158. **Round-celled sarcoma.** The small-round-celled sarcomata are very soft rapidly-growing tumours. They chiefly occur in the connective tissues of the locomotive and skeletal system; as also in the skin, testis, ovary, and lymphatic glands. They are usually milky white on section, and not infrequently contain softened or cheesy patches. A milky juice can be got by scraping the cut surface. Their structure is very simple: it consists almost entirely of round-cells and vessels (Fig. 48). The former are

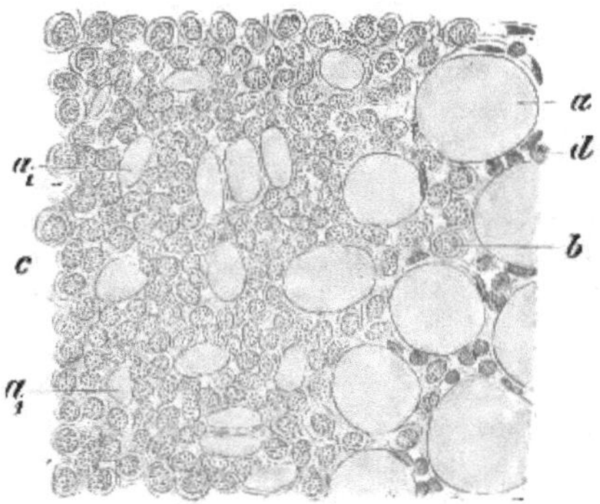

FIG. 48. SECTION THROUGH THE MARGIN OF A SARCOMA AFFECTING THE INTER-MUSCULAR CONNECTIVE TISSUE. (*Carmine staining*: ×300)

a normal muscle-fibre
a_1 atrophied muscle-fibres
b round-cells intruded between the muscle-fibres
c fully developed tumour-tissue
d round-cells resembling white blood-corpuscles

small and fragile, have but little protoplasm, and enclose a rounded or slightly oval vesicular nucleus (Fig. 48 *c*). This nucleus seems more highly developed than it is in ordinary lymphoid cells.

The intercellular substance is scanty, and fibro-granular in texture. The vessels appear as thin-walled channels between the groups of cells. In the case of an invaded muscle, such as that in the figure (Fig. 48), the tumour seems to consist of an aggregation of round-cells (Fig. 48 *b c*) seated in the intermuscular connective tissue. Lymphoid elements are not infrequently found mingled with the tumour-cells: their nuclei (Fig. 48 *d*) are easily distinguished by the fact that they take a deeper staining than the other elements.

A second variety of small-round-celled sarcoma is the so-called **lymphosarcoma**. It is a sarcoma whose structure somewhat resembles that of a lymphatic gland. There is a kind of reticular stroma (Fig. 49 *a*), made up in part of anastomosing ramifying cells (Fig. 49 *b*); and this contains a multitude of round-cells in its meshes. If a small piece of the tumour be first shaken up in a test-tube with some liquid, so that the cells drop away, the structure can then be easily made out under the microscope.

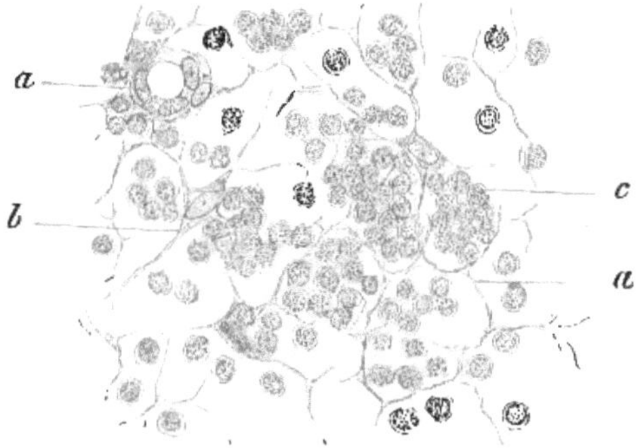

FIG. 49. SECTION OF LYMPHOSARCOMA FROM THE NASAL MUCOUS MEMBRANE.

a reticulum (the *a* to the left points to a blood-vessel with subdividing cells)
b cells of the reticulum
c round-cells

The tumour has the same general appearance as the commoner small-round-celled variety. Both forms are highly malignant, partly because of their rapid growth, partly from their tendency to give rise to secondary growths, which may affect the entire body.

Lymphosarcoma most commonly originates in lymphatic glands, and in the lymphadenoid tissue of the mucous membranes. It may however arise elsewhere. When it attacks a lymphatic gland, it may be distinguished from mere hyperplastic lymphoma by its rapid growth, and by its tendency to overpass the limits of the gland, and to form metastases.

159. Large-round-celled sarcomata are made up of cells considerably larger than those of the varieties just described. They occur in the same localities. They are not quite so soft in texture. Their cells are often uniformly large, and have an abundant protoplasm and large oval vesicular nuclei (Fig. 50). Many of the cells are binuclear, a few are multinuclear. The intercellular substance is arranged in a kind of network, interspersed with fusiform and ramified cells. Together they form an alveolar reticulum in whose spaces lie the large epithelium-like round-cells. On account of these characters BILLROTH has described the tumour as a 'large-celled alveolar round-celled sarcoma.' The vessels have usually very thin walls.

In the other varieties of large-round-celled sarcoma, the cells are very unequal in size. Fig. 51 represents a section of a mammary sarcoma in which the cells are for the most part round; but their sizes vary greatly, and there is a partial admixture of elongated cells, as well as of multinuclear giant-cells (*e*). If this last be taken as characteristic, the tumour may be called a giant-celled or **myeloid sarcoma** (Art. 160).

The large-round-celled sarcomata are generally less malignant than the small-celled kinds; but they likewise may form metastases. The patient from whom the tumour represented in Fig. 50 was taken died from metastatic growths.

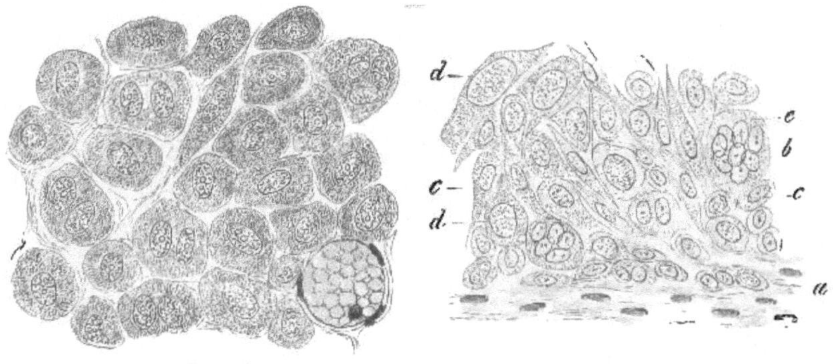

FIG. 50. FIG. 51.

FIG. 50. SECTION FROM A FUNGATING LARGE-ROUND-CELLED SARCOMA.
(*From the skin of the leg: carmine staining:* ×400)

FIG. 51. SECTION OF A SARCOMA OF THE MAMMA CONTAINING VARIOUSLY FORMED CELLS. (*Bismarck-brown staining:* ×300)

a fibrous tissue
b cells of the sarcomatous tissue
c smaller cells
d cells with hypertrophied nuclei
e multinuclear cells

160. **Spindle-celled sarcoma** (including forms with ramified multiform cells, and fibrosarcoma). Sarcomata consisting of spindle-shaped or ramified cells are among the most common of all

tumours. They are usually much firmer in texture than the round-celled forms. On section they look greyish or yellowish-white, and translucent; if the vessels are full of blood they may accidentally be tinged with red. They are generally speaking much less malignant than the round-celled sarcomata, but this depends somewhat on where they are seated.

Sarcomata in which spindle-cells predominate are called briefly spindle-celled sarcomata: they are divided into large-celled and small-celled varieties. The cells may be more or less isolated by teasing out fragments of the tumour-tissue, and in this way very long spindle-cells may occasionally be found (Fig. 52). They lie side by side in the tumour, and group themselves into bundles. In a section these bundles may be seen cut through lengthwise, crosswise, or slantwise; which shows that they run in diverse directions through the growth.

The grouping of the spindles into definite bundles is often very striking; but sometimes there is no such grouping, the spindles all lying parallel to the same direction throughout a considerable area. Sometimes also the arrangement of the spindles seems to depend on the direction of the vessels, the bundles forming a kind of sheathing to each vessel.

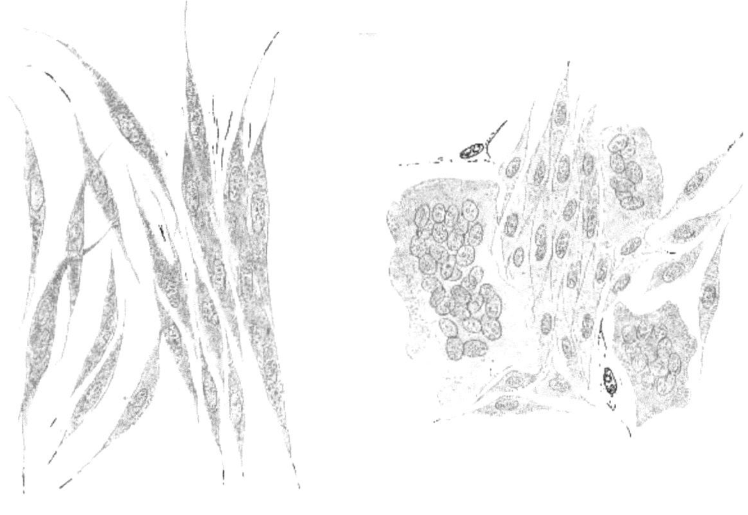

FIG. 52. FIG. 53.

FIG. 52. SPINDLE-CELLS FROM A LARGE-SPINDLE-CELLED SARCOMA OF THE CHEEK. (*Teased preparation*: ×400)

FIG. 53. SECTION FROM A GIANT-CELLED SARCOMA ORIGINATING IN THE MEDULLA OF THE TIBIA ('MYELOGENIC' SARCOMA). (*Haematoxylin staining*: ×400)

The intercellular substance may be very scanty, or altogether imperceptible in a section. In other cases it is abundant, and shows a kind of fibrillated structure. The cells are then poorer in protoplasm; so much so in fact that there is often none to be seen around the nucleus, and the cell-processes seem to start from the nucleus itself ('nuclear fibres'). Such tumours are firm and coarse-grained, and approach the fibromata in texture. They are called **fibrosarcomata.**

Sarcomata whose cells are of several diverse forms are equally common. Their cells are spindle-shaped, pyramidal, prismatic, stellate, or altogether irregular (Fig. 53). Each cell seems in fact to take the form of the space which is left to it to fill. Sarcomata of this kind, as also the spindle-celled kind, usually contain a larger or smaller number of giant-cells (Fig. 53). These tumours are perhaps more properly described as giant-celled or myeloid sarcomata than those referred to in Art. 159. They chiefly affect the osseous system.

The vessels of a sarcoma have generally walls which are quite distinguishable. In some cases however they have the appearance of canals excavated in the substance of the tumour, the tumour-cells themselves bounding the lumen of the vessel. Here it would seem as if the tumour had in part arisen from multiplication of the cells in the original vessel-wall.

161. **Sarcomata of peculiar types.** Sarcomata do not usually exhibit any special structure, or any resemblance to a

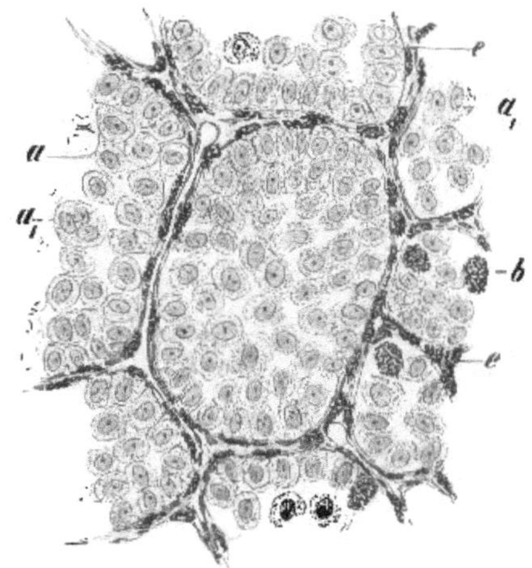

FIG. 54. SECTION FROM A MELANOTIC ALVEOLAR SARCOMA OF THE SKIN.

(*Haematoxylin staining*: ×300)

a uninuclear, a_1 multinuclear epithelial-like tumour-cells
b pigment-cells
e stroma enclosing blood-vessels and pigment

glandular type. The cellular elements, even when they seem to resemble epithelial cells, are dispersed uniformly throughout the intercellular substance, as in the connective tissues. There are however exceptions to this in special cases. There are sarcomata which have a structure resembling that of gland-tissue, or of epithelial new growths. This appearance of structure is due in part to the epithelial look of the cells, but chiefly to their aggregated arrangement in groups separated by fibrous septa. Such tumours are described as **alveolar sarcomata**. Fig. 54 represents a section from an alveolar sarcoma of the skin.

The cells *a* exactly resemble epithelial cells: they are grouped into masses, and sharply distinguished from the fibrous framework (*e*) in which they are embedded. This latter contains the blood-vessels, or rather the framework is chiefly made up of a network of blood-vessels; but no vessels enter the cell-groups. This is another point of structure in common with the epithelial growths.

Tumours of this kind occur chiefly in the skin, but they are also met with in the bones, lymphatic glands, and pia mater. In the case of the skin they originate in warts and pigment-spots, which generally contain such groups or nests of cells (Arts. 156 and 398).

The way in which the alveolar structure is developed can often be clearly made out, especially in tumours of the central nervous system. The normal intervascular tissue is transformed into masses of sarcoma-cells, while septa are formed between the cell-masses by the fibrous tissues lying along the course of the vessels. In other cases it looks as if a plexus of pre-existing or new-formed vessels took on as it were an investment of cells, and this grew thicker and thicker till at length the intervascular spaces were entirely filled up. Accordingly we find this form of growth described as plexiform angiosarcoma. It has also been described, and not infrequently, as **endothelioma**. On this view the cell-nests arise by proliferation from endothelial cells. This certainly happens when masses of cells are formed from the endothelial covering of the subarachnoid meshwork and pia mater: the masses afterwards group themselves into 'nests'. Sometimes the proliferous endothelial cells of the pia mater are aggregated into small spherical nodules of a peculiar lustrous appearance. The tumour into which the membrane is transformed then contains small shining pearly bodies, made up of laminated layers of squamous or tabular cells. Such tumours have been called **cholesteatomata** or pearly tumours.

The expression 'plexiform angiosarcoma' is due to WALDEYER (*Virch. Arch.* vol. 55). The vessels of the brain, lymphatic glands, serous membranes, and testis possess what is called a perithelium: that is, the adventitia is invested with endothelial cells. Proliferation begins in the cells of this perithelium, and the vessel is thus invested with a stratified covering. See KOLACZEK, *Deutsche Zeitsch. f. Chir.* IX; MAURER, *Virch. Arch.* vol. 77; NEUMANN, *Arch. d. Heilk.* 1872; KLEBS, *Prager Vierteljahrsschr.* 1876.

It is still a matter of dispute whether the cholesteatomata are really endotheliomata of the pia mater (EPPINGER, *Prager Vierteljahrsschr.* 1875). They may possibly belong rather to the dermoid tumours (Art. 178). Similar growths are met with in the middle ear (WENDT, *Arch. d. Heilk.* 14, 1873; LUCAE, *Arch. f. Ohrenheilk.* (New Series) 1, 1874). Some regard them as tumours, others (with WENDT) as inflammatory products.

162. Sarcomata which contain deposits of pigment are described as **melanosarcomata** (Fig. 54). The pigment is black or brown, and lies partly in the tumour-cells, partly in the fibrous matrix and vessel-walls. It occurs chiefly in the form of amorphous granules; but there are generally a number of diffusely stained cells as well. Melanosarcomata are malignant.

When the pigmentation is not extreme the tumour has on section a brownish grey look, or it may only show patches of brown or black. In more marked cases the section is uniformly black. Very often the secondary growths are more intensely pigmented than the primary tumour, and this is also the case in growths that have recurred after resection. Tumours of this kind develope in tissues like the eye and pia mater, which normally contain pigment-cells, or in pigmented pathological formations. The black pigment-spots (melanomata) of the skin are of this latter class: it has already been mentioned that they contain peculiar clusters or nests of cells (Fig. 54).

We do not know in what way the pigment is formed (Art. 67). It is not to be confounded with the brown pigment derived from extravasated blood. Patches stained with this blood-pigment are sometimes found here and there in a sarcomatous growth, but the true melanotic pigment is something quite distinct.

Psammomata, like melanosarcomata, are growths which arise in certain definite tissues, and but rarely anywhere else. They are sarcomatous, fibrous, or myxomatous tumours originating in the brain and its membranes, more particularly in the choroid plexus and pineal gland, and containing a multitude of chalky concretions. These have the same structure as the grains of the normal brain-sand (*acervulus cerebri*). They are made up of concentric calcareous strata, and form spherical or dendritic aggregations. They may be so abundant as to give the tumour a stony feel.

We may here just mention the variety of sarcoma called **chloroma.** It is a cellular tumour, whose section has a light green or dirty brownish green tint. The colour soon fades on exposure to the air. Nothing is known of the nature of the colouring-matter. Chloromata occur chiefly in the periosteum of the skull. See HUBER, *Arch. d. Heilk.* 1878.

163. Some very peculiar forms of tumour are produced when sarcomatous tissue undergoes partial hyaline or mucoid degeneration; or when sarcomatous and myxomatous formations combine. They are generally included under the term **cylindroma**, though this may also be applied to tumours of another species in which epithelial cells are involved (Art. 173, Fig. 72).

The ordinary soft cellular sarcomata have now and then a more translucent appearance than usual, and yield on section a turbid slimy juice. These have already begun to undergo mucoid change, as may be recognised by the swollen appearance of the cells, and the formation of drops of liquid within them. When the tissue has been hardened the change is not so easily made out. The cells then seem shrunken (Fig. 55 *b*), and separated from the stroma (*a*) by a clear zone. Sometimes a few distended and transparent nuclei are observed, their protoplasm having become mucoid and so vanished.

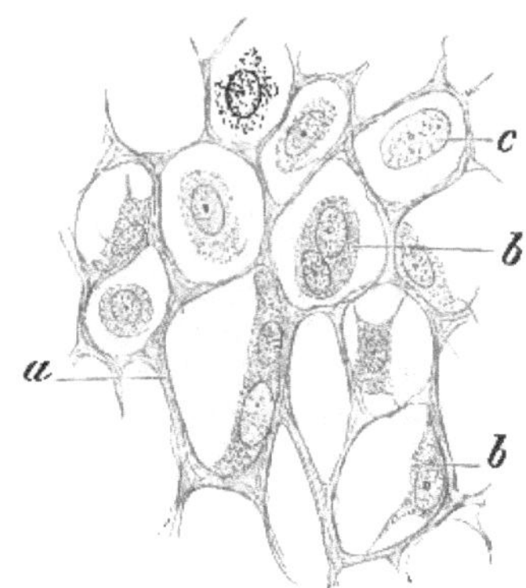

FIG. 55. SARCOMA MYXOMATODES. (*Haematoxylin staining*: × 400)

a stroma
b sarcoma-cells separated from the stroma by a clear zone (in part due to hardening in chromic acid and alcohol)
c swollen nucleus which has lost its protoplasm

This mucoid change may at times extend throughout the entire substance of the tumour; or it may be confined to scattered patches, separated by unchanged cells. Isolated hyaline spherules are occasionally noticed among the cells. Such partially degenerate sarcomata we may describe as **myxomatodes.**

The tumours in which sarcomatous and mucous tissue are found combined have on section either a hyaline or an opaque dirty white appearance. The mucous tissue is partly composed of a network of ramified and anastomosing cells (Fig. 56 *a*), in addition

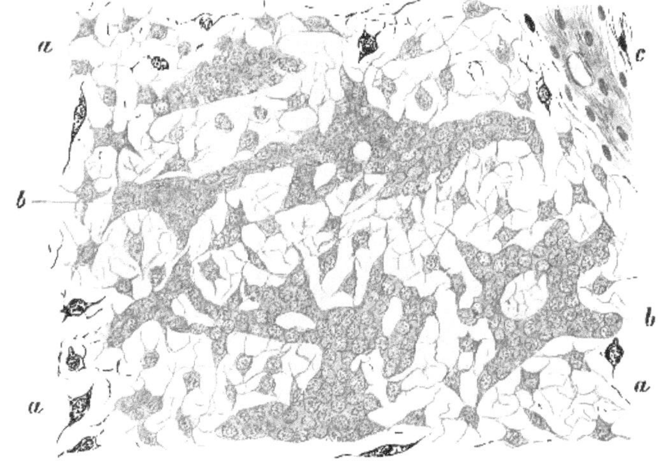

FIG. 56. SECTION OF MYXOSARCOMA (CYLINDROMA). (*Carmine staining*: × 250)
a mucous tissue *b* strings and clumps of cells *c* fibrous tissue

to a mucoid basis-substance. Within this tissue lie also branching clumps and strings (*b*) made up of closely compacted cells. These strings are very irregular in form and anastomose in all directions; they give the tumour a very peculiar texture. Its general structure justifies the name of **myxosarcoma**, which has been applied to it. It forms, as has been said, a subdivision of the class of cylindromata. It is not clear, from a histological point of view, in what way the clumps and strings of cells are formed. They seem to have no relation to the ramifications of the vessels, for these are seen to be unchanged, and run through parts where the fibrous tissue has undergone no degeneration.

A third variety of cylindromatous tumour, also somewhat translucent and in part gelatinous, is characterised by the hyaline degeneration which affects the walls of its vessels and the tissue around them. If one of these vessels be isolated, it is seen to be invested with a more or less abundant deposit of hyaline substance (Fig. 57 *a*). To this sheath are attached similar hyaline appendages not traversed by vessels. Outside the hyaline sheaths, alternating with them in fact, are nests and strings of cells which here and there seem fastened or anchored to the hyaline masses (Fig. 57 *b*). The strings of cells have much the same look as

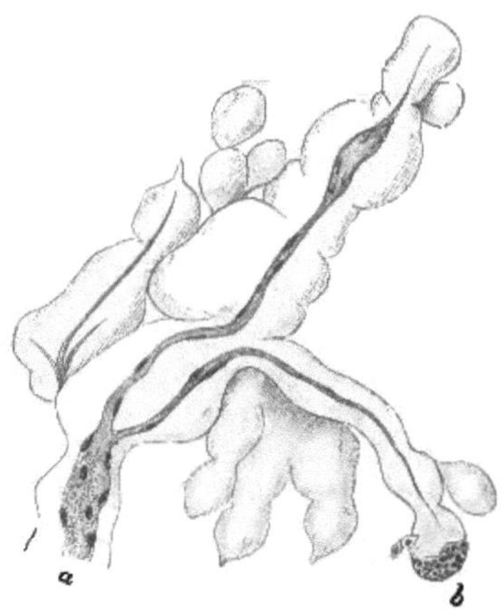

FIG. 57. BLOOD-VESSELS WITH HYALINE SHEATH AND APPENDAGES FROM A CYLINDROMA.

(*From* SATTLER'S '*Cylindrome*' 1874: × 200)

a small vessel
b patch of epithelial-like cells on one of the hyaline appendages

those shown in Fig. 56, and we infer that the tumour in question is allied to the myxosarcomata just described. The homogeneous appendages are the result of hyaline degeneration of the vessel-walls, or of the neighbouring tumour-cells; and this hyaline degeneration is either identical or connected with mucoid degeneration. The fact that actual mucous tissue (like that in Fig. 56) is occasionally found mingled with the hyaline masses tells in favour of this view.

This form of cylindroma may therefore be regarded as a peculiar variety of myxosarcoma, in which the mucoid change is chiefly confined to the vessels, and in which the formation of new vessels is an essential feature. To emphasise the important part played by the vessels in this neoplasm, we might call it **angiosarcoma myxomatodes**.

Such growths have been found principally in the lacrimal glands, salivary glands, and in the brain. They occur however elsewhere, as in the lip, placenta, adipose tissue, &c.

Cylindroma is a term due to BILLROTH (*Untersuch. über die Entwick. d. Blutgefässe* 1856). Such tumours, characterised by gelatinous masses and reticula, have since then been very variously interpreted. KÖSTER described them as cancroids (*Virch. Arch.* vol. 40); SATTLER (*Ueb. d. sogen. Cylindrome* Berlin 1874) as alveolar sarcomata, in which the cell-masses derived by proliferation from the adventitia had been transformed into hyaline cylinders; EWETZKY (*Virch. Arch.* vol. 69) as plexiform angiosarcomata with hyaline degeneration of the fibrous stroma, or of the adventitia of the vessels. R. MAIER (*Virch. Arch.* vol. 14, and *Lehrb. d. allg. path. Anat.*) found cylindromata in the placenta and dura mater: he regarded the presence of an abundance of hyaline mucous tissue persisting for a long period unchanged as characteristic of the tumour. This tissue may develope out of cells or out of intercellular substance, fibrous tissue, cartilage, or tunica adventitia.

Various tumours have been described as cylindromata which certainly do not all belong to the same species. A number of them belong to the sarcomata. Within this group we may, as we have said, distinguish two main forms; first, the combined sarcoma and myxoma, and secondly, the sarcoma with hyaline or mucoid degeneration extending to the cells, but chiefly affecting the sheaths of the vessels. Between these two, however, many transitional forms are found.

l. Mixed tumours of the connective-tissue group.

164. We have already referred to various tumours in which combinations of different tissues present themselves. In one sense no tumour can be said to consist of a single kind of tissue only. In a new growth of any size we must always have new vessels, for instance. And tumours whose characteristic element is not fibrous tissue—such as chondromata, osteomata, sarcomata, myomata, and myxomata—always contain a very considerable quantity of fibrous tissue as an accessory.

We do not speak of such cases as examples of mixed tumours, because the accessory tissue is as it were put out of sight by the characteristic element: it is entirely subordinate. But if the second tissue comes into the foreground and affects the texture of the growth in a perceptible way, we must indicate this in our terminology. This is done by applying to the name of one neoplastic tissue the name of the other as a qualifying term; or by simply combining the two names into a compound word. Thus, as in gliomata and fibromata, the blood-vessels may be remarkable by their abundance, size, and dilatations; we then speak of the growth as a glioma (or fibroma) telangiectodes or cavernosum. A morbid combination of adipose tissue with mucous tissue is called lipoma myxomatodes or lipomyxoma; a combination of cartilage and sarcoma—chondrosarcoma; and so on. It is not rare for three or more kinds of neoplastic tissue to be found within the same tumour. A growth which starts in fascia or intermuscular fibrous tissue may consist, for example, of fibrous, sarcomatous, mucous, and adipose tissue; there may even be vascular changes here and there which give it a telangiectatic character. Such a combination is not very surprising. The neoplastic proliferation may itself result in the development of several diverse tissues—or, what is more common, the tissues of the connective group become transformed the one into the other. We showed, for example, in Arts. 90—92, that cartilage readily passes into mucous tissue, which is also frequently produced from fibrous or adipose tissues. Sarcomatous tissue may easily be the result of proliferation of the cartilage of a chondroma, or the fibrous tissue of a fibroma; and conversely, sarcomatous tissue may equally well be transformed partially into osseous tissue. Tumours originating in bone are very apt to show a tendency to bone-formation. There are two forms especially in which this often occurs—namely, osteoid chondroma, a combination of cartilage and bony tissue; and osteosarcoma, a combination of sarcoma and bony tissue.

165. **Osteoid chondroma** (or osteochondroma) chiefly affects the larger long bones. If no sarcomatous proliferation has modified it, it usually forms a hard tumour seated on the bone or embracing it. It often reaches an enormous size; and cannot be cut with the knife, unless a patch of unaltered cartilage be hit upon. When sawn through, the cut surface has the look of dense white continuous bone: on closer examination this is seen to be interspersed with streaks and islands of more translucent cartilage. Fig. 58 shows well the general texture of the growth and its matrix, and its relation to the bone. The section represented is taken from a tumour of the humerus. The tumour was very firm and bony, and surrounded the bone so as to double its diameter. It was found on dividing the bone longitudinally that the medullary spaces were filled with firm tumour-tissue of the same structure as the periosteal growth. The original bone was only recognisable in the region of its cortical layer. Fig. 58 represents a section taken at right angles to the axis of the bone, and including the periosteal growth, the cortical layer, and a part of the altered cancellous tissue.

We find instead of periosteum a mass of cartilaginous tissue (*g*) interspersed thickly with bony trabeculae (*h*). These run generally at right angles to the surface of the original bone, but anastomose freely. Small lacunae and canals are seen throughout the cartilage; they contain a few blood-vessels and a small amount of fibrous tissue. The cortical layer (*a*) is still distinguished by the concentric stratification of the lamellae. Many of its Haversian

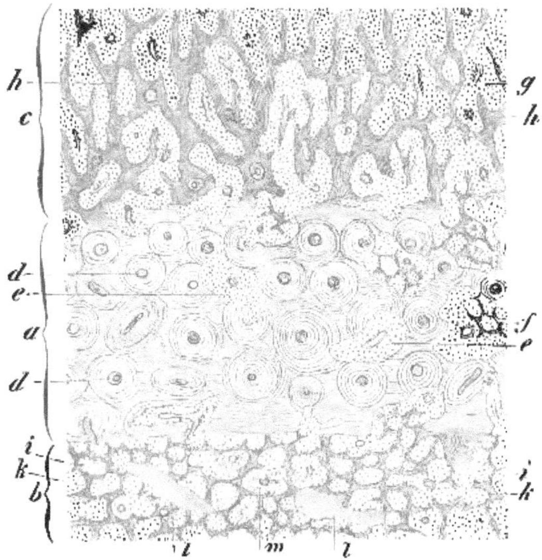

FIG. 58. SECTION FROM AN OSTEOID CHONDROMA OF THE HUMERUS.

(*Magnified by means of a simple lens: double-staining with haematoxylin and carmine*)

a cortical layer
b medullary spaces or cancelli
c periosteal growth
d normal Haversian canals
e Haversian canals distended with cartilage, which at *f* contains a core of new bone
g cartilage developed from periosteum, which at *h* contains bony trabeculae
i cartilage developed from medullary tissue, which at *k* contains bony trabeculae
l original trabeculae
m remnants of medullary tissue

canals are dilated and filled up (except for a small lumen in which the blood-vessel runs) with masses of cartilage. These masses sometimes contain trabecular cores of new-formed bone (*f*). Instead of the marrow, which should fill the interior of the bone (*b*), we find vascularised cartilage also containing numbers of trabeculae. The genesis and primary seat of the growth may thus be made out at once from this preparation. Cartilaginous proliferation has been set up in the periosteum and in the medullary tissue, and the product has subsequently been partially transformed into bone.

Osteosarcoma has an exactly analogous appearance. The difference is merely that sarcomatous tissue fills the spaces between the trabeculae instead of cartilage. The trabeculae are at the same time more delicate and less numerous. The seat of the tumour (as is the case too with osteoid chondroma) is often confined to the periosteum. The bone is then more or less eroded.

References :—MÜLLER, *Müller's Arch.* 1843; VIRCHOW, *Die kr. Geschwülste* I; RINDFLEISCH, *Path. Hist.* II; WILKS and MOXON, *Path. anat.* London 1875; PAGET, *Surg. Path.* Lect. 33. A summary of cases and some beautiful drawings of sarcomatous tumours connected with bone will be found in BUTLIN'S *Sarcoma and Carcinoma* London 1882.

CHAPTER XXVII.

EPITHELIAL TUMOURS.

166. The tumours we have hitherto treated of have been developed out of tissues belonging to the connective-tissue group; in other words, out of tissues derived from the mesoblast. The tumours we have now to deal with contain in addition **epithelial elements**, that is to say, structures derived from the epiblast and hypoblast. These epithelial elements are in fact the structures which give its special character to the class. The tumours of the class are therefore very fitly comprehended under the one title of epithelial neoplasms. All of them consist of epithelial cells on the one hand, and of vascular connective tissue on the other. The latter tissue goes to form the framework or stroma in which the epithelial elements are embedded. The type or plan of their construction is that of the simple gland, and they maintain the resemblance throughout many of the phases of their development. They thus call to mind in many ways the various glands of the body; though the degree of resemblance differs much in the different forms.

Some of them are built exactly on the plan of some particular gland: the new-formed tissue corresponds to a definite glandular type. Tumours of this kind we call **adenomata.**

Another group never reach this perfection of structure. They exhibit as it were only the first stage of the gland-making process. Epithelium and fibrous tissue interpenetrate each other in an inchoate way. The process is never carried higher, but the crude formation is repeated and reproduced indefinitely. By multiplication of the epithelial cells we have produced nests and clusters and strings of cells, and these are embedded in connective tissue whose elements are likewise multiplying. The result is a neoplasm consisting of a fibrous network or framework, in the meshes of which are lodged a multitude of variously-shaped epithelial cells. But there is no orderly arrangement of these epithelial cells. In the adenomata they tend to clothe the walls of the alveoli in a regular way, leaving open a central lumen as in the acinus of a gland. In the tumours now considered the cells remain in compact irregular masses. Epithelial tumours of this kind, in which the glandular type is most imperfectly followed, are described as **carcinomata** or true cancers.

Adenoma and carcinoma are generally malignant. They tend to invade the surrounding tissues; and, by the channels of the lymph or of the blood, are apt to affect distant regions and produce metastases. But the degree of malignancy varies greatly; it depends not only on the histological structure of the growth, but to an even greater extent on its locality.

The definition we have given of adenoma and carcinoma is based partly on their histology, partly on their mode of genesis. From the morbid anatomist's point of view this is the only correct mode of definition. Tumours containing none but mesoblastic cells may and do correspond in their general structure with others, in which undoubted epithelial cells form the characteristic element; and for this reason a merely anatomical method of diagnosis would be insufficient. If carcinoma be defined as an alveolar tumour composed of a fibrous network containing nested cells, it is impossible to separate between carcinoma and alveolar sarcoma. It is owing to this purely anatomical mode of definition that we have had controversies as to whether carcinoma really depends upon epithelial proliferation, and whether cancers may not have their origin in fibrous structures. Such controversies become irrelevant if we base the distinction on histogenetic grounds. A tumour is to be called carcinomatous only when the epithelial elements take an active part (as above described) in its formation. A connective-tissue tumour which has ostensibly the same structure, but whose mode of genesis is entirely different, is to be distinguished as an alveolar sarcoma.

a. Adenoma.

167. **Adenoma** is a tumour constructed after the type of a secreting gland. The definition might at first sight tempt us to term every glandular enlargement, in which the elements are abnormally multiplied, an adenoma. This would however be incorrect. Adenoma is a true neoplasm, characterised physiologically by its impotence to produce the normal gland-secretion, and anatomically by its want of relation to the tissue in which it is seated. A gland enlarged by over-growth, or over-work, or chronic inflammation, cannot be described as an adenoma. It is a hyperplasia: and if it be the true gland-tissue and not merely the fibrous framework which is excessively developed, the physiological activity of the gland is thereupon increased.

We must regard in the same way the tumour-like growths which occasionally develope in mucous membranes, chiefly as a result of chronic inflammation. They are mere localised proliferations, rising above the general surface as nodular, polypous, or papillary outgrowths. The fibrous tissue is the first to increase, and this leads to some increase of the epithelium, chiefly because the local submucous swelling involves an increase of the mucous surface. If any glands are present (as in the intestine or uterus), they also undergo change. If their ducts become blocked, they may become distended with secretion, and form larger or smaller cysts. Other glands may enlarge by increase of their stroma; and lastly there may be in some an active growth and increase of the specific gland-tissue.

It is easy to demonstrate that such new-formations of fibrous and glandular tissue do take place. The most suitable objects for examination are perhaps the papillary or villous growths which form on the inner surface of glands undergoing cystic degeneration (Fig. 59 *c*). These are sometimes so abundant that the cyst seems quite filled up with the new tissue.

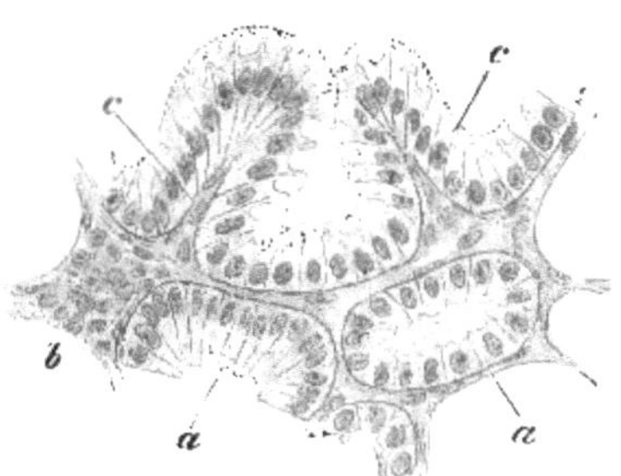

FIG. 59. PAPILLARY GROWTHS INSIDE A CYST.

(*From a gastric polypus: haematoxylin staining:* × 300)

a gland-tubules with cylindrical epithelium
b stroma infiltrated with cells
c papillary growths into a cyst, covered with mucoid epithelium

Such an overgrowth of the mucous membrane, in which the local glands are simultaneously enlarged, is best described as a glandular hyperplasia.

168. True adenoma is generally distinguishable from glandular hyperplasia by obvious characteristics. Its consistence, colour, and structure all mark it off plainly from the surrounding tissue.

Adenomata are usually knot-like growths arising within the substance of glands, or in glandular epithelial or epidermal tissues. In the first case it is generally a part only of the gland that is transformed into tumour-tissue. In the mucous membranes and skin the tumour is likewise circumscribed. When an entire organ like the ovary is included in the growth, it is easy to make out by the alteration in the structure that it is an adenoma, and not the result of simple hypertrophy. Adenomata are often pale soft and marrowy: in other cases they are dense and coarse.

Microscopic examination will obviate any doubt, which mere inspection may leave, as to the nature of a questionable adenoma. The structure of the neoplasm is always different from that of the affected tissue. It always corresponds with the type of some normal tissue; but this is not the type of the matrix in which it lies. Adenoma of the intestine may be made up of ramified and convoluted tubules—not of lieberkühnian crypts. Adenoma of the liver may be made up of tubular glands instead of lobules. Adenoma of the mamma is at once distinguished from the normal gland-tissue by the mode in which the epithelial cells are reproduced and arranged, and by the structure of the neoplastic acini.

The difference between normal and neoplastic gland-tissue is perhaps most marked of all in the case of the ovary. Ovarian adenoma is apt to grow to an enormous size, and very often imperils the life of the patient afflicted with it. It usually takes the form of a multilocular **cystoma** or cystadenoma, as it is called; and is made up of a multitude of small and large cysts. These contain a ropy, clear or turbid, and variously tinted liquid. Their inner surface resembles that of smooth mucous membrane. The walls are chiefly of a fibrous texture: but here and there occur masses of tissue with a soft marrow-like section and white or pink in colour, which resemble parenchymatous gland-substance. These masses exemplify the early stages of the tumour's development: they consist of a fibro-cellular stroma, containing glandular tubules lined with tall cylindrical epithelium (Fig. 60). Some of the

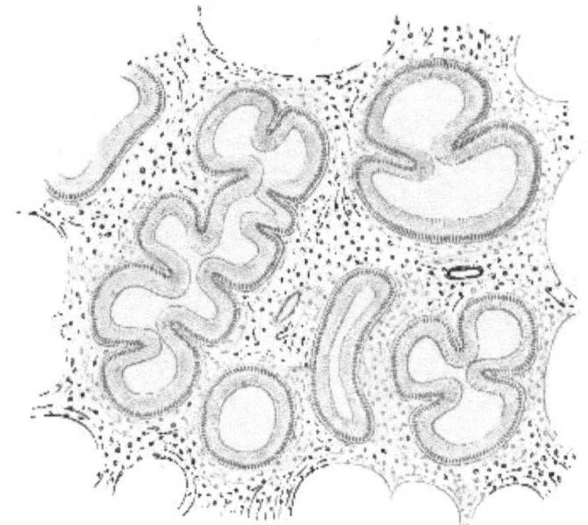

FIG. 60. SECTION FROM A PAPILLIFEROUS CYSTADENOMA.
(*Haematoxylin staining*: ×40)

tubules are dilated. This dilatation is the first step towards the formation of a cyst; it is the result of an accumulation of secretion. When small cysts are thus formed, the fibrous tissue round them often proceeds to grow into the cavity in the form of papillary protuberances (Fig. 60). These papillary growths, which often develope in vast numbers, give to this variety its specific name of papilliferous cystadenoma.

169. All adenomata have not the same grave significance, whether we regard the affected organ or the system generally. Ovarian adenoma destroys the organ and jeopardises life by its size; but it forms no metastases and does not invade neighbouring structures. Adenoma of a sweat-gland or sebaceous gland remains as a local tumour, never reaching any great size. But the case is different with the adenomata of the alimentary canal, namely those of the stomach, large or small intestine, and rectum. Each of these tends to invade and destroy the surrounding parts, and to form

metastases. They are as malignant as the malignant carcinomata. In order to indicate this fact in their distinctive name, they have been called destructive adenomata, or **adenocarcinomata**. Their malignancy is manifested even in their local behaviour. Fig. 61

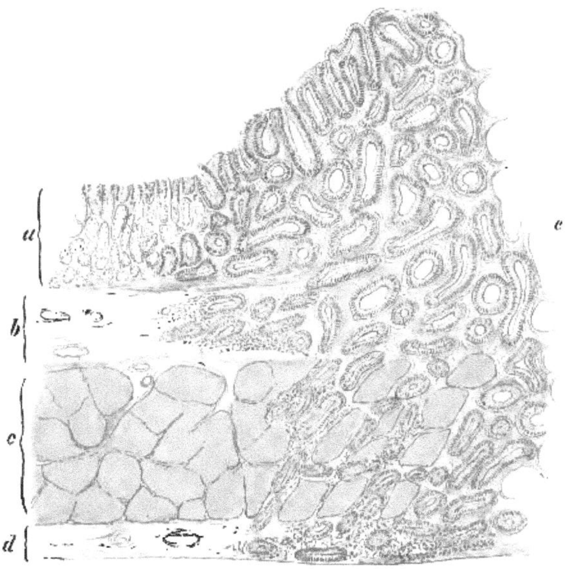

FIG. 61. SECTION THROUGH THE ADVANCING MARGIN OF A DESTRUCTIVE ADENOMA OF THE STOMACH.

(*Haematoxylin staining:* ×25)

a *mucosa*
b *submucosa*
c *muscularis*
d *serosa*
e neoplasm which starting from the *mucosa* has invaded the other layers. Small-celled infiltration here and there accompanies the formation of the neoplastic tubules.

represents a section through the advancing margin of a small destructive adenoma of the stomach; it is remarkable for the great size of its glandular tubules and of the epithelial cells which line them.

The figure (Fig. 61) shows that the neoplastic tubules are first developed in the *mucosa*, the normal constituents of the mucous membrane simultaneously disappearing. Starting thence the neoplasm invades the *submucosa* (*b*). It intrudes itself along the intermuscular septa between the muscle-bundles of the *muscularis* (*c*): and finally extends along the serous layer (*d*). Here and there through the fibrous tissue may be seen heaps of small cells: this indicates that proliferation is going on in this tissue likewise.

This invasion of the neighbouring tissues is the first step towards the formation of metastases. Clearly the lymph-spaces of the tissue are certain to be encountered by the advancing growth, and when this happens the path of infective transport stands open.

Destructive adenoma is a soft marrowy tumour, taking the form either of a papillary or fungous outgrowth, or more commonly of a level and extensive thickening of the mucous membrane. The new tissue frequently breaks down and ulcerates. The ulcers have a soft infiltrated base and raised rampart-like edges, or the surrounding tissue is beset with nodular growths.

b. *Carcinoma.*

170. If we define **carcinoma** as a growth characterised by epithelial multiplication (Art. 166), and not agreeing with any normal glandular type, we must at the same time lay stress on the fact that this epithelial multiplication is no merely accessory or subordinate feature. It is the essential and distinguishing character of the neoplasm.

Simple non-typical multiplications of epithelium are by no means uncommon; but they are not necessarily to be interpreted as carcinomatous. Subepidermic granulomatous tumours of the skin (Art. 132 Fig. 37) will often exhibit in their superficial layers clusters and rolls and strings of epithelial cells altogether diverse from any normal mode of grouping; and the same may be observed in skin-wounds which are in process of repair by epidermal growth and multiplication. So too in glands altered by inflammation, and in fibrous tumours occurring in glands, the glandular epithelium may begin to multiply and lead to the formation of epithelial masses that are altogether non-typical or atypical in appearance. Formations of this kind are not to be classed with the carcinomata. They lack the power of growing indefinitely and of infiltrating the surrounding tissues. They are incapable of raising themselves to the rank of the independent tumour, that is nourished like a parasite at the expense of the organism, and invades the tissues to their destruction. They can only extend where a free surface is open to them, due either to antecedent inflammation or to the formation of a true tumour. In wounds or subepithelial granulations, these proliferous growths have no more significance than the covering of an abraded surface with new epithelium. The epithelium forms only in places where the underlying tissue is so arranged as to leave free surfaces or open fissures, and the process amounts, in a word, merely to the 'skinning-over' of internal surfaces.

The mode in which true carcinoma developes and extends is quite different. The epithelial new-formation is not limited to free or bared surfaces; it actively invades the contiguous connective tissues. Thus we may have a cutaneous cancer or epithelioma, which consists essentially of cellular prolongations of the interpapillary promontories of the malpighian layer, penetrating and ramifying in the fibrous tissue of the corium (**Fig.** 62 *f*). These prolongations go on growing and multiplying, and ultimately

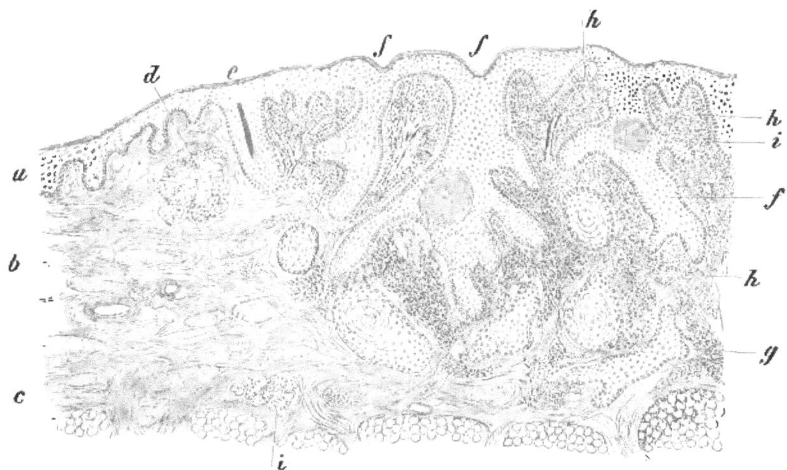

FIG. 62. SECTION FROM A CUTANEOUS CANCER OR EPITHELIOMA.

(*Aniline-brown staining*: ×20)

a epidermis
b corium
c subcutaneous areolar tissue
d sebaceous gland
e hair-follicle
f cancerous ingrowths from the epidermis
g deep-set cancerous cell-groups
h proliferating fibrous tissue
i (*above*) cell-nest or epidermic globe
i (*below*) sweat-gland

infiltrate the corium over a more or less extensive area, taking the form of detached strings and nests of cells (*g*). In this case then, we may regard the carcinoma as an epithelial infiltration of the corium starting in the superficial epidermis. The share taken by the corium itself is not always the same. At first we are generally unable to detect in it any histological change whatsoever. The fibrous stroma in which the epithelial cells are lodged is furnished by the unaltered corium alone. In other cases, and in later stages (Fig. 62 *h*), a perceptible amount of cell-multiplication and occasionally of vascularisation takes place. It almost looks as if the fibrous tissue were endeavouring, by compensatory growth on its own part, to counteract the invasion of its borders by the epithelium.

In tumours formed in the way we have described, the intruded masses of epithelial cells are spoken of as **cancerous cell-nests**, and the separate cells as **cancer-cells**. The fibrous framework in which they lie, made up partly of pre-existing and partly of new-formed fibrous tissue, is called the **cancerous stroma**.

171. The development of cancer in glands is essentially similar to that which starts in squamous epithelium or epidermis. Thus

in the glands of the uterus, we have cancer commencing with active growth and multiplication of the cylindrical epithelial cells. The single layer of cylindrical cells is transformed into a series of stratified or disorderly masses of epithelium (Fig. 63) piled upon

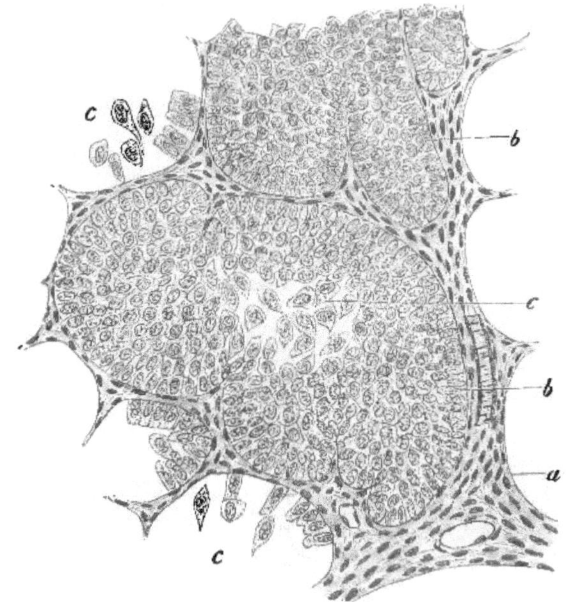

FIG. 63. SECTION FROM A CANCER OF THE UTERINE GLANDS.
(*Haematoxylin staining*: × 250)
a stroma *b* cancerous ingrowths or loculi *c* isolated cancer-cells

each other. The size of the gland (*b*) is thus considerably increased, and soon its typical structure is overlaid and lost by the substitution of great cell-masses and cancerous cell-nests or loculi. The cells retain their cylindrical form only at the borders of these groups. This represents the first stage. In the second, the surrounding tissue is invaded and infiltrated by cancerous cell-nests.

A section from the advancing margin of a mammary cancer (Fig. 64) shows at one view the various steps of the process; a low magnification is all that is necessary. The first stages in the formation of the mammary cancer are essentially the same as those observed in uterine cancer, though the peculiarities of the matrix bring about certain minor variations. The primary aberration is an excessive multiplication of the glandular epithelium. This is followed by general epithelial infiltration. The small and scattered acini of the mamma are replaced by cancerous cell-nests of various form and size (*e*), embedded in a scanty stroma. Starting from these as primary foci, the infiltration of the connective tissues (*gf*) extends far and wide, beyond the region of the gland-tissue itself. The fibrous bundles are thrust asunder by the multiplying cells, which link themselves into fusiform or rounded masses, or into long ramifying strings and bands. Spreading upwards these invade the corium; single cell-nests may even be found immediately underlying the epidermis (*g*). Within the substance of the nipple (*a*) also, we may discover numerous cancerous patches (*h*) in the fibrous tissue between the galactophorous ducts (*d*). In the figure we note that the only uninvaded part of the gland is near its edge. Even here however the groups of round-cells scattered through the connective tissue (*k*) show that the structures are not altogether in their normal condition.

To sum up all that we learn from this preparation concerning the extension of the cancer we may say—that the process consists in infiltration of the connective tissue with epithelial cell-nests: that this is accompanied or succeeded by inflammatory or proliferous changes in the connective tissue: and that these ultimately result in fibrous hyperplasia.

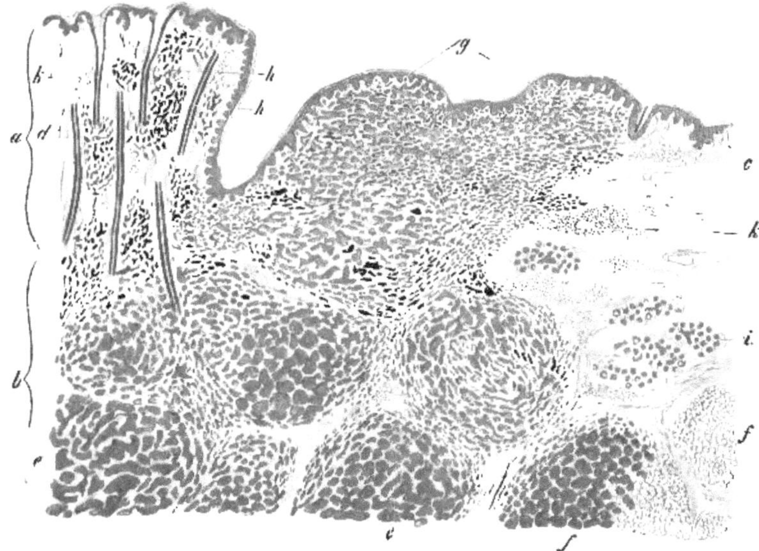

FIG. 64. SECTION THROUGH A MAMMARY CANCER.

(*Magnified by means of a simple lens*)

a nipple *b* mammary tissue
c skin *d* galactophorous ducts
e cancer-tissue replacing the gland-tissue
f fat-lobules, normal or undergoing cancerous change
g cancerous skin
h cancerous cell-nests in the nipple
i normal acini
k infiltration of fibrous tissue with round-cells

We are chiefly indebted to THIERSCH (*Der Epithelialkrebs* 1865) and WALDEYER (*Virch. Arch.* vols. 41, 55) for the discovery that a large class of tumours (other than the adenomata) existed, in which epithelium formed an essential constituent. THIERSCH demonstrated that cancer-cells are derived from epithelium, drawing his arguments principally from cases of cutaneous cancer or epithelioma. WALDEYER extended his researches to organs of every kind. Many subsequent observations have proved—that a considerable number of tumours which were believed by VIRCHOW and others to originate as connective-tissue growths do really originate in epithelial growth and multiplication. The class of connective-tissue tumours has thus been greatly diminished. The great majority of the alveolar tumours included by VIRCHOW under the general term carcinomata must now be ranked as epithelial tumours. See BILLROTH'S *Surg. Pathology* 3d ed.; LÜCKE, in *Billroth u. v. Pithas Handbuch* vol. II; SCHRÖN, *Contrib. alla anat. della cute umana* 1865; and, for criticism of the 'epithelial theory' of carcinoma, PAGET'S *Surg. Path.* Lect. 35. KÖSTER'S attempt (*Die Entwickelung der Carcinome* 1869) to disprove the participation of the epithelium in a large class of alveolar tumours, and to derive the cell-nests from the proliferous endothelium of the lymphatics, has not proved successful.

This being the case, it will be best in future to designate the various tumours not according to their structure merely, but also with respect to their genesis. Carcinoma will then imply not only an alveolar structure, but an epithelial origin also. The mode of genesis is the distinctive and definitive character: the alveolar structure is merely a result of contingent or non-essential factors.

172. From the description we have given, it will be manifest that the so-called cancer-cells are nothing other than proliferous epithelial cells; and we may therefore expect them to exhibit epithelial characteristics. Accordingly we find that they preserve throughout the traces of their descent. They are comparatively large, and have large vesicular nuclei containing nucleolar corpuscles: and they have certain habits of grouping peculiar to the parent structures. Cutaneous cancers (epitheliomata) contain cells exactly like those of the Malpighian layer, and they may undergo cornifying processes analogous to those which are normal in the case of the epidermis. Cancers starting in the intestinal mucous membrane are provided with cylindrical epithelium. But this maintenance of the ancestral cell-type has its limits.

When strings or wedges of epithelial cells penetrate the fibrous tissues, it invariably happens that the tightly packed elements affect each other mutually, and chiefly as regards their form (Fig. 65). We may see how this occurs by considering a section of one of these conical epithelial wedges—which from their appearance have been called '**bird's-nest bodies**'

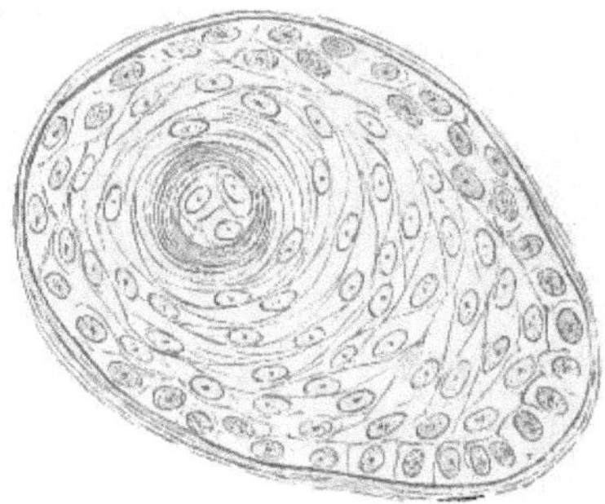

FIG. 65. BIRD'S-NEST BODY OR 'CONCENTRIC GLOBE' FROM AN EPITHELIOMA (× 250)

(concentric or epidermic globes). When the cells are isolated it is found that there are scarcely two alike in shape. This multiformity of the cells of cancer has long been a familiar fact; it has even been exalted into a characteristic feature. It obtains in squamous epithelioma and in cylindrical carcinoma, starting in the cylindrical epithelium of intestine or gland. The original type is only in a few cases preserved pure and unmodified.

At the same time we must not look upon this multiformity as anything peculiar to cancer. Multiform cells may occur in other tumours—in the sarcomata, for instance. All we can say is—that in virtue of the peculiar mode of cell-multiplication in the carcinomata, multiform cells are especially apt to be produced in them. What is true of their alveolar structure is also true here. In consequence of their mode of development we always find that cancers are alveolar; but other tumours whose genesis is entirely different may nevertheless exhibit the same structure.

173. **Varieties of carcinoma** have been distinguished according to their site and place of origin, the form and texture of the cells, the arrangement of the cells, and the mode of epithelial infiltration dependent thereon, and finally the abundance and texture of the fibrous stroma. Many of these distinctions have now ceased to have any real significance. The title given to certain cancers of the skin or mucous membrane—namely, epithelioma or epithelial cancer—is now useful only as indicating conveniently their seat and histological structure. Formerly the title implied a contradistinction between cancer of the epithelia and cancer of the connective tissues. Other terms like medullary, simple, or scirrhous, applied to various structural varieties of cancer chiefly originating in the glands, have also only a limited application; inasmuch as an individual cancer may not have exactly the same structure throughout all its parts, or in all its successive stages.

Generally speaking, the form of the cancer depends on the structure of the matrix in which it is seated. A certain group of forms are found to recur perpetually in each particular organ. It would seem most natural *a priori* to divide the carcinomata into two groups—those, namely, which start in investing or surface epithelium, and those which start in glandular epithelium. Such a division might be preferable from a theoretical point of view; but it is not always practicable, as it demands rather minute histological investigation. An epithelioma starting in a sebaceous gland has generally the very same appearance as one starting in a hair-follicle or in the epidermis. In cancer of the intestine, it would often be a matter of very great difficulty to decide whether the disease started in the simple lining epithelium, or in that of the crypts of Lieberkühn. For this reason it is advisable to classify the carcinomata under a few main types, distinguished by sufficiently well-marked anatomical differences. The following are the most important.

(1) **Squamous epithelial cancer.** The chief representative of this class is epithelioma or cutaneous cancroid (Fig. 62). This gives rise to warty and nodular tumours, or to diffuse thickenings of the skin. It is characterised by the occurrence in it of large epithelial nests, made up of large multiform squamous cells. Ulcers are very often formed by the breaking down of the new tissue.

If the section of an epithelioma be scraped, a gritty mass is obtained consisting mainly of nests and single cells. The nests often take the form of globes, in which the cells are arranged concentrically like the coats of an onion (Fig. 62 *i*). These at times become horny, forming what are called epithelial pearls. Epitheliomata in which these pearls are a distinct feature have been called horny or corneous cancroids. The tumour-cells of epithelioma are descendants of the superficial epidermis, and also of the epithelia of the hair-follicles and sebaceous glands. Squamous epithelial cancers occur in all the mucous membranes covered with squamous epithelium—in the mouth, pharynx, oesophagus, bladder, vagina, etc.

(2) **Cylindrical epithelial cancer.** This has its seat in mucous membrane, chiefly that of the intestine, but also in that of

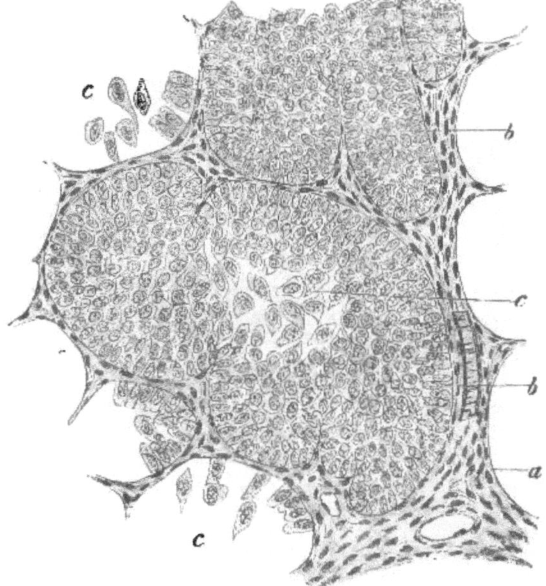

FIG. 66. GLANDULAR CANCER OF THE UTERUS. (*Haematoxylin staining:* ×250)
a stroma *b* cancerous nests or loculi *c* isolated cancer-cells

the uterus. It forms soft nodulated tumours which start in the columnar epithelium of the glands.

In consequence of active multiplication among the epithelial cells the glands become distended into more or less globular nests (Fig. 66). By mutual compression the cells assume very various forms, retaining their columnar character only at the periphery. Sometimes an unoccupied space or lumen remains at the centre. The cell-nests having thus the appearance of gigantic gland-acini, the tumour has also been described as adeno-carcinoma: we reserve this term for the destructive adenoma described in Art. 169.

Glandular cancer of a like kind, with a coarse alveolar stroma, occurs in glands like the kidney and mamma, as well as in mucous membrane. In them it likewise starts in overgrowth and multiplication of the glandular epithelium. The difference between this variety and the last consists simply in the absence of tall columnar epithelial cells among the other constituents. This is due to the fact that the epithelium in which the growth originates is spheroidal rather than columnar.

(3) **Simple carcinoma** is a term often applied to a variety usually originating in glands, and forming rather firm nodulated tumours. In section these have generally a light greyish translucent look. The stroma and the cell-nests are often sharply distinguished from each other by the difference of their colour;

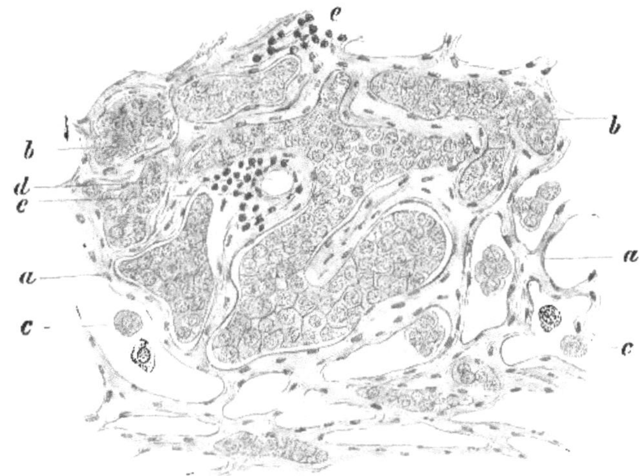

FIG. 67. SECTION FROM A SIMPLE CARCINOMA OF THE MAMMA.

(*Haematoxylin staining:* × 200)

a stroma
b nests or loculi
c single cancer-cells
d blood-vessel
e fibrous stroma infiltrated with small cells

especially when the cells have already undergone partial fatty change, and so look white or yellowish-white and opaque. By scraping the section we can often obtain a fairly abundant milky juice. The tumour has a somewhat coarse fibrous framework (Fig. 67 *a*), containing alveoli of various sizes and shapes filled with masses of epithelial cells. It particularly affects the mamma, and occurs also in the stomach, pancreas, and kidneys.

(4) **Medullary** (or encephaloid) **cancer**. When the cells are very abundant and the stroma delicate and scanty, the consistence of the tumour may become remarkably soft and semi-fluid. Such forms occur chiefly in mucous membrane, but also in the ovary, kidney, testis, etc. They are described as medullary or encephaloid cancers. They resemble very much the softer adenomata and sarcomata. An abundant milky cancer-juice may be expressed from the cut surface: it contains numerous cells and free nuclei, with fatty detritus and free oil-globules.

(5) **Scirrhus**, or scirrhous cancer. In this the cell-groups are small and scanty and the stroma coarse and dense. The tumour feels firm or even hard, and looks very much like a dense fibroma.

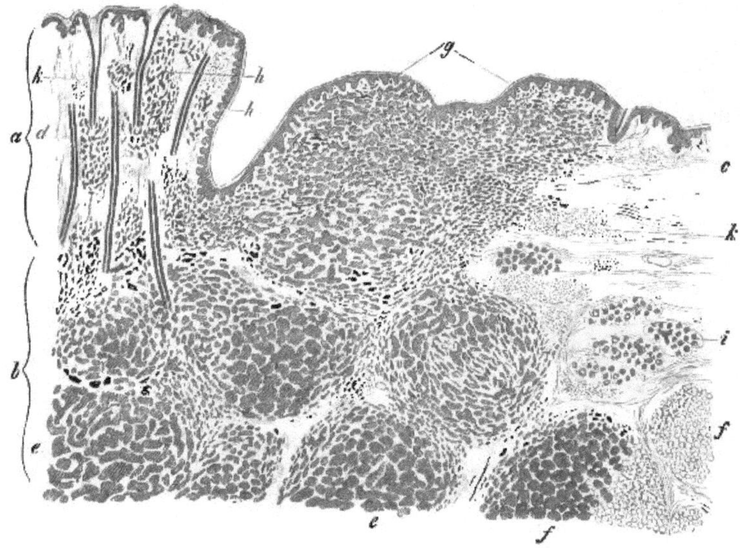

FIG. 68. SIMPLE CANCER OF THE MAMMA (SCIRRHOUS IN PARTS).
(*Magnified by means of a simple lens: same as Fig. 64*)

a nipple
b mammary tissue
c skin
d galactophorus ducts
e cancer-tissue replacing the gland-tissue
f fat-lobules, normal or undergoing cancerous change
g cancerous skin
h cancerous infiltration of the nipple
i normal acini
k infiltration of fibrous tissue with round-cells

There is no sharp line to be drawn between scirrhus and simple cancer. Within one and the same growth we may find a part having the texture of scirrhus, and another resembling simple cancer (Fig. 68). The question is merely whether the stroma or the cellular elements predominate. The characteristic hardness of scirrhus is found at spots where the fibrous stroma is not so much alveolated as interspersed with small fusiform cell-nests (Fig. 68 *g h*).

The cancer-cells often perish by fatty degeneration, and are then absorbed. The coarse fibrous stroma is left, looking like a deposit of firm scar-tissue. Cancers which have become hard and fibrous in this way are found not only in the mamma but also in the stomach, testis, ovary, and kidney.

(6) **Colloid** (otherwise gelatinous or alveolar) **cancer** occurs as a definite tumour or a diffuse infiltration. It is most frequently found in the alimentary tract and in the mamma, more rarely in the ovary or other organ. It is characterised by the translucency of its substance. The stroma seems to contain masses of jelly rather than the usual more or less opaque cell-nests. The transparent glassy look may be apparent even on the outside of the tumour. This is true, for instance, in the case of colloid cancer of the mucous membrane, which usually forms semi-transparent papillary or fungous excrescences. In the mamma the colloid character becomes apparent only on cutting through the tumour. It often happens that the whole tumour is not alike; some parts being translucent, others greyish or reddish like the more ordinary forms.

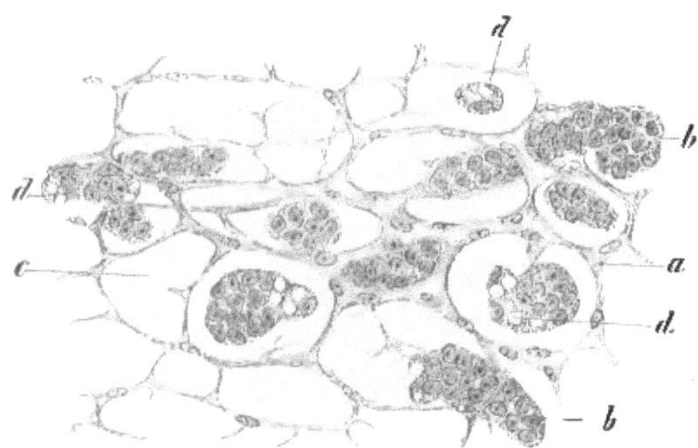

FIG. 69. COLLOID CANCER OF THE MAMMA.

(*Haematoxylin staining:* ×250)

a stroma
b cancerous cell-nests
c empty alveoli
d cells containing globules of colloid substance

The colloid or gelatinous texture of the tumour is due to mucoid or colloid change affecting the cancer-cells (Fig. 69).

It begins with the formation of clear globules in their interior (*d*). The cells then perish, and the globules coalesce with each other and with larger gelatinous lumps already formed. In this way a large homogeneous colloid mass is ultimately built up. It is not uncommon for all the cells over a wide area to perish in this manner, so that the stroma is the only formed constituent remaining. In other spots, cell-groups may still be found encircled by colloid masses (Fig. 69 *b*): in others again there is no colloid substance at all.

(7) **Carcinoma myxomatodes.** A cancerous tumour may likewise assume a gelatinous texture in consequence of mucoid change affecting the stroma (Fig. 70). With this metaplasia of the fibrous tissue there may also be associated a mucoid degeneration of the cancer-cells (Fig. 70 *d*): and this may increase considerably the transparent and gelatinous appearance of the growth. The connective-tissue cells of the stroma may also

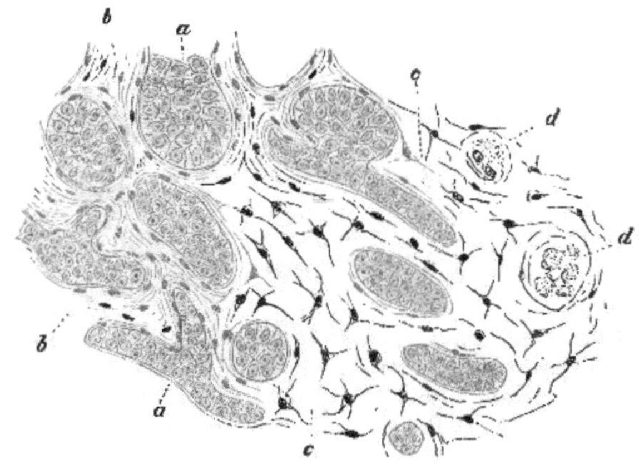

FIG. 70. CARCINOMA MYXOMATODES OF THE STOMACH.
(*Haematoxylin staining*: ×250)

a cancerous loculi
b fibrous stroma
c mucoid stroma
d mucoid cancer-cells

perish, so that we are often unable to find any traces of cell-structure over wide areas. The favourite seats of this variety are the same as those of colloid cancer.

(8) **Cylindroma carcinomatodes** is a very rare variety of cancer, characterised by the formation of homogeneous spherules within the cell-nests (Fig. 71).

These spherules, which are possibly to be regarded as masses of colloid substance, press asunder the other cells of the group (Fig. 71 *b*). If a considerable number of spherules form within the same loculus, the cells may be compressed into slender trabeculae (*c*), and so come to form a kind of anastomosing network. This variety

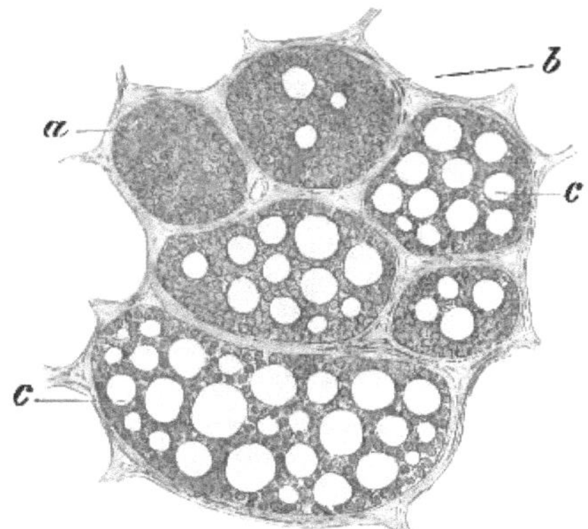

FIG. 71. SECTION FROM A CYLINDROMA CARCINOMATODES.
(*Carmine staining*: × 150)

a unaltered loculus or cell-nest
b cell-nests with a few hyaline spherules
c cell-nests reduced to a honeycombed reticulum by the formation of numerous hyaline spherules

has been described as a cylindroma (ZIEGLER has only once met with it, and then in the lacrimal gland). To distinguish it from the sarcomatous kind (Art. 163), it has been called carcinomatodes.

(9) **Giant-celled** (or myeloid) **cancer** is a form in which some of the cancer-cells attain an inordinate size. All parts of the cell—protoplasm, nucleus and nucleolar corpuscles—contribute to this enlargement. They become at the same time remarkably transparent, and the general aspect is much as if the cell had imbibed a great quantity of water, and had in consequence swollen out enormously.

(10) **Melanocarcinoma** is a sufficiently distinct variety to deserve mention. It gives rise to grey, brown, or black tumours. The pigment is contained partly in the cancer-cells, partly in the stroma. It is seldom met with; being much rarer than melanotic sarcoma.

References:—WALDEYER, *Virch. Arch.* vol. 55; RINDFLEISCH, *Path. Histology* vol. I; LÜCKE, Art. *Geschwülste* in *Hand. d. Chirurgie v. Pitha u. Billroth* II; PERLS, *Allg. Path.* 1877; PAGET, *Surg. Path.* Lects. 30—35; LEBERT, *Des maladies cancéreuses* Paris 1851.

174. The **extension of a cancerous growth** is not at an end when the organ originally attacked is infiltrated throughout. Cancer pays small heed to the boundaries between the various

tissues. Sooner or later (latest of all in encapsuled organs like the kidney), the cancerous process invades the neighbouring tissues. Some of these, chiefly the specific tissues like glandular epithelium, muscle, bone, etc., disappear before the advancing growth. Fibrous tissue on the other hand is usually excited to proliferation, and new tissue and blood vessels may thus be formed and converted into cancer-stroma. Now and then other proliferations are set up in the neighbourhood of the tumour: and in this way, for example, new bony growths may be formed.

In addition to this peculiar power of invasion, cancer has also in a high degree the power of originating **metastases** or **secondary growths.** The germs which give rise to these metastases are the cancerous epithelial cells, which are carried off to remote places by the blood or lymph. The first development of the secondary nodules starts in these, when they have found a suitable nidus. An epithelial germ may reach the liver, for instance, and become wedged in one of the terminal radicles of the vena portae. If it finds adequate nutriment there, it begins to grow. It subdivides and multiplies, and thus a cell-nest is presently formed (Fig. 72) which distends the capillary vessel, and by compression causes the liver-cells to dwindle and atrophy. By the aid of the fibrous elements of the vessels, which proceed to multiply and so furnish a fibrous stroma and accessory vessels, a secondary nodule

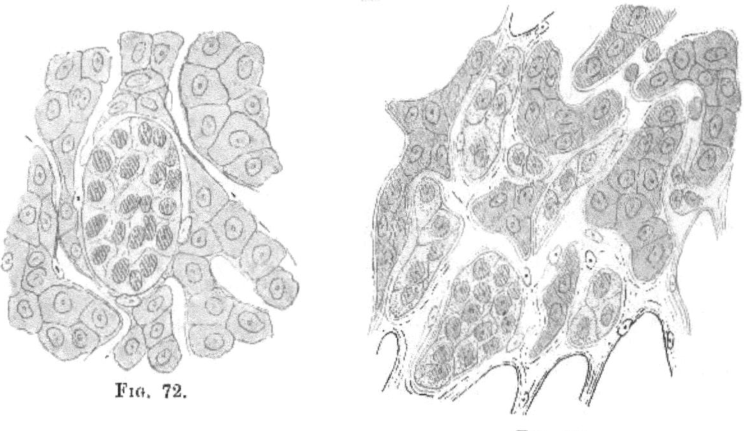

FIG. 72.

FIG. 73.

FIG. 72. SECTION PASSING THROUGH A CANCEROUS EMBOLUS OF A HEPATIC CAPILLARY.
(From a case of primary adenocarcinoma of the stomach: haematoxylin staining: × 300)

The cancer germs have just begun to develope into a secondary nodule.

FIG. 73. METASTATIC DEVELOPMENT OF CANCER IN A HEPATIC CAPILLARY.
(The primary focus was in the pancreas: fibrous tissue as well as cell-nests have been formed within the capillary: × 250)

is at length evolved, whose structure resembles in all points the structure of the parent nodule. The hepatic lobules are either pushed aside and compressed, or they are interpenetrated by strings of cancer-cells starting from the nodule. This is the result of the mode of growth of the nodule. It grows chiefly at its periphery, and extends along the open capillary channels (Fig. 73). In this way the capillaries themselves are one after another replaced by cancer-tissue. As this latter extends, the liver-cells gradually disappear.

The epithelial elements of the secondary nodules are to be regarded as, without exception, the progeny of the original cancer-cells transplanted from the parent growth. The fibrous tissue in which they are embedded is furnished by the connective-tissue elements of the blood-vessels.

The origin of the cancer-cells in secondary nodules has been the subject of as much discussion as the genesis of the primary growth. Even now a certain amount of disagreement exists on the question. RINDFLEISCH, KLEBS, GUSSENBAUER, WEIL, and others, maintain that the connective-tissue cells, and especially the endothelia of the blood-vessels and lymphatics, take an active share in forming the cancer-cells of the metastatic growths. GUSSENBAUER (*Langenbeck's Arch. f. Chir.* XIV) and WEIL (*Wien. med. Jahrb.* 1873) go so far as to say that even striated and non-striated muscle-fibres may be stirred up (in a manner infected) so as to produce cancer-cells. SIMON, CREIGHTON, MOXON, and others in this country, have put forward like theories: they are accustomed to speak of a 'spermatic' influence exerted by the transported germs upon the tissue-elements of their new seat (*Trans. Path. Soc.* 1874).

ZIEGLER is unable to find any satisfactory evidence for such a view. He made numerous investigations bearing on the question, and under his guidance FRONISTA examined a multitude of secondary growths in various organs; but no certain grounds for the theory were ever discovered. Active changes in the fixed cells were often very beautifully shown; but wherever it was possible to trace the fate of these cells it was found that they merely went to form the type of tissue which they would reproduce in normal circumstances. The osteoblasts of the periosteum and marrow form bone or fibrous tissue; endothelial cells likewise produce only connective tissue. It is not however to be inferred that these investigations absolutely and certainly exclude the possibility of a cancerous transformation of the products of connective-tissue proliferation. When a tissue has undergone extensive proliferous changes, nothing certain can be made out from it regarding the origin or the fate of individual cells. The cancerous embolus acts like a foreign body. Round it are set up inflammatory infiltration of leucocytes on the one hand, and multiplication of the fixed cells on the other. Both processes result in fibrous hyperplasia, which in many cases goes to form a new stroma for the growing nodule. The same processes are thus repeated here as occur in the fibrous structures of the primary focus. It is therefore well to hold by the doctrine of REMAK and GOODSIR—at least until it is certainly disproved—that as the descendants of the different embryonic layers are never transformed into each other in normal circumstances, so also under pathological conditions no such metaplasia can occur. Even the transformation of one epithelial formation into another suggested by some (RINDFLEISCH, *Path. Histology* Art. 531; PERLS, *Virch. Arch.* vol. 56; etc.) has not been established. When carcinomata of the liver are examined the liver-cells are seen to dwindle and perish, but not to change to cancer-cells. Even in cases where mammary cancer penetrates the corium and reaches the epidermal layers of the skin, it is always possible to distinguish clearly between the cancer-cells and the true cutaneous epidermis.

175. Carcinoma is very prone to undergo retrogressive change. In the juice scraped from the cut surface of a cancer we may nearly always find cells which are fatty or disintegrating. This is especially the case in soft quickly-growing tumours. If the fatty change is extensive the affected spots look white and opaque, and by and by break down into a creamy pulp. The disintegrated cells may also become condensed into cheesy masses. More commonly, however, we find that a part of the cells become absorbed. In tumours lying beneath the surface of an organ or raised above its general level, a central depression or dimple may thus be formed. The tumour is then said to be **umbilicated**. In cancers with a dense stroma, in which the disappearance of the cells is accompanied by hyperplasia of the fibrous elements, we may find the original growth replaced by a dense coarse deposit of fibrous tissue containing few if any cancerous cell-nests. This transformation is specially frequent in the case of mammary and gastric scirrhus.

Mucoid degeneration has already been discussed (Art. 173). Amyloid degeneration of the stroma has frequently been observed.

The necrotic disintegration of cancerous growths, and the consequent formation of **cancerous ulcers**, deserve special mention. Tumours of great size may in this way be wholly destroyed. In intestinal cancer, for example, it is no rare thing to find after a certain time nothing but an ulceration, replacing the original tumour, and bearing hardly any resemblance to it. If the ulcerative process is not far advanced, the remains of the tumour may be recognised as nodules or papillary excrescences rising from the base or border of the ulcer. In later stages the base may be smooth and clean, consisting simply of firm fibrous tissue; while the edges rise like ramparts, or are beset with papillary or nodular growths. Now and then these may disappear in like manner, and the ulcer appears as a non-cancerous sore with an indurated base. Even on section it may not always be possible with the unaided eye to decide whether the tissue still contains cell-nests or not. We must in such cases have recourse to the microscope.

Cutaneous or epitheliomatous cancers, like those of mucous membrane, may also ulcerate; and so too may cancers of the mamma or other subcutaneous glands. The surface of these breaks down, and great putrid or foetid ulcers are the result.

The seat of an ulcer is always the seat of a more or less intense inflammatory infiltration. Sometimes this results in vigorous granulative proliferation, the granulations rising above the surface as fungous excrescences. They are distinguished from ordinary granulations by the cell-nests they contain. From this granulation-tissue ordinary cicatricial tissue may be elaborated. A sort of local healing and recovery may thus result—from the destruction of the tumour, and the formation of granulative and cicatricial tissue. The growth may seem to have altogether disappeared. But this healing is only local and relative, and it does not last. Microscopic examination shows that the cancerous invasion of the deeper structures still persists. The formation of secondary growths, even after the surface ulceration is scarred over, testifies to the fact that the malignancy of the process is not removed with the removal of the primary growth.

176. Adenoma and carcinoma may be combined with other neoplastic formations; that is to say, the stroma may be composed of other than fibrous tissue. In the first place it must be remembered—that as cancer invades successive tissues, the most various structures may in turn be utilised to form its stroma. Thus when a uterine cancer reaches the muscular coats of the organ, we find that the stroma of the tumour contains smooth muscular fibres. When secondary nodules form in the liver, we often see liver-cells, atrophied no doubt but still recognisable, in the trabeculae of the stroma. The new-formed tissues which actually originate in the stroma are to be distinguished from such pre-existing formations. In the former case we may find that not only fibrous tissue but even cartilage or sarcomatous tissue has been developed. Such neoplasms are described as complex or **mixed tumours**. They are most common in the testis and parotid gland. They resemble the simple carcinomata in their general relations.

CHAPTER XXVIII.

AETIOLOGY OF TUMOURS.

177. Our knowledge of the aetiology of tumours is still very defective. What we have to say on the subject is, generally speaking, largely hypothetical.

We might at first be inclined to regard a tumour as the result of a local overgrowth of tissue, and to look for the conditions of its development among those which determine ordinary hyperplasia. But facts soon appear which tend to show that the processes are not parallel. There is, first, the histological diversity of the tumour (Art. 136) from the matrix in which it grows. Secondly, there is the associated impairment or extinction of the physiological function of the matrix-tissue. These facts do not suggest a mere over-active growth *in situ*. The anatomical facts are thus against our regarding tumours as localised hyperplasias. It follows that we cannot expect to discover the efficient causes of tumour-growth among the factors which give rise to such hyperplasias.

Nor can we fairly compare the tumours with the inflammatory new-formations. Tumours may indeed contain foci which are infiltrated with leucocytes. But these are of secondary significance. The entire process of neoplastic histogenesis shows that it is something quite different from the formative processes which originate in inflammation. We thus exclude at once the possibility of attributing the growth of a tumour to a traumatic lesion, at least in any immediate or direct way. Clinical experience bears this out; for if now and then we have tumours developed in a substratum of tissue which has been injured and has undergone inflammatory change, it is on the whole a rare occurrence, and does not prove that such injury would of itself suffice to set up tumour-formation in previously healthy tissue.

This being the case, we are perforce constrained to admit that other factors must be sought, if we are to explain the genesis of tumours.

If we did not know that tumours may develope at the most various periods of life—nay, that many forms are wont to appear only in advanced age, it might perhaps suggest itself to look for their aetiological factors in the embryo—to regard them in fact as local malformations. But the peculiar modes of occurrence referred to, and the observation that tumours originate in tissues which before looked perfectly normal, would scarcely make us regard such an embryonic theory as very probable beforehand.

COHNHEIM has very recently propounded an **embryonic hypothesis** of another kind. We are not to refer the actual development of the tumour itself to the embryonic period, but are to attribute its appearance in later life to the persistence of germinal embryonic tissues in the otherwise mature organism (COHNHEIM, *Allg. Path.* I). A tumour takes its rise in what we might call a belated rudiment—a focus of formative embryonic tissue, which has not been utilised in elaborating the normal tissue of the part—and so has lingered on unchanged. COHNHEIM therefore defines a tumour as—an atypical new-formation starting in a latent embryonic rudiment. The tumour-germs, consisting as they do of embryonic cells, may be very small and so elude observation. It is even conceivable, he thinks, that the germinal cells may be quite unrecognisable among the ordinary physiological elements of the part. They may linger on for a long time inactive. It is only when they are favoured by the external conditions—such as the supply of nutriment, and their relation to the surrounding tissues—that they begin to multiply and to form a tumour. In this way it becomes possible that a traumatic lesion may set up the active change. In most cases however the awakening impulse is beyond our power to discover.

We cannot deny that COHNHEIM's hypothesis would explain satisfactorily many of the peculiarities of tumours. Those growths, for example, whose structure reminds us so strongly of earlier developmental stages of particular tissues, would be acquitted of their (at present) unaccountable heterology. It also tells in favour of the theory—that a class of tumours does actually exist, of which we can say with certainty that they date their origin from the embryonic stage. At the same time we may well question whether our knowledge of the subject justifies us in attributing an embryonic origin to all tumours, or whether we should accept the theory only with considerable limitations.

COHNHEIM bases his view mainly on the arguments—that many tumours have been shown to be hereditary; that many exist at birth or at least develope in infancy; that they show a preference for sites where in earlier developmental stages some complication of structure occurred, *e.g.* for the places where diverse epithelial formations pass one into the other (lips, anus, stomach, cervix uteri), or for parts where the entire process of development is highly complex (genital apparatus). Finally, he holds that the atypical structure of tumours generally is in favour of his account of them.

It must be granted that these arguments speak strongly for the hypothesis.

They at least make it highly probable for certain classes of tumours. But they do not suffice to prove its applicability to all.

The view that tumours arise in consequence of injury, especially of frequently repeated irritation, is very widely accepted (VIRCHOW, *Die krankhaften Geschwülste;* KRÖNLEIN, *Lang. Arch. f. klin. Chir.* XXI; KOCHER, Art. *Krankheiten des Hodens, Handb. d. spec. Chir. v. Pitha u. Billroth;* BÖGEHOLD, *Virch. Arch.* vol. 88). COHNHEIM has justly objected to this view—that the number of cases of tumours in which antecedent injury has been demonstrated does not reach more than 14 per cent. of the whole number, and is by some given as 7 per cent. (BOLL, *Das Princip des Wachsthums* Berlin 1876; S. WOLFF, *Zur Entstehung von Geschwülsten nach traum. Einwirk.* In. Diss. Berlin 1874; VON WINIWARTER, *Beiträge z. Statistik d. Carcinome* Stuttgart 1878). From this we may infer that an injury may perhaps give rise to a tumour; but that neither injury nor inflammation is at all a necessary antecedent.

178. We are acquainted with a considerable number of forms of **congenital tumour**, whose origin can be referred with more or less certainty to the embryonic period. Of these it is however to be remarked—that their structure and composition are only in part analogous to those of the post-embryonic growths hitherto discussed. Many of them possess a structure entirely peculiar to themselves, so that they cannot be classed with any of the preceding tumours. They are therefore regarded by all authorities as special and peculiar formations, and are distinguished as teratomata.

Teratomata or teratoid tumours (Art. 13) are congenital growths, which are remarkable for the heterogeneity of their constituent elements. They may be large even at birth, or they may grow from small beginnings to a large size after birth. They may contain fibrous tissue, cartilage, bone, muscle, skin, hair, nerves, gland-tissue, and simple cellular or embryonic tissue. At times they may have the look of complex histioid tumours; but the combinations they present are usually much more various and heterogeneous than in any ordinary histioid growth. We even meet in them with structures which recall the appearance of some normal organ—the differences lying chiefly in the rudimentary nature of the outward shape or configuration, and the abnormal site. Sometimes the various tissues are grouped into something like orderly disposition, giving one the impression of a more or less organised foetus.

Teratomata, when externally visible, are usually placed at parts of the trunk corresponding to those at which double monstrosities cohere. These are chiefly—the lower end of the spine, the head, and the neck. Internal teratomata are usually connected with the genital apparatus.

Such teratomata are some of them true double monstrosities. One foetus has been surrounded and enclosed by another, and so has become stunted and ill-developed (Art. 13). The remainder are due to some misdevelopment of the tissues within a single foetus.

Dermoid cysts form a special class of teratomata. They are cysts whose inner surface has the same structure as the normal skin; but they occur in places where no skin is ever found normally. Their commonest seat is in the generative organs, especially in the ovary. More rarely they are found in other parts, such as the peritoneum, neck, and around the orbit. The smallest examples form little cysts which, as in the ovary, are distinguishable from their contents. The contents are usually greasy, semi-solid, yellowish-white, and interspersed with hairs. The wall is thicker, firmer, and whiter, than that of the Graafian follicles. Under the microscope it is seen to be composed of a corium and epidermis: it may even contain hair-follicles and sebaceous glands, or more rarely sweat-glands. Now and then an adipose layer, like the subcutaneous fat, is found beneath the corium. In rare cases, flat or irregular fragments of bone or cartilage and even teeth are found beneath the cutaneous layer. The teeth may also be found free within the cyst. Very rarely the cyst-wall contains muscular or nervous tissue. The larger dermoids, *i.e.* those reaching from the size of a walnut to that of the fist, are sharply marked off from the surrounding tissues by a fibrous capsule. They enclose large quantities of oily or greasy detritus, interspersed with fair or reddish hairs.

Dermoids are found in young individuals as well as old. Some are found even in the new-born. They grow very slowly. Judging by the special character of their lining membrane, these formations would seem to be derived from the same rudimentary elements as the external skin. They are probably due to aberrant germinal cutaneous cells from the epiblast, which have somehow wandered to an abnormal site, and there have at a later stage begun to develope after their kind.

References on the subject of teratomata and dermoid cysts:—Art. 13; KOHLRAUSCH, *Müller's Arch.* 1843; LEBERT, *Gaz. méd. de Paris* 1852; REMAK, *Deutsche Klinik* 16, 1856; HESCHL, *Prager Viertelj.* 1860; LÜCKE, *Handb. d. Chir. v. Pitha u. Billroth* II; HAFFTER, *Arch. d. Heilk.* XVI, 1875; PANUM, *Virch. Arch.* vol. 72; KLEBS, *Handb. d. path. Anat.*; DANZEL and MARTINI, *Arch. f. klin. Chir.* XVII; WALDEYER, *Arch. f. Gynäk.* I; WILSON FOX, *Journ. of Anat.* 1865; GORDON, *Med. chir. Trans.* XIII; PAGET, *Surg. Path.* Lect. 23.

179. Besides the teratomata there are other tumours more nearly allied in structure to the ordinary forms, which are either congenital or appear so soon after birth that their origin may with more or less certainty be referred to the embryonic period. The best-known examples are the **congenital angiomata** and **pigment-spots** (beauty-spots, moles) in the skin. The former have already been discussed (Arts. 148—150). Of the latter we have merely to say—that they appear as brown or black slightly raised patches in the skin, and are composed of tissue exactly resembling alveolar sarcoma (Fig. 54) covered over with epidermis.

We may likewise mention in this connexion—certain cutaneous fibromata; enchondromata of the skull, spinal column, and fingers; myxomata of the jaws; renal adenomata and cancers; and cystic adenomata seated on the sacrum and communicating with the central canal of the spinal cord.

The number of really congenital tumours observed is by no means great. Cases of tumours appearing in the earlier years of infancy and referable to embryonic conditions are more numerous. Of this kind are the sarcomata of infancy; especially the form of myosarcoma of the kidney referred to in Art. 153. It is not impossible that some of the ovarian adenomata may date back to the embryonic period. If we consider carefully the scanty details we possess of congenital tumours, taken in conjunction with the familiar facts of post-embryonic tumour-formation, we must admit that the support which COHNHEIM'S theory derives from this side of the subject is not very great.

It must not however be forgotten that this theory requires the existence—not of congenital tumours—but only of congenital rudiments of tumours. As to these latter our knowledge is unfortunately very small. It is almost entirely confined to the pigmentary and vascular naevi we have mentioned. They may be regarded, and with equal justice, either as germinal rudiments of tumours, or as developed growths. The former view is justified by the fact—that in later life it is not uncommon for these structures to develope into true malignant tumours.

Tumour-germs in bone were discovered some years ago by VIRCHOW (*Berlin. acad. Monatsbericht* 1875). He showed that islands of cartilage, which remain untransformed in the general ossifying process, may in later life become the starting points for the formation of chondromata.

Nothing certain is known of embryonic epithelial germs, such as may subsequently develope into tumours. Their existence may be surmised in the case of early epithelial tumours of the ovary, kidney, or intestine; but it has not been demonstrated. The frequently observed accessory glands occurring in connexion with the pancreas, mamma, thyroid, etc. are not to be regarded as mere germinal rudiments, inasmuch as they contain fully developed gland-tissue.

From what we have said, then, it will be seen that the histological evidence for the existence of embryonic germinal tissue in the fully developed organism is very slender.

ZIEGLER describes a tumour of some interest which he found in the small intestine seated in the *submucosa;* it was as large as a pea, and was made up of minute cysts. It should probably be regarded as a local misformation, rather than a deposit of germinal tissue. Its cysts contained papillary excrescences covered with columnar epithelium; and small gland tubules were found in the cyst-walls. It is conceivable that, from a misformation of this kind, a true tumour might at some time or other begin to develope.

References on congenital tumours:—VIRCHOW, *Die krank. Geschwülste;*

DUZAN, *Du cancer chez les enfants* Paris 1876; AHLFELD, *Arch. f. Gynäk.* XVI; ROHRER, *Das primäre Nierencarcinom* Zürich 1874; MAAS, *Berl. klin. Woch.* 47, 1880; C. VOGT, *Ueber angeb. Lipome* In. Diss. Berlin 1876; CHIARI, *Jahrb. d. Kinderheilk.* XIV; WEIGERT, *Virch. Arch.* vol. 67 (renal adenoma).

Many authorities are of opinion that COHNHEIM's theory is strongly borne out by the experiments of ZAHN (*Sur le sort des tissus emplantés dans l'organisme*, International Med. Congress, Geneva 1873) and LEOPOLD (*Virch. Arch.* vol. 85). They took bits of cartilage from a living foetal rabbit, and transplanted them into the peritoneal cavity and anterior chamber of the eye of an adult rabbit. The cartilage continued to grow, while pieces of cartilage taken from animals after birth were merely absorbed. This scarcely seems sufficient ground for COHNHEIM's generalisation. The faculty of growing after transplantation is not manifested by all foetal tissues: many or most of them are dissolved and absorbed by the disintegrating action of the fixed and migratory cells of the new matrix (LEOPOLD, *Arch. f. Gynäk.* XVIII). These experiments only show that foetal cartilage has the power of persisting and even of growing for a time—in spite of defective nutrition, and the absorbent action of the cells of the other tissues.

180. The inadequacy of the evidence for the existence of germinal embryonic rudiments in the adult tissues makes it appear a somewhat bold step to ascribe an embryonic origin to all tumours whatsoever. The observed and recorded cases do not justify us in saying more than that some tumours arise in rudimental structures, which were histologically distinguishable from the normal tissues before the tumour began to grow. And even in saying so much we must not interpret the term embryonic too literally. Embryonic formations are such as possess a structure resembling that of undeveloped tissue—an indefinite structure preceding the definitive or specialised structure. Tissues that are merely misdeveloped, pieces of tissue (such as epithelium or gland-tissue) displaced from their proper seat and transplanted elsewhere, as in the case of accessory glands and dermoid cysts, are not what we understand by embryonic tissues.

The class of tumours referable to embryonic rudiments will be somewhat enlarged, if we enlarge the signification of the term embryonic so as to include under it all tissues in process of active and energetic growth.

So long as an organ continues to grow, so long are multitudes of new cells formed in it. These formative cells may be called embryonic, inasmuch as they continue to multiply actively and so are nearer akin to the cells of the embryo than to those of mature tissue. In this way osteoblasts and osteoclasts and the proliferating cartilage of growing bone, the cells of the enlarging uterus in pregnancy, the tissue of the mamma preparing for lactation, all might be described as embryonic. If the hypothesis be thus extended, a whole series of tumours will certainly be comprehended under it. When, for instance, a tumour developes in the mamma or uterus in connexion with parturition, or a sarcoma or enchondroma forms in bone, periosteum, or marrow during ossification, it is not difficult to believe that the same cells which are building up the normal tissue may also give rise to the tumour.

But if we extend the meaning of the term embryonic so as to include all this, where are we to stop? Growth, *i.e.* restoration and replacement of what is being used up, continues throughout life. Surface epithelium is cast off and is regenerated; glandular epithelium is used up and replaced; even bone, though it seems so stationary, is exposed to changes at all stages of life—it is being resorbed by the osteoclasts and built up again by the osteoblasts.

If all post-embryonic processes of growth are to be styled embryonic, we cannot refuse to give the same title to all the processes of new cell-formation that occur during life. If this be granted, embryonic tissue becomes exactly the same as that which VIRCHOW called proliferous tissue, *i.e.* tissue capable of proliferation. We gain nothing by the mere substitution of one name for another: in the present case we lose something, for we are no longer able to distinguish in expression between embryonic and post-embryonic formation. For this reason it is better to confine the term embryonic to tissues which actually originate in the embryonic period.

The fact that we really know nothing of the persistence of true embryonic tissue—or in other words, that it has not been histologically demonstrated—is acknowledged by COHNHEIM. He seeks to explain the fact by supposing that the embryonic foci are very small and hard to distinguish; or even that the germinal cells may be mingled with the normal elements and so not distinguishable at all. It is not easy to imagine how embryonic cellular germs can possibly remain unchanged in the midst of mature tissue. COHNHEIM and MAAS (*Virch. Arch.* vol. 70) have shown that living tissue, such as periosteum, when introduced into another tissue like the lung, may continue to grow for a time; but afterwards it is absorbed and destroyed by the tissue in which it lies. An embryonic germ seems to have but three courses open to it. It may remain embryonic: in this case it is as it were alien to the tissue in which it lies, and will be absorbed like an organic foreign substance. It may assimilate itself physiologically as well as anatomically with the surrounding tissue, taking part in its physiological function and working with it: in this case it loses its embryonic character. Or thirdly, it may develope into an independent formation, interpolated as it were into the general system: in this case it forms what we call a congenital tumour (naevus, adenoma, sarcoma).

HASSE has attempted to give COHNHEIM's hypothesis a morphological basis (*Die Beziehungen der Morphologie zur Heilkunde* Leipzig 1880). The morphologist distinguishes two kinds of substances within the organism: one kind undergoes a series of transformations, the other provides for the formation of new tissue. The latter he describes as 'embryonic substance'. It is represented by cells which have undergone little or no transformation, and are the more apt to multiply the less their original character and structure has been modified—the nearer they stand to the formative cells of the embryo. From these cells only can new tissue be formed. Tumours are especially likely to be developed at spots where these 'embryonic cells' are abundant and unmodified. HASSE's distinction between proliferous and non-proliferous tissue-elements is perfectly just (Arts. 84—89): and any one may if he chooses call the former embryonic (as do French writers especially). In this case however the antithesis, on which COHNHEIM lays so much stress, between the cells of the embryo and the proliferous elements of the organism after birth, simply ceases to exist.

181. It is plain from the above that we do not think the hypothesis tenable which refers all tumours whatsoever to pre-existing embryonic germs. Anatomical investigation forces us rather to the conclusion that tumours may arise in tissues that are in very different states—embryonic, growing, mature, or retrogressive.

What is then the efficient cause of the formation of a tumour? It is as yet impossible to give any precise answer to this question. It is highly probable that the causation of the various classes of tumours is not subject to one law only, but to several.

The entire behaviour, anatomical and biological, of tumours justifies us in regarding them as formations more or less emancipated from the matrix-tissue. It is true they draw their nutriment from the organism, and cannot continue to grow without its support. In other respects, however, they behave like independent growths isolated from the rest of the organism. It is in this independence or quasi-isolation that the aetiological difficulty really lies. How does the neoplasm thus assume properties distinct from those of its surroundings? We believe that the phenomenon is ultimately due to some change affecting individual elements of a tissue, whereby they are rendered dissimilar to their neighbours. The change is manifested especially in this—that the normal checks to the indefinite growth of the proliferous cells (Arts. 78—83) are inoperative or inadequate; either because the formative and productive energy is increased, or because the restraining influence of the surrounding structures is diminished, or from both causes together.

In the case of tumours appearing in the organism during the stage of development, it is most natural to suppose that the originating cause lies in an increased local growth due to intrinsic conditions: or, it may be, in a disturbance and diversion of the developmental process from its normal course. What the ultimate factors determining these deviations may be we know as little as we do the causes of gigantic overgrowth or local dwarfing of a limb or organ. When the anatomical and physiological relations of the affected tissue are altered to a certain extent by this local change, it would seem as if the tissue had no longer the power to maintain the normal direction in which its development should proceed. The altered relations (such as misplacement, etc.) seem to involve the withdrawal of the limiting and directing influence exerted on the growing tissue by its environing structures. The result is the development of a tissue of abnormal type, a local misformation in the histological as well as the anatomical sense. The tumours whose genesis is probably of this kind are chiefly the connective-tissue growths of childhood. Among epithelial tumours we may also perhaps include the few observed cases of renal and intestinal cancer, and of ovarian adenoma, in infants.

It is thus not impossible that tumours of the developmental

period may arise from causes similar to those which give rise to local malformations in the stricter sense of the term. Arrest of the process by which osteoblastic cells are transformed into bone might thus, for example, give rise to an abnormal formation of tissue such as cartilage, in other words, to enchondroma; or by encouraging an over-abundant cellular growth, to sarcoma.

Tumours arising in a mature tissue are to be explained only by supposing some antecedent alteration over a more or less extensive region of the tissue. This alteration must be of such a kind as to favour the emancipation of the subsequent neoplasm from its matrix-tissue, without at the same time diminishing the neoplasm's own productive power. This last indeed must rather be increased. In this way we may perhaps explain the operation of a traumatic lesion in inducing the growth of a tumour. In special circumstances it is conceivable that such a lesion may fulfil both the essential conditions we have named.

In the case of the connective-tissue growths of later life, it would seem as if increased cell-activity were always a necessary condition for their development. This must presumably always be a condition of tumour-formation in tissues whose cells are replaced but slowly or not at all. The primary impulse which excites the cells to active growth may be derived from some change either in the cells themselves, or in the intercellular substance.

With regard to epithelial tumours, anatomical investigation shows that increased cell-production is not an indispensable prerequisite. In the carcinomata of later life, for instance, it would appear that the origin of the neoplastic growth is to be looked for, not so much in any increased activity on the part of the cells, as in a change of mutual relation between the several constituents of the tissue. THIERSCH has pointed out—that in old age this latter effect may be due to certain retrogressive changes which then make their appearance. In the corium, for instance, such changes lead to a loosening of its texture, and so modify the relations of the epithelial cells to the fibrous tissue. This modification may make itself felt in one of two directions. In the first place, the epithelium, always in process of decay and replacement, may in the course of its physiological growth and multiplication penetrate to regions which are normally devoid of epithelium. Loosening and displacement affecting the fibrous basis of an organ may give rise to something like fissures or spaces with free surfaces, and into these the contiguous epithelium may readily penetrate and grow. The first sproutings or outgrowths of glandular or lining epithelium may conceivably take place in this manner. We might fairly expect that the fibrous structures would as it were rise up against the intruder, and attempt to eliminate it as a foreign substance. This may well happen in many cases, and then the further advance of the process will be checked. In other cases it does not happen, probably because the invaded tissue is no longer in its normal or healthy state. We have indeed evidence of vascular alteration, infiltration of leucocytes, and even of new-formation of vessels and fibrous tissue; but this, the normal eliminating process, is feeble and sluggish, and is inadequate to deal with the intrusive epithelium. The vascular changes and the increased afflux of nutriment tend rather to react favourably upon the epithelium, and to foster its reproduction. It becomes gradually more and more active—and so the foundation of a carcinoma is laid.

It seems not improbable that the process of neoplastic development does in fact occasionally pursue this general course. In other instances, it may well be that the fibrous basis-substance has a certain intrinsic predisposition favouring the formation of cancer, while the primary impulse which brings this into play is afforded only by some increase of formative activity on the part of the epithelial cells.

The instructive discussion on the nature of cancer reported in the *Trans. Path. Soc.* 1874 should be consulted in this connexion. For an exposition of the constitutional theory, which makes cancer a specific blood-disease, see PAGET, *Surg. Path.* Lects. 34, 35. See also PAGET and MOORE, *Holmes's Syst. of Surg.* vol. I; WILKS, *Guy's Hosp. Rep.* 1872.

SECTION VII.

PARASITES.

CHAPTER XXIX.

GENERAL CONSIDERATIONS.

182. A **parasite** is a living organism inhabiting another living organism, and deriving its nutriment either from the tissues or from the food-supply of its host. The parasites inhabiting man are some of them animal, and some of them vegetable. If they inhabit the superficial parts of the skin or mucous membrane they are called **ectozoa** (or epizoa), if animal, and **epiphytes**, if vegetable: if they inhabit the deeper structures they are **entozoa** and **entophytes**, respectively. The parasitic animals occurring in man belong to the classes of Arthropoda, Scolecida (embracing the Platyelminthes and Nematoidea), and Protozoa. The vegetable parasites are all of them Fungi, and belong to the subdivisions Schizomycetes (bacteria), Blastomycetes (yeasts), and Hyphomycetes (moulds).

The various parasites are of very various importance. Many of them produce no perceptible injury to the tissue in which they lie. Others produce very serious local changes, but have no power to extend their influence to remote tissues. Others invade the system, so to speak, and migrating in various directions produce multiple local affections. Many are conveyed throughout the body by the blood or lymph, in which case serious general affections and frequently death itself are the result. The great majority of parasites, and especially the vegetable parasites, increase and multiply within the body, often to an enormous extent. Others, chiefly the animal forms, pass only a part of their existence within the body. The local changes they produce are generally confined to the mechanical compression and destruction of tissue, and to the setting up of inflammation. They affect the system as a whole by abstracting nutriment and oxygen from it, and by giving rise to multitudes of centres of disturbance; while many of them generate actual poisons. The Schizomycetes or Bacteria play the most important part of all. It is they of all the parasites that have most power of exciting general or systemic affections. The Blastomycetes and Hyphomycetes, fungi akin to the yeast-fungus and mould-fungus respectively, exert a merely local influence. The animal parasites become dangerous in virtue of their size or multitude, or by penetrating into vital organs.

Parasitism is an extremely common mode of life throughout the organised world. Innumerable plants and animals are parasitic either for a season or for the whole course of their life. Accordingly there are few living organisms that are not inhabited by parasites. A plant or animal which merely inhabits the body of an organism is not necessarily a parasite. The term is only applicable to organisms nourished at the expense of their host.

CHAPTER XXX.

THE SCHIZOMYCETES OR BACTERIA.

Morphology, Development, and Classification.

183. The Schizomycetes or Schistomycetes, frequently included under the general term **Bacteria**, belong to the Protophytes—the smallest and simplest of all plants. Many of them are so small that they approach the limit of visibility, even when the highest powers of the microscope are used. When they occur in animal tissues they are to be distinguished only with great difficulty, and by special methods. Special reagents or staining processes must be employed; sometimes certainty is only reached by experimental cultivation of the products of disintegration of the tissue in question. That they do occur in animal tissues is now established beyond all doubt. Their growth and multiplication have been experimentally demonstrated.

The Bacteria are all of them unicellular organisms devoid of chlorophyll: they are often however aggregated into larger or smaller colonies. COHN has classified them according to their form into **Sphaerobacteria** (globular cells), **Microbacteria** (minute rod-like cells, Bacteria proper), **Desmobacteria** (larger rod-like or filiform cells, Filobacteria), and **Spirobacteria** (twisted or spiral cells). Movements are noticed in the three latter forms; their protoplasm is therefore contractile. Neither potash, ammonia, nor dilute acids destroy them, so it is probable that they possess a bounding membrane. Bacteria grow longitudinally: new cells are formed by transverse subdivision. These remain in connexion with each other, or become detached.

VON NENCKI'S researches (*Journ. f. prakt. Chem.* 1879, *Beiträge zur Biologie der Spaltpilze* 1880) go to show that the bacteria are composed of a peculiar albuminoid body which he has called mycoprotein. They contain only the minutest quantities of bodies resembling cellulose.

The above classification of the Bacteria is taken from COHN (*Beiträge zur Biologie der Pflanzen* vol. I; *Q. Journ. M. S.* 1873, 77, 79), and his work has been mainly followed in the next four paragraphs. He makes the following remarks on the general question of classification:—"I have come to the conclusion that the Bacteria are as capable of exact specific classification as other plants. They lie at the limit of microscopic visibility. In the minuter forms it is therefore impossible to make out either structure or organisation. The size and shape of the cells, and the mode in which they are combined into colonies, are then the only *differentiae:* of these however it is not always easy to say whether they indicate original specific distinctions, or whether they depend on external conditions and lie within the limits of variability of one and the same species. Size is the easiest feature on which distinctions may be based, though even this is by no means easy to determine in the minuter forms. Differences in the mode of reproduction are only discoverable in the higher forms, such as the Bacilli. The genera of Bacteria have not the same significance as those of the higher plants. They are based chiefly on the characters of the vegetative cell-forms, not on the reproductive features. Every form distinguished by prominent or obvious characters is provisionally furnished with a generic name: smaller deviations serve to designate the species. It is thus not at all impossible that some of such species and genera may really represent different developmental stages of one and the same fungus." Since this utterance of COHN's a great number of researches have been made into the growth and multiplication of the Bacteria. KOCH especially has devoted himself to the subject (*Mittheil. a. d. kaiserl. Gesundheitsamte* Berlin 1881). After long-continued experiments on cultivation, in which bacteria were bred in nutritive gelatine ('the dry process') he has reached the conclusion—that each species of bacteria possesses characteristic and easily recognisable peculiarities in respect of structure, form, size, and mode of growth of its colonies on the gelatine.

The Schizomycetes have been very variously named by different authors. PASTEUR speaks of them as *végétaux cryptogames ou microscopiques, animalcules, champignons, infusoires, torulacées, bactéries, vibrioniens, monades, mycoderma, microbes, microsphères, bactériens, bactéridies, etc.* In Germany the terms *Pilze, Monaden, Vibrionen, Mikrozyma* and (by KLEBS) *Mikrospora* and *Monadine* have been used. BILLROTH introduced the term *Coccobacteria*. In England we have corresponding terms, with others like *monads, zymes, microzymes* (SANDERSON), *microphytes, microparasites, saprophytes, germs, etc.*

184. The **Sphaerobacteria** are the smallest of all bacteria. Under the microscope they appear as bright round or ovoid spherules of scarcely measurable size. Two genera are distinguished: *Micrococcus* (Fig. 74, 1) and *Sarcina* (Fig. 74, 15).

The spherules known as micrococci exhibit no perceptible organisation, but it is highly probable that they are differentiated into cell-membrane and cell-contents. They are found in liquids and in tissues either isolated, or arranged like strings of beads or 'chaplets' (Fig. 74, 1*b*), or grouped in colonies (zoogloea, Fig. 74, 2). On examination it is found that in these colonies or zoogloea the separate spherules are united by a gelatinous intercellular substance. COHN affirms that this is nothing but the swollen and thickened cell-membrane. VON NENCKI affirms that it consists of mycoprotein.

With regard to their growth and increase, it is made out that the individual cells first elongate and then subdivide transversely. If the subdivided cells remain conjoined the result is a *diplococcus* (BILLROTH). If the process of subdivision goes on, the new cells remaining attached and in line, chains or chaplets are produced. If large numbers of spherules remain after subdivision within the swollen and continually enlarging membrane, the result is a mass of zoogloea.

The genus *Micrococcus* includes several species. These are distinguished partly by their morphological and partly by their physiological characters. In the first place the micrococci are of various sizes. When cultivated on a proper soil they form colonies of various types. Many of them as they multiply produce yellow, red, blue, green, or brown colouring matters. Lastly, the effects produced in the soil or liquid in which they grow are various; nor do they all flourish on the same kind of nutriment. It is still doubtful whether the micrococci are motile. The oscillatory movements observed in them are probably to be regarded as Brownian or pedetic movements. KLEBS believes that the zoogloea are contractile.

The genus *Sarcina* is very clearly marked. The globular cells divide crosswise, and the daughter-cells usually remain combined in tetrads (Fig. 74, 15). Various species have been distinguished according to the size of the cells.

BILLROTH and KLEBS assert that micrococci may grow into rodlets or bacilli. It is not to be denied that some bacterial spherules become transformed into rods (Art. 185), but COHN is probably right in maintaining that *Micrococcus* is a definite genus of constant form. ZIEGLER has cultivated *Micrococcus luteus*, a bacterium which developes on boiled eggs exposed to the air and forms yellow zoogloea; and though the experiments were carefully made to that end, he could never obtain bacilli, but always micrococci. Experiments on parasitic micrococci seem equally to indicate that there is a genus of bacteria which forms globular cells only. It is not yet certain whether or not the micrococci produce spores. KOCH thinks it unlikely. See also EWART, *Proc. Roy. Soc.* XXVII.

185. The **Microbacteria** are classed together as a single genus *Bacterium*. The principal species are *Bacterium termo* (Fig. 74, 3), and *Bacterium lineola* (Fig. 74, 5). The first appears in the form of minute cylindrical rods, 0·5 to 1·5 micromm. in length, and appearing bright or dark according to the mode of illumination. Sometimes they remain at rest, sometimes move about more or less actively. From their manner of subdivision they are often found coupled in pairs; they do not usually form chains or chaplets; but are often grouped as zoogloea (Fig. 74, 4), which are remarkable for the great abundance of the gelatinous intercellular substance. *B. termo* is very generally found in putrefying matters. *B. lineola* resembles *B. termo*, but it is larger in every way. It is found in water, in infusions, on potatoes, etc. The cells, which are from 3·8 to 5 micromm. in length, contain a clear bright substance interspersed with fine granules. In other respects the bacterium resembles *B. termo*; it swims about actively, moving forwards and backwards in curves, rotating, or oscillating. At times it remains motionless. It forms continuous pellicles on the surface of liquids containing it.

When micrococci or microbacteria have exhausted the nutriment contained in the liquid in which they live, they fall to the bottom as a powdery precipitate.

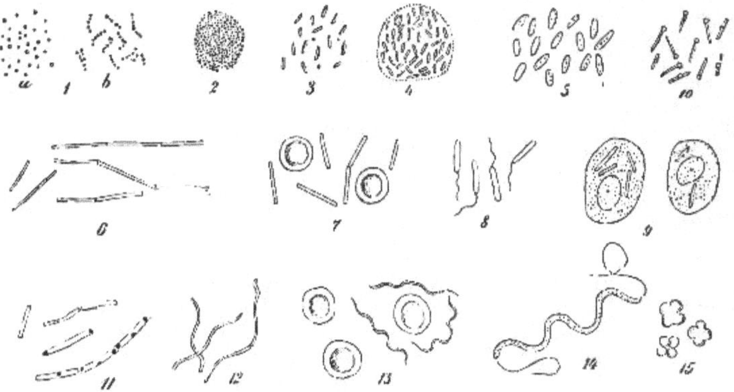

FIG. 74. VARIOUS FORMS OF BACTERIA (× 500 *in each case*)

1, *Micrococcus septicus; a* separate, *b* in chaplets. 2, *Micrococcus diphtheriticus* forming a zoogloea-mass. 3, *Bacterium termo.* 4, Zoogloea of *B. termo.* 5, *Bacterium lineola.* 6, *Bacillus subtilis.* 7, *Bacillus anthracis*, with red blood-cells. 8, Flagellate bacillus from the mouth. 9, *Bacillus leprae* (ARMAUER HANSEN). 10, Bacillus with terminal and medial spores, from a putrefying liquid. 11, *Bacillus malariae* (KLEBS), with spores. 12, *Vibrio serpens* (COHN). 13, *Spirochaeta Obermeyeri* ('spirillum' of relapsing fever). 14, *Spirillum volutans* (COHN). 15, *Sarcina ventriculi.*

As has been indicated in Art. 184, BILLROTH, HALLIER, and KLEBS maintain that the microbacteria represent merely a developmental stage in the life-history of the micrococci. BILLROTH (*Unters. über Coccobacteria septica* Berlin 1874) believes that all bacteria belong to a single species of plants, the members of which are composed partly of round and partly of rod-like segments varying greatly in size. The round segments are the cocci, the rod-like segments bacteria. Each form may pass into the other on occasion; though they so far breed truly that for some generations cocci produce only cocci, and bacteria only bacteria. According to size we may distinguish them as micrococci, mesococci, and megacocci, and microbacteria, mesobacteria, and megabacteria. Megacocci may break up into micrococci. The plant which passes through all these stages BILLROTH calls *Coccobacterium septicum.* In the process of multiplication it developes a gelatinous envelope or gliacoccus. When this occurs at the surface of a liquid so that a pellicle is formed, he calls it petalococcus or petalobacterium. Masses of cocci enclosed in a cylindrical sheath of gliacoccus are called ascococci (VAN TIEGHEM, *Bull. Soc. Botanique* 1880). Coupled spherules are diplococci; chains or chaplets of spherules, streptococci: and in like manner he describes diplobacteria, and streptobacteria. RAY LANKESTER (*Q. Journ. M. S.* 1873) also inferred from certain experiments of his that COHN's forms are not really distinct. HABERKORN (*Bot. Centralb.* 10, 1882) maintains that COHN's four divisions merely represent diverse species of a single genus. BILLROTH's view of the specific unity of all the bacterial forms has been discredited by later researches (*cf.* TIEGEL, *Virch. Arch.* vol. 60; LISTER, *Trans. Roy. Soc. Edin.* 1875).

KLEBS (*Arch. f. exp. Path.* IV) divides the globular and rod-like bacteria into *Microsporina* and *Monadina.* He defines the *Microsporina* as small micrococci which in the resting state form well-defined and compacted balls, the several spherules being regularly deposited in layers and surrounded by only a small quantity of gelatinous matter. The peripheral spherules grow into minute motile bacteria, which tend to move away from the mass, and thus further the diffusion of the organisms through the nutrient liquid. The highest stage of their development is reached in the formation of a matted tuft of unbranched filaments. The monadina form loose balls, from which motile monads or vibrios break away. These grow into rodlets which are relatively short and broad; and these again subdivide; they probably increase also by conjugation. They then pass into a resting state, and lie quietly alongside each other. Lastly they break up into spherules; it is rare for them to form tufts or clusters. They require oxygen, and thrive better on albumen than on gelatine.

It is not yet certainly known whether *Bacterium termo* produces spores or not. It has been described as possessing *flagella* by DALLINGER and DRYSDALE (*Month. Mic. Journ.* XIV), and by KOCH (*Beiträge zur Biol.* 1877).

186. The **Desmobacteria** (or Filobacteria) are cylindrical rodlets of varying length; some of them are thick, and some slender and delicate. COHN describes a straight form which he calls *Bacillus*, and a wavy or curved form which he calls *Vibrio*. *Bacillus* increases by transverse subdivision, and frequently forms a long string (Fig. 74, 6) commonly referred to as a *leptothrix* (HALLIER). It is not always easy to make out that the string is made up of distinct rodlets. In other cases bacilli form swarms. Many bacilli pass through both a resting state and a swarming state. Many are provided with a flagellum or cilium, which acts as an organ of locomotion (Fig. 74, 8). The best representatives of this genus at present known are *B. subtilis* (Fig. 74, 6), *B. anthracis* (Fig. 74, 7), *B. tuberculosis* (Fig. 80), and *B. leprae* (Fig. 74, 9). The various specific forms are distinguished by their general size, and by the relation of their length to their breadth. Some of them are cut off square at the ends, others are rounded off or pointed. Even more marked differences than these become apparent when the various forms are cultivated in nutrient liquids. 'Cultures' of this kind have been made by COHN, KOCH, KLEBS, BREFELD, PRAZMOWSKI, LISTER, NAEGELI, BUCHNER, KLEIN, and many others, and we have thus come to know something of the life-history of many of the varieties. COHN bred the *B. subtilis* in hay-infusions; KOCH the *B. anthracis* found in the blood and tissues of animals suffering from splenic fever; and also the *B. tuberculosis* (Art. 206).

The life-histories of the different species differ in many details; but they usually agree in their main features. Features which thus constantly recur are—the longitudinal growth of the rodlets, their transverse subdivision and abstriction, and the formation of spores or gonidia. The life-history of *B. anthracis* is briefly as follows.

If the anthrax-bacillus be observed under proper conditions, it is found in a short time to grow lengthwise to a very considerable size (Fig. 75 *b*). Within twenty-four hours a string or filament is formed (Fig. 75 *c*), which may be ten or twenty times as long as the original rodlet. In ten or fifteen hours more the clear contents of the filament become granular. Then appear at regular distances small darker bodies, which grow in a few hours into larger highly refracting spores (Fig. 75 *d*). The

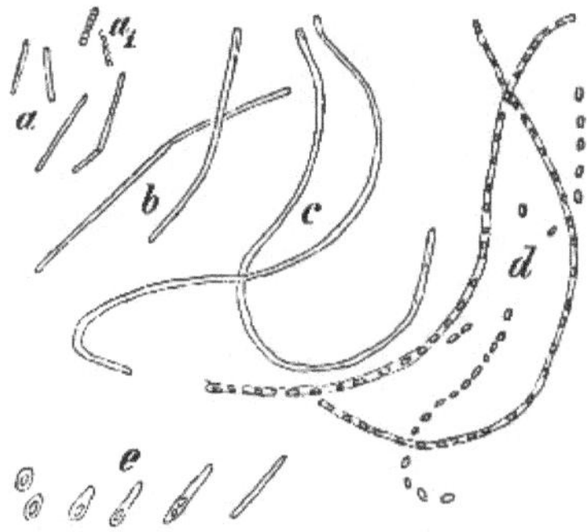

FIG. 75. DEVELOPMENT OF *BACILLUS ANTHRACIS*. (*From* KOCH: × 400)

a bacilli from the blood
a_1 dead bacilli
b bacilli cultivated for three hours,
c for ten hours,
d for twenty-four hours; spores are forming and the filaments are breaking up
e germination of spores

filaments afterwards break up, and the spores are set free. In favourable circumstances these spores may germinate and develope into bacilli exactly like those originally taken from the blood.

According to KOCH, each spore consists of a bright body surrounded by an envelope of clear protoplasm. As the spore germinates the latter grows into a rodlet (Fig. 75 *e*). The researches of KLEIN, BREFELD, PRAZMOWSKI, EWART, and others do not corroborate this account. They make out that the spore consists of protoplasm enclosed in a membrane. The rudimentary bacillus is developed not from the peripheral layer of the spore, but from its protoplasmic centre.

In addition to this mode of increase by spore-formation observed in cultivated bacilli, the rodlets multiply by transverse subdivision. This is especially the case in the blood of living animals.

As we have said, all bacilli have the power of forming spores. It is not however essential to the process that long filaments should be formed. Many bacilli produce spores without having undergone any marked increase in their length. The number of spores in each rodlet varies from one to three. They may occupy either a terminal or a medial position (Fig. 74, 10 and 11).

Anthrax-bacilli cultivated on gelatine are never motile (KOCH): they always form flakes or tufts made up of long wavy tress-like or twined filaments. The bacilli of hay-infusion grow out into long filaments in very young colonies only. When they become more mature and cause the gelatine to liquefy, they are seen in active movement at the centre of the colony, while round its periphery they stand in regular array all perpendicular to the surface and penetrating the firmer gelatine. The colony then looks as if it were surrounded by an aureole of rays. Other bacilli form colonies looking like tufted roots of trees: others again spread out in one plane and form mosaic designs.

COHN's and KOCH's researches are published in the *Beiträge zur Biologie d. Pflanzen* vol. II, and *Mittheil. a. d. kais. Gesundheitsamte* Berlin 1881: BREFELD's are in the *Botan. Zeitung* 1878, and in *Botan. Unters. über Schimmelpilze* 1881: KLEIN's, SANDERSON's, and EWART's in the *Quart. Journ. Micros. Science* 1878. PRAZMOWSKI asserts (*Unters. über d. Entwick. einiger Bacterien* Leipzig 1880) that the germination of the spores of *B. subtilis* follows a different course to that of *B. anthracis*. The mature spore is oval, highly refracting, sharply defined, and surrounded by a transparent zone. On germination the spore becomes pale, and loses its lustre and its sharp contour. At each pole a kind of shading appears, the spore meanwhile beginning to move in a tremulous manner. After a time the contents escape laterally in the form of a minute cylindrical shoot, which grows into a rodlet; and this latter then proceeds to subdivide.

PRAZMOWSKI has also made out the life-history of the so-called *Clostridium butyricum* (PASTEUR's *vibrion butyrique*, VAN TIEGHEM's *Bacillus amylobacter*). It forms rodlets 9—10 micromm. long, which are seen alternately at rest and in moving swarms. Before fructification they increase in thickness and become more fusiform or pear-shaped. On germination the spore swells and begins to jerk about. The membrane at one end is absorbed, the germinal cylinder escapes, and as it grows proceeds to subdivide as before.

KERN describes a bacillus under the name of *Dispora Caucasica* (*Biolog. Centralb.* 5, vol. II) much resembling *B. anthracis*; it is however distinguished from the latter by its always exhibiting terminal spores at each end of the rodlets. When cultivated in milk this bacillus sets up a peculiar fermentation, which produces an agreeable drink much used in the Caucasus.

BREFELD distinguishes an external spore-membrane or exosporium which is thrown off in germination, and an internal or endosporium which becomes the envelope of the germinal cylinder.

With regard to the term *leptothrix* it is to be noted that all filaments or strings so named do not necessarily represent developmental stages of a bacillus. The filaments formed by algae, for example, are also spoken of as *leptotriches*.

187. The **Spirobacteria** are divided into two genera—*Spirochaeta* (Fig. 74, 13) with long flexible close-wound spirals; and *Spirillum* (Fig. 74, 14) with short stiff open spirals. For the pathologist, *Spirochaeta Obermeyeri* (13) and *Spirochaeta denticola* are the most important species of the first genus. The former (often referred to simply as 'spirillum') is constantly found in the blood of patients suffering from relapsing fever, during the paroxysms. The latter is found in the mouth and nose of persons who may be quite healthy or suffering from nasal catarrh. The length of the former is twice or thrice the diameter of a red blood-cell. It moves with extraordinary agility through the blood, and is therefore hard to see unless it be somehow fastened down or restrained. No structure has been made out in it.

No details are known of the life-history of *Spirochaeta*. It plainly increases very rapidly within the body. It probably produces resting-spores.

The largest of all bacteria, *Spirillum volutans*, belongs to the *Spirilla* (Fig. 74, 14). Apart from its size it is distinguished by its granular protoplasm and its pair of flagella. It sometimes moves about actively, sometimes lies quiescent. It is occasionally found in drinking-water. Two smaller forms, *Spirillum tenue* and *Spirillum undula*, also belong to this genus (Art. 207).

Biology of the Bacteria.

188. **Conditions of life.** All bacteria require to be supplied with certain definite nutritive substances if they are to develope normally. The requisite substances are partly inorganic, and partly organic (carbohydrates and albuminoids). The inorganic components are derived from salts containing sulphur, phosphorus, magnesium, and potassium. The requisite carbon and nitrogen are mainly derived from animal and vegetable matters. But bacteria have also the power of assimilating nitrogen from ammonia, urea, or even nitre, provided only the other mineral substances needed are also present, and in addition some appropriate organic carbon-compound, such as sugar.

These nutritive substances must be presented to the bacteria associated with a certain amount of water. None of the bacteria can develope without water, though many of them may be without it for a time and still continue to live. This is especially the case with bacterial spores. If the water contains no proper nutriment, or if the nutriment is already used up, the bacteria cease to develope, and after a time die outright. But here, as when water is lacking altogether, it is possible for the bacteria to maintain life for a time. The spores are still more tenacious of life, and can hold out almost indefinitely. Free oxygen is absolutely necessary to the development of many of the bacteria: others can do without it if they are otherwise favourably placed, and in circumstances where they can set up fermentation. The former kind, *e.g.* *Bacillus anthracis* and *B. malariae* (KLEBS), have been called by PASTEUR **aërobious** fungi. The latter, of which *Bacterium termo* and *Clostridium butyricum* are the best-known examples, are **anaërobious**. Pure oxygen is said to kill bacteria outright.

NÄGELI gives minuter details of the conditions of life of the various bacteria (*Die niederen Pilze* Munich 1877, and *Untersuch. über die nied. Pilze* 1882). PASTEUR, JOUBERT and CHAMBERLAND have papers in the *Gaz. méd. de Paris* 1876 on the relations of bacteria to oxygen. PRAZMOWSKI asserts that so far as concerns *Clostridium* oxygen is not merely unnecessary but positively harmful. *B. anthracis* on the other hand dies if deprived of oxygen, breaking up into rounded fragments. PASTEUR again affirms that the bacillus which gives rise to the 'Pasteurian' septicaemia in rabbits, dies if exposed to the air. According to KOCH (*Mittheil. a. d. k. Gesundheitsamte* Berlin 1881), the anthrax-bacillus perishes if it is allowed to become dry;

while the spores may be preserved for years in the dry state. They may even be kept moist for a time without losing their power to germinate or to produce the specific infection.

189. The **temperature** of the nutrient medium has great influence upon the development of bacteria. If the temperature be lowered, the effect is generally to slow and to weaken the vital processes, and ultimately to put an end to them altogether. As the temperature is raised on the other hand, these processes become more and more active until a certain maximum is reached: carried beyond this point they rapidly and suddenly cease, in most instances not to revive again. The maximum temperature which can be borne by fungi varies in the different species; a few are capable of growth at 70° to 74° C (VAN TIEGHEM). The development of all kinds is stayed at a temperature of 5° C. They become stiff and immobile, but are not absolutely killed even by very extreme degrees of cold. The *rigor frigoris* sets in at different temperatures in different species; in the case of *B. termo* at 5° C, of *B. anthracis* at 15° C. For *B. anthracis* the temperature most favourable to development is 30°—40° C; at 42° C development ceases. *B. termo* developes best between 30° C and 35° C.

All bacteria and all bacterial germs are killed by boiling-hot water or steam, after exposure for a certain time. The spores are much more resistent than the bacteria. In dry air both may endure much higher temperatures. Spores, for instance, are not destroyed at a temperature of 140° C until after three hours' exposure. *B. termo* perishes at 65° C, if the temperature be kept up for a considerable time.

Researches on the effect of temperature on the bacteria and their spores have been made chiefly by EIDAM (*Cohn's Beiträge z. Biologie d. Pflanzen* vol. II), KOCH, WOLFFHÜGEL, GAFFKY, and LÖFFLER (*Mitth. a. d. k. Gesundheitsamte* Berlin 1881), VAN TIEGHEM (*Bull. Soc. Bot.* 1881). The following are the chief results arrived at.

Bacterium termo passes into *rigor frigoris* at 5°, into *rigor caloris* at 40°. At 45° the ordinary putrid decomposition of albuminoids ceases to go on (EIDAM).

Bacillus anthracis multiplies the more slowly as the temperature is lower, within certain limits. Between 30° and 40° growth and spore-formation are completed in twenty-four hours. At 25° this time is increased to thirty-five or forty hours. At 23° the spore-formation occupies forty-eight or fifty hours: at 20° seventy-two hours: at 18° it takes five days, at 16° seven days. Below 15° growth and spore-formation cease (KOCH). Spores are still formed at a temperature of 42°. See also SANDERSON and EWART, *Q. Journ. Mic. Sci.* 1878.

Bacteria without spores when exposed to hot air cannot endure a temperature much over 100° for so long as an hour and a half. The spores of bacilli are only destroyed after three hours' exposure to a temperature of 140°. In the case of objects exposed to heat with a view to disinfection, it is noteworthy that the temperature penetrates very slowly. Objects of moderate size such as bundles of clothing, pillows, etc. are not completely disinfected even when exposed for three or four hours to a temperature of 140° (WOLFFHÜGEL). Anthrax-bacilli perish when exposed to boiling water for two hours; when exposed to steam in a closed space ten minutes suffices. On the other hand the peculiar bacillus found in garden-soil is not destroyed by this exposure. Superheated steam at 105° kills all bacterial germs. A jet of steam is more powerful than steam in a closed chamber. It will kill all kinds of germs in ten to fifteen minutes, and it readily penetrates the articles to be disinfected (KOCH, GAFFKY, LÖFFLER). When using boiling water for disinfecting purposes, care must be taken that the heat is kept up long enough, *i.e.* until all the parts are warmed up to 100°.

The effect of temperature in modifying the virulence of pathogenous bacteria will be referred to later on.

190. Another factor of importance in regard to bacterial development is the **presence of foreign** or non-nutritive **substances** in the nutrient liquid. Many substances (like corrosive sublimate, bromine, iodine, and some acids) have a very powerful effect even in small quantity. They put an end to growth and fermentive action, or kill the organisms outright. Other substances have no injurious effect unless present in considerable quantity.

The fermentive action of the fungi leads to the formation in the nutrient liquid of substances which, when they reach a certain degree of concentration, may ultimately put a stop to the growth and multiplication of the fungi themselves. In alcoholic or lactic fermentation, for instance, the gradually accumulating alcohol or lactic acid ultimately brings the fermentive process to a standstill.

If nutritive matters be present in excess (or if, in other words, the supply of water be inadequate), the growth and multiplication of the fungi ceases in like manner. This is the reason why conserves of fruit made with sugar do not ferment, why condensed milk does not turn sour, and why dried or salted meat does not putrefy. By withdrawing water, or by adding substances which dissolve in the organic liquids, we are able to increase the proportion of solids to liquids in organic substances such as provisions, and so preserve them from decomposition by fungi. The quantity of water necessary for the development of fungi like bacteria and the yeast-plant is greater than in the case of the mould-fungi.

HORWATH'S and REINKE'S researches (*Pflüger's Arch.* XVII, XXIII) show that constant agitation of the liquid hinders the development of bacteria, and may even check their multiplication altogether.

A further factor of importance in bacterial development is the presence of lower orders of fungi in the nutrient liquid. As higher plants often encroach on and interfere with each other, so it is possible for bacteria, yeast-plants, and moulds to interfere and compete with each other for nutriment (NAEGELI). A bacterium, which is thriving and multiplying in a given liquid, may be checked and ultimately killed merely by introducing another fungus which is still more at home in the liquid. Thus if we introduce into a nutrient liquid containing sugar the germs of a number of fungi of different classes, the bacteria alone will multiply and set up lactic fermentation. If a half per cent. of tartaric acid be now added, the yeast-fungi alone will proceed to multiply, and alcoholic fermentation will begin. Add now from four to five per cent. of tartaric acid, and mouldy growths appear. The tartaric acid does not kill the other fungi; it merely favours one more than the others. Thus it is that in grape-must it is only the yeast-fungi which flourish, though other germs are certainly present. Only when the sugar is all used up have the bacteria a chance to multiply, and then they set up acetous fermentation. Mould-fungi may then develope in the presence of the vinegar, and they consume the acetic acid. Lastly, when this is done, the bacteria reappear and set up putrefaction.

Even among the Bacteria themselves a like mutual interference and struggle for existence is observed. Micrococci may be thrust aside by microbacteria. Bacilli may be killed by *Bacterium termo*, when the supply of oxygen is insufficient for both.

It is also a point of importance, when there are various kinds of fungus-germs present, to know which kind is most abundant. If the soil be equally well adapted for two or more forms, the form represented by the majority of germs will have the advantage.

KOCH and WOLFFHÜGEL have made very careful investigations into the action of various substances on the life and multiplication of bacteria. (*Mittheilungen &c.* 1881). The subject has also been treated by BUCHHOLTZ (*Arch. f. exp. Path.* IV), SCHOTTE and GÄRTNER (*Deutsche Viertelj. f. öff. Gesund.* XII 1880), NÄGELI (*Die niederen Pilze* Munich 1877 and 1882), ROBERTS (*Phil. Trans.* 1874), HAMLET (*Journ. Chem. Soc.* 1881), and many others. The following results of investigation are worthy of note.

Corrosive sublimate has the most powerful effect on bacteria: an aqueous solution of 1 : 20,000 kills the spores of bacilli in ten minutes. A solution of 1 : 5,000 is thus a certain disinfectant, even when the time of exposure is very short. Mercuric sulphate is somewhat less active. KOCH finds that an aqueous sublimate-solution of 1 : 300,000 puts a stop to the germination of bacterial spores.

Sulphurous acid does not take a high place as a disinfectant. Bacteria clinging to dry objects are killed by twenty to thirty minutes' exposure to an atmosphere containing 1 vol. per cent. of sulphurous acid. Spores of *B. subtilis* and *B. anthracis* are still capable of development after ninety-six hours' exposure to an atmosphere containing 5 to 6 vols. per cent. of sulphurous acid. Even when moist they are very hard to kill with it. It is thus an altogether untrustworthy disinfectant, and all the more because it has little power of penetrating compact masses or bundles (WOLFFHÜGEL, BUCHHOLTZ, SCHOTTE and GÄRTNER, KOCH, BUCHNER).

Carbolic acid in 5 per cent. solution will kill the spores of the anthrax-bacillus in twenty-four hours. A 3 per cent. solution will not do so in the same time. The bacilli however are killed in a few minutes even by a 1 per cent. solution. A solution of 1 : 400 checks the development of bacterial spores. Vapour of carbolic acid at ordinary temperatures is without effect; at 55° C it kills spores in two or three hours (KOCH, *loc. cit.*; DE LA CROIX, *Arch. f. exp. Path.* XIII). Chloride of zinc in 5 per cent. solution has no effect on anthrax-spores—even when they have lain in it for a month (KOCH).

Iodine, bromine, and **chlorine** are far more active than sulphurous acid. Bacilli cease to grow in presence of iodine in the proportion of 1 : 5,000, and of bromine of 1 : 1,500. Steam from bromine-water kills spores in twenty-four hours, from chlorine-water in two days. Iodine-water and chlorine-water kills spores in one day, a 5 per cent. solution of chloride of lime in ten days.

Benzoic acid, sodium benzoate, potassium chlorate, and quinine have little effect on spores. The following substances even in dilute solution have a restraining influence on bacterial development—allylic alcohol; oils of mustard, peppermint, turpentine, and cloves; thymol; chromic, picric, hydrochloric, and salicylic acids; quinine. The effect is perceptible in solutions of 1 : 300,000 for oil of peppermint, of 1 : 800 for quinine, of 1 : 75,000 for oil of turpentine.

All disinfecting agents should be used in aqueous solution. In alcohol or oil they are either inactive or enfeebled. Bacillus-spores still retain their power to germinate after lying for months in absolute alcohol. In water and in glycerine they may lie for weeks undestroyed.

Bacteria become less able to resist heat in presence of small quantities of acid. They are made more resistent by alkalies. For the effect of light on their development see ENGELMANN, *Rev. internat. Sci. biol.* 1882.

191. **Influence on the nutrient liquid.** In the first place the bacteria, as they grow and multiply, withdraw from the nutrient liquid the elements they require for building up their cells. These elements are chiefly nitrogen, carbon, hydrogen, and oxygen, as also the mineral constituents mentioned in Art. 188. In the next place they set up marked chemical changes in the nutrient liquid. It is bacteria which superinduce putrid decomposition in albuminoid bodies; they transform sugar into lactic acid (as in soured milk); lactic acid into butyric acid (as when sourkrout ferments, or butter becomes rancid); sugar into a gum-like slime (as in 'slimy' or 'long' wine); and alcohol into acetic acid. Large quantities of material may in this way be very rapidly transformed.

When albuminoids undergo putrid decomposition, we have formed peptones and similar bodies; a certain putrid principle or poison (PANUM), and bodies resembling ferments; sepsin (BERGMANN and SCHMIEDEBERG); nitrogenous bases, like leucin and tyrosin; amines like methylamine, ethylamine, propylamine; fatty acids, like formic acid, acetic acid, propionic acid, butyric acid, valerianic acid, palmitic and stearic acids, lactic acid, succinic acid, etc.; aromatic matters, indol, phenol, cressol, pyrocatechin, hydroquinone, hydroparacuminic acid, and paroxyphenylacetic acid (VON NENCKI, SALKOWSKI, BRIEGER); and lastly sulphuretted hydrogen, ammonia, carbonic anhydride, and water. These products are the result partly of hydration, partly of reduction, and partly of oxidation.

The immediate cause of the process is unknown. NAEGELI (*Die niederen Pilze* 1877), PASTEUR, LISTER, and others regard the decomposition as the direct result of the vegetation of the bacteria. Decomposition and fungus are inseparable: the one ceases when the other is removed. Processes of this nature, set up by bacteria, are best distinguished as **fermentations**. Considered with respect to their property of setting up fermentation, bacteria are often described as 'formed' or 'organised' ferments. Bacteria have also the power of setting free certain substances which have a decomposing action like themselves, but are capable of separation from them, and are known as 'unorganised' ferments. Such unorganised ferments can, for instance, change lactose into fermentable sugar, transform starch and cellulose into grape sugar, and render soluble coagulated albumen and other insoluble albuminoids. In consequence of such changes milk may undergo alcoholic fermentation, wood may become soft and rotten, damp bread turn sour, and insoluble albuminous matters be transformed into a putrid ammoniacal slime.

Under the influence of bacteria are also developed certain bitter, acrid, and nauseous products of whose composition nothing is known (as when milk turns bitter). Now and again colouring matters are produced by them, red, yellow, green, blue, and violet. So bread may become covered with a blood-red film of *Micrococcus prodigiosus* ('bleeding' bread). Bandages and pus in wounds become blue from the presence of *Micrococcus cyaneus.* Boiled eggs exposed to moist air are often quickly covered over with a yellow film of *Micrococcus luteus.*

The hypotheses proposed to explain fermentation, especially the alcoholic fermentation, have been very various. Some of them attempt to connect the process intimately with the vital activity of the cells which give rise to it; others seek to separate them. LIEBIG describes the process as a molecular motion transmitted by matter (the unformed ferment) already in a state of chemical motion (*i.e.* in the act of decomposing) to other matters composed of elements in loose combination. HOPPE-SEYLER and TRAUBE (*Pflüger's Archiv* XII 1875, and *Physiologische Chemie*) imagine that the cells secrete certain unformed ferments, which produce decomposition by mere contact (or catalytically), without themselves taking part in the chemical changes they set up.

PASTEUR (*Annal. de Chimie et de Phys.* 58, 64; *Comptes Rendus*, 45, 46, 47, 56, 80; *Studies on Fermentation* London 1879; DUCLAUX's *Ferments et Maladies* Paris 1882) regards fermentation as immediately dependent on the activity of the living cells. Fermentation begins only when the supply of free oxygen to the cells is restricted. They then begin to abstract oxygen from the compounds contained in the nutrient liquid, and so disturb their molecular equilibrium.

NÄGELI's physical (or molecular) theory (*Abhand. d. bayr. Akad. math.-physic. Cl.* XIII, p. 76, 1879) supposes that the natural motions of the molecules and atoms of the various constituents of the living cell-protoplasm are transmitted mechanically to the fermenting matter. The protoplasmic constituents remain chemically unchanged, but the molecular equilibrium of the fermenting matter is disturbed, and disintegration results. NÄGELI's theory emphasises strongly the dependence of the fermentive process on the life of the cells, and is thus in harmony with our general view that all vital processes are ultimately cellular.

The power of exciting fermentive decomposition in nutrient liquids is very probably possessed not merely by bacteria and yeast-cells but also by the cells of higher organisms, as of man. VOIT (*Physiologie des Stoffwechsels* Leipzig 1881) refers the disintegration of the soluble albumen circulating through the system to fermentive action of the tissue-cells. PASTEUR has shown that in proper conditions fruits and leaves may exhibit fermentive properties.

The chemical changes occurring in the putrid decomposition of the albuminoids have been studied by NENCKI, SALKOWSKI, BRIEGER, and HILLER. See HILLER, *Die Lehre von der Fäulniss* Berlin 1879; NENCKI, *Zersetzung der Gelatine und des Eiweisses bei der Fäulniss mit Pancreas*

Berne 1874, and articles in the *Journ. für prakt. Chemie*, *Journ. für physiol. Chemie*, and *Bericht. d. deutsch. chemisch. Gesell.* 1876—82; SALKOWSKI, articles in the *Bericht. d. d. chem. Ges.* and *Zeitsch. f. physiol. Chem.* of the last year or two; BRIEGER, *Zeitsch. f. physiol.* Chem. II, III, IV, and *Zeitsch. f. klin. Med.* III; GAUTIER and ÉTARD, *Comptes Rendus* 1882.

The quantity of oxygen present has an important influence on the products formed in bacterial decomposition. PASTEUR asserts that fungi which grow in presence of oxygen set up chiefly oxidative changes. Those which can multiply in the absence of oxygen give rise to non-oxidative decompositions. HOPPE-SEYLER (*Ueb. d. Einfluss des Sauerstoffes auf Gährungen* Strasburg 1881) supports this view by his observation that when oxygen is abundantly supplied to the yeast-plant the disintegration of sugar into alcohol and carbonic anhydride is retarded, and volatile acid bodies are produced in abundance. If bacteria in an albuminous liquid be well supplied with oxygen, products like indol, hydroparacumaric acid, and sulphuretted hydrogen (which are largely formed when oxygen is wanting), entirely disappear. The oxygen oxidises them as they are produced; the primary products of the fermentation at once undergo further change.

On pigment-producing bacteria see COHN and SCHROETER, *Beiträge z. Biol. d. Pflanzen* vol. I.

192. Fermentation and putrefaction can only take place in the presence of the corresponding fungi, and the amount of decomposition produced depends on the quantity of fungi present. It does not however follow that each kind of decomposition is due to a single specific fungus, nor that one fungus may not give rise to more than one kind of decomposition. We cannot as yet define with certainty the kinds of decomposition which correspond to each species of fungus. We know however that ordinary putrid decomposition occurs under the action of *Bacterium termo;* while COHN asserts that micrococci do not give rise to putrid change, but to changes of another kind. The butyric fermentation is said to be chiefly due to the presence of *Clostridium butyricum.* Anthrax-bacilli generate ammonia in the nutrient liquid. In most putrefying substances we find bacteria of several species.

NAEGELI affirms that it is possible by cultivation so to alter the properties of a bacterium that it no longer has the power to produce the changes originally associated with it; while it assumes the power of calling forth fermentations of a different kind. Thus the bacterium which produces the lactic acid fermentation may, he says, be cultivated in saccharated extract of meat in such a way that at first it produces in milk an ammoniacal decomposition only; and it does not resume its power of generating lactic acid until after several generations. If this be so we may perhaps infer that within certain limits the physiological properties of a bacterium may be transmuted: or at least that, by change of condition, one or other of several potential functions may be called into activity. The statements have not however been sufficiently confirmed.

We have said that fermentation and putrefaction are always due to fungi; but we do not thereby deny that other kinds of decomposition may affect organic substances in which fungi play no part. Such changes do in fact occur. They usually take the form of slow oxidation or combustion, in which carbonic anhydride, water, and (in nitrogenous substances) ammonia, are formed. Such slow changes are set up when organic matters are in contact with water and atmospheric air. They also of course occur in the living organism. In dead organic matters the process corresponds in part to what is called 'dry rotting' or 'mouldering'.

BRIEGER (*Zeitsch. f. klin. Med.* III) thinks that the various aromatic products of the putrefaction of albumen are equally well obtained whether it is set up by the addition of sewer-mud or of pancreas. The essential factors are the duration of the putrefactive process, the temperature, and the amount of oxygen present. The albuminoids undergo the same changes in the intestine as they do in artificial putrefaction brought about outside the body. The same series of changes are also set up in putrid pleurisy and bronchitis, and in pulmonary gangrene.

193. **Bacteria without and within the body.** If the facts already cited be duly considered, it will appear very probable *a priori* that the diffusion of the bacteria is enormously wide. Matters on which they can grow and thrive are found almost everywhere. We might especially expect to find them wherever dead organic substances occur, either in solution or at least associated with a certain amount of water. This expectation is fully confirmed by experience. Bacteria are found in all waters whether flowing or stagnant, in all liquids that can ferment or putrefy, and in all vegetable and animal tissues that are sufficiently moist.

KOCH'S researches have shown that the surface soil or mould is extraordinarily rich in bacterial germs. It is surprising to learn that these are chiefly the germs of bacilli; but micrococci are also found. In soils soaked with midden-runnings the micrococci are more numerous than the bacilli. If the soil become very dry, the micrococci disappear while the bacilli persist. This is due to the fact that the resting-spores of bacilli are very tenacious of life. The micro-organisms present diminish rapidly as we go deeper. At the depth of a metre they seem entirely absent. Spring-water coming from a depth contains hardly any.

But we have by no means exhausted the field of their distribution. When liquids containing fungi are violently shaken or broken into spray, the fungi pass into the air. This happens also when such a liquid dries up, or when a solid nutritive substance is broken up or disintegrates. If in the latter cases no substances are present which agglutinate the bacteria into a compact mass, they may pass into the air in immense numbers. Owing to their extreme smallness and lightness (NAEGELI estimates the weight of small moist bacteria at one ten thousand millionth (10^{-10}) of a milligramme) they are carried about by the faintest breath of air. In this way they must of course very often reach and rest on bodies which can offer them no nutriment. But they must also often fall on a fit soil, and then proceed to grow and multiply afresh. Circumstances in general are in fact so favourable to the bacteria that we find them or their germs almost everywhere; but chiefly where the presence of organic matters, moisture, and warmth go to favour their multiplication.

NÄGELI (*Die niederen Pilze* Munich 1877) asserts that fungi can only pass into the air when their nutrient liquids dry up. SOYKA (*Münch. acad. Sitzungsber., math.-phys. Cl.* 1871) has shown that bacteria may be swept out of liquids that contain them by gentle air-currents. BUCHNER (*Ueb. d. Beding. d. Ueberganges von Pilzen in d. Luft u. üb. d. Einathmung derselben, Zur Aetiol. d. Infectionskrankh.* Munich 1881) disputes SOYKA's conclusions. He maintains that even strong currents of air are insufficient to sweep bacteria from a liquid: and that even in the case of dried-up masses containing fungi, the fungi are not set free unless the surface is actually broken. ZIEGLER agrees rather with BUCHNER's view.

NÄGELI further thinks that very slight upward air-currents are enough to prevent floating bacteria from settling down. The condensed watery vapour that surrounds them tends to maintain their buoyancy. Friction also retards their fall. See SOYKA, *Ueb. Canalgase als Verbreiter epidem. Krankh.* and *Ueb. Richtung und Stärke d. Luftzuges in Sielen, Deutsche Viertelj. f. öffent Gesundh.* XIV, 1882; and *Ueb. d. Natur und d. Verbreitung d. Infectionserreger, Zur Aetiol. d. Infectionskrankh.* Munich 1881; NÄGELI, *Untersuch. üb. nied. Pilze* Munich 1882.

WERNICH (*Cohn's Beit. z. Biol. d. Pflanzen* III) has shown that air-currents may sweep off bacteria from moist fungus-masses adhering to the surface of solid bodies. Researches on the bacteria and bacterial germs found in the air have been published by COHN (*loc. cit.*), MIQUEL (*Des bactéries atmosphériques, Gaz. méd. de Paris* 30, 1880), WERNICH (*Virch. Arch.* vol. 79), TYNDALL (*Floating-matter of the air* London 1881); CUNNINGHAM (*Microscopic exam. of air* Calcutta 1874) gives an excellent summary of previous observations. On bacteria and their germs in the soil, see KOCH (*loc. cit.*), and CECI (*Arch. f. exp. Path.* XV).

194. Consideration of the wide-spread occurrence of the bacteria and their peculiar vital properties will already have raised the question whether these micro-organisms may not have the power of exciting more or less grave disturbances in the human system, provided they obtain an entrance into it. We have seen that almost all fluids contain bacteria or their germs, unless they are actually poisonous or are 'sterilised' by appropriate means, such as by boiling. Micro-organisms are also frequently found in solid organic matters. In view of this it would seem that we cannot avoid swallowing numbersof bacteria with our food. Moreover we frequently eat articles which are in a state of partial putridity or fermentation (such as cheese and milk): in this state they of course contain numerous bacteria. The alimentary tract must thus be reached by enormous multitudes of bacteria together with the products of decomposition which they set up.

This is however by no means the only way in which we come into intimate relation with these organisms. The air always contains a greater or lesser number of them. In breathing we draw them into the lungs, and they settle in the bronchi or alveoli.

Lastly, all parts exposed to the air come into contact with bacteria, the unwounded skin as well as the wounded or abraded skin.

What becomes of all these organisms? The greater number undoubtedly pass out of the body again. It is hardly possible that any can penetrate into the deeper tissues through the uninjured skin. Those which settle on the mucous membranes are certainly for the most part not absorbed, but are thrown off after a longer or shorter time. This is however not always the case. Experience shows that, in special circumstances, bacterial invasion of the system may actually start from the mucous membrane.

What is the exception in the case of mucous membranes is the rule in the case of matters inhaled into the lungs. Experiment shows that fine corpuscular or particulate matters are very quickly taken up by the lymphatic capillaries of the lungs, and are so carried into the lymphatic glands, or it may be into the blood. Wounded surfaces are in like manner quick to absorb such corpuscular bodies.

Resuming what we have said, we may put it generally that bacteria of various forms may reach not only the surfaces of the body which are directly accessible from without, but also at times the deeper structures, if circumstances favour their penetration.

The question whether bacteria occur in the healthy body seems easily answered from such general considerations, though it is one which has been much disputed. Bacteria are perpetually entering the body with the food we eat and the air we breathe. They must therefore be at times found in the tissues, especially in places where access is direct. The fact that they are not easy to demonstrate is readily explained. It must be only a small number that can multiply in the tissues they have penetrated; the majority must quickly perish. See NENCKI, *Journ. f. prakt. Chemie* 1879; WEISSGERBER and PERLS, *Arch. f. exp. Path.* VI; ROSENBACH, *Deutsche Zeitsch. f. Chir.* XIII: LEUBE, *Zeitsch. f. klin. Med.* III; STERNBERG, *Stud. Biol. Lab.* Baltimore 1881; LISTER, *Trans. Roy. Soc. Edin.* 1875. LEUBE, LISTER, ROBERTS, and others have been unable to find living bacteria in healthy urine. This would indicate that the greater part of the bacteria which penetrate into the body are destroyed.

195. If the bacteria were inert corpuscular elements incapable of multiplication, we should have little more to say concerning their significance to the human organism. We should merely have to point out that they are in part taken into the body at certain points, are carried about hither or thither within it, are deposited here or there as innocuous substances, and sooner or later are destroyed or cast out again through the liver, kidney, or other secreting organ. As a fact this is what really happens with regard to some of the bacteria. Even when they pass through the bronchial glands from the lungs into the blood, they have no more significance than any other like minute foreign matters, such as occasionally circulate in the blood without causing disturbance. These are simply deposited and destroyed, or excreted. Thus the *Micrococcus luteus* may be introduced in considerable quantity beneath the skin of a rabbit, without inducing any serious affection either of the tissue or of the system generally. The bacteria which are thus innocuous may easily be indicated from previous considerations. They are such as cannot find within the human body the conditions favourable to their development.

This is unfortunately not the case with all bacteria. There are some which find their appropriate soil in the perfectly healthy organism, and in it they grow and multiply. Others are unable to settle in a perfectly healthy body; they can only develope when the physico-chemical constitution of the tissues is morbidly altered so as to correspond with their requirements.

The forms of bacteria that have the power of gravely affecting the system, whether it be healthy or diseased, are described as **pathogenous bacteria**.

It is manifest from the above that the determination of the vital properties and conditions of the different bacteria is a matter of the greatest importance. This knowledge would enable us to combat earlier the development of bacterial disease, and the injury it produces. It would further give us the necessary hints for preventing its invasion; for we should know where to seek the bacteria and how to destroy them or render them harmless. Our knowledge in this respect is unfortunately still defective. There are but few species of bacteria whose life-history we know with any exactness of detail.

196. The factors which determine the invasion and the course of development of bacteria within the human body are two. On the one hand the bacteria must be endowed with certain vital properties of a special kind: on the other hand there must be a predisposition on the part of the system.

Our present knowledge does not yet allow us to specify accurately the properties which an infective bacterium must possess. We can only say in general—that it must find within the body and in proper combination all the conditions necessary for its growth and multiplication. Thus the temperature of the body must be such as favours its development; it must be able to abstract fit nutriment from the tissues in which it settles; it must nowhere encounter substances which check or injure it.

Investigations into the bacterial affections have shown that very slight chemical changes in the constitution of a tissue are often enough to determine whether a given bacterium can develope in the tissue or not. In other words the significance of this factor of predisposition is greater than it may have appeared at first sight. Now and then of course the predisposition is due to very obvious alterations in the tissues. For instance, we find that many cases of bacterial invasion depend on the formation of a local necrosis or wound, in which the fungus can settle and develope. In other cases some grave disturbance of the circulation may lead to a failure of resistence on the part of the tissue. These instances are however matched by others in which the anatomical basis of the predisposition is beyond our power to discover. We know, for example, absolutely no reason why—of two individuals exposed to the infection of measles, scarlatina, small-pox, typhus, or tuberculosis—the one should be taken with the disease and the other left. The factors which decide the matter in such cases are plainly such as at present escape our notice, either from their apparent slightness, or because they are not such as our tests can discover. Yet they doubtless consist in very real and very special differences in the condition of the tissues. Many of the bacteria can only come to development within the human body on rare occasions, as their usual habitat is without it. Others only meet with fit conditions for their existence and growth within the body, and do not multiply at all without it.

The respective parts played by the inherent properties of the bacterium and the predisposition of the tissues to invasion have been illustrated by many observations both clinical and experimental. If a mass of bacteria of different forms be introduced into an animal's body, some of the forms develope and lead to certain tissue-changes, others perish inert. If a similar mass be injected into an animal of a different kind, the bacteria which develope are not the same as in the first instance. KOCH (*Aetiologie der Wundinfectionskrankheiten* Leipzig 1878, *Traumatic Infective Diseases* London 1880) has shown that there is a fungus which brings certain death to one species of mouse, while it is entirely inactive when introduced into another species of mouse. Mice are highly susceptible to the infection of anthrax; rats enjoy an almost perfect immunity. The poison of 'rabbit-septicaemia' kills rabbits and mice with unfailing certainty; guinea-pigs and rats are unaffected by it; sparrows and pigeons again are highly susceptible. The *spirillum* of human relapsing fever will develope only in monkeys among the lower animals. Animals of the same species but differing in age have different degrees of susceptibility. Young dogs are easily infected with anthrax, old ones are not (KOCH). We cannot at all tell on what circumstances immunity of this kind can possibly rest. Similar examples are easily obtained (Arts. 204, 206). The majority of the infective disorders are in fact limited each to a few species of animals or to a single one.

Differences also exist in respect of the diffusion of the bacteria through the body. The fungus, which in one kind of animal brings about a fatal general disease, may in others produce a merely local and non-fatal disturbance. Even the point of entrance of the bacteria into the body has its importance. A rabbit inoculated with bacteria in the back of the neck may die, while inoculation of the ear is followed by a simple local affection.

ROSSBACH states (*Centralb. f. med. Wiss.* 5, 1882) that injection of papayotin into the vessels is followed by a rapid development of micrococci in the blood, so that in two hours the blood in the heart is found to be swarming with them. The fact is doubtful, but if it be confirmed, it would seem to show that the composition of the blood is so altered by the unorganised ferment that germs can proceed to develope in it which before were unable to do so: in other words, that the action of a chemical substance has called forth a special predisposition.

ROSENBERGER (*Centralb. f. med. Wiss.* 4 and 41, 1882) observed a like result after the injection of sterilised septic blood. The animals died of septicaemia, bacteria being developed. If the injected liquid were really sterilised, we can only interpret the observation as showing that the septic matter so altered the blood and liquids of the animals as to make them predisposed for the development of micro-organisms. The experiments do not however seem quite free from objection. In 1869 SEMNER communicated similar results, which he obtained with the use of sepsin prepared from yeast (*Viertelj. f. wiss. Veterin.* XXXII).

BOSER maintains that the most essential condition for the settlement of bacteria in the body is their adaptation to the quantum of mineral salts present in the blood and tissues. This can hardly be a sufficient condition.

197. The healthy organism is always beset with a multitude of **non-pathogenous bacteria**. They occupy the natural cavities accessible from without, and especially the alimentary canal. They feed on the substances lying in their neighbourhood, whether brought into the body or secreted by the tissues. In so doing they set up chemical changes in these substances.

While the organs are acting normally, these fungi work no mischief to the tissues in which they lie, or to the system generally. The products of decomposition set up by such non-specific micro-organisms are either harmless, or are conveyed out of the body before they begin to be active.

Settlements of this kind may however become of importance, if the bacteria proceed to develope to any unusual extent. This happens when the contents of the natural cavities in question remain unchanged for any great length of time, or when (as in catarrh) the normal secretion undergoes some alteration. The products of bacterial fermentation may then accumulate to an excessive amount, and products may also be formed which do not normally occur. Thus when the contents of the stomach are not passed on, and become as it were stagnant, an abnormally acid fermentation may be set up. If the chyme is retained over-long in the small intestine, the aromatic products of albuminoid putrefaction will gather in excessive quantity. So too we may have decomposition in the stagnating secretions of the bronchi, prepuce, etc. All these changes react harmfully on the tissues and may set up inflammation, not infrequently ending in suppuration and necrosis. Moreover the system in general may suffer by absorption into the blood of the soluble products of decomposition.

The latter contingency is not to be lightly regarded. Though we may partake with impunity of many fermenting or decaying substances as food, we must not think that all the products generated by the non-pathogenous fungi are equally harmless. Highly poisonous substances are formed in many of the bacterial decompositions. One of the most speedily fatal of diseases, septicaemia, is due to poisoning of the system with the products of bacterial putrefaction, or sepsis. 'Cadaveric alkaloids' the poisons of decaying fish, sausage, cheese, mussels, etc. are very probably the chemical products of special forms of putrefaction. We unfortunately know but little, in some cases we know nothing, of the substances which have this poisonous character. BERGMANN and SCHMIEDEBERG have, it is true, prepared their so-called 'sepsin' and PANUM his 'putrid poison,' from decaying substances; but we do not know the composition of these bodies, and they are certainly not the only poisons of the kind.

Putrid or septic poison may be absorbed by wounds as well as by mucous surfaces. Septicaemia, which has just been cited as an instance of septic poisoning, is generally due to wound-infection.

It is due to the absorption of products of bacterial decomposition formed in a wound contaminated by bacteria (Art. 204). This is especially apt to happen when necrosed tissue exists in the wound, for this affords the bacteria a suitable soil for their development.

The poisonous action of putrid matters is fully discussed by HILLER in *Die Lehre von der Fäulniss* Berlin 1879. He gives full references to the literature of the subject. HILLER lays special stress on the fact that in the septic process it is not simply the bacteria themselves that do mischief, it is the products of their action which act so as profoundly to alter or even to destroy outright the tissues exposed to them. If the infection become generalised, it is almost always due to intoxication of the system with unorganised chemical substances.

PANUM'S paper just alluded to is in *Virch. Arch.* vol. 60; BERGMANN'S is a work called *Das putride Gift und die putride Intoxication* Dorpat 1866. WOLFF (*Virch. Arch.* vol. 81) has lately taken up the question. On the absorption of putrid matters by the alimentary canal see SALKOWSKI *Centralb. f. med. Wiss.* 46, 1876, and *Berichte d. chem. Gesells.* X, 1877; NENCKI and BRIEGER, *ibidem*; BRIEGER, *Zeitsch. f. phys. Chem.* II, *Zeitsch. f. klin. Med.* III; BOLLINGER, *Ueber Fleischvergiftung, intestinale Sepsis, und Abdominal-typhus, Zur Aetiol. d. Infection.* Munich 1881.

It is possible that harmless colonies of bacteria may become dangerous if they are removed from their normal seat to other regions. Thus the saliva, when it contains bacteria, may excite violent inflammation if it reaches the bronchi or alveoli of the lungs.

198. **Pathogenous bacteria** have the power of settling, not merely in the ingesta and secretions or in dead tissue, but also in living tissue. This happens chiefly in the mucous membranes and in the lungs. The uninjured skin is protected against invasion by the horny epidermis.

Many of the bacteria can settle in perfectly healthy mucous membranes. In the case of others we must imagine that they do not find a proper soil for their development, unless the mucous membrane is injured or altered. Of course injury or alteration of this kind may serve to make the outer skin, or any other accessible tissue, the starting-point of a bacterial invasion (wound-infection). All that is necessary is that a bacterium should reach a spot that affords the conditions for its development. If this occur, it multiplies and forms colonies or swarms. These may, according to the species of the fungus and the nature of its soil, remain in aggregation forming heaps or masses, or may spread through the tissues. Such a settlement is never without effect on the tissues concerned. The bacteria may force their way into the substance of the constituent elements, and especially into the tissue-cells, which are sometimes found to be crammed with bacteria.

The effect of the invasion is not always at once apparent, even under the microscope. The cells attacked by the fungi often appear quite uninjured: in other instances they are seen to be altered. The epithelial cells swell up (Fig. 76 *c*) and liquefy, or degenerate into flaky homogeneous lumps, or turbid denucleated masses. Often they break down into granular detritus. The nucleus is broken up, or swells and disappears (Fig. 76 c). The fibrous elements of the connective tissue degenerate like the epithelial cells. The ground-substance alters at the same time. It becomes turbid, loses its structure, and ultimately dissolves.

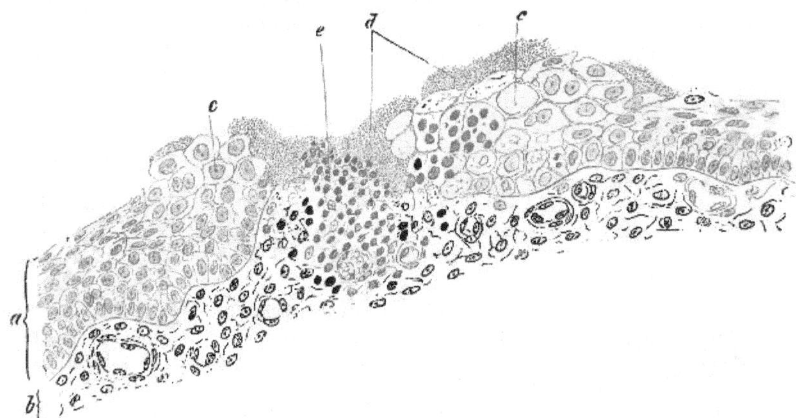

FIG. 76. SECTION CONTAINING COLONIES OF MICROCOCCI FROM THE VOCAL CORD OF A CHILD. (×200)

a epithelium
b connective tissue of the mucous membrane
c swollen degenerated and denucleated epithelial cells
d layer of micrococci
e inflammatory small-celled infiltration of the degenerated epithelium and of the fibrous structures

In general terms we may say—that local settlements of bacteria will sooner or later bring about degeneration and necrosis of the affected tissue. When this may occur, and how widely it may spread, are circumstances depending on the nature of the bacteria and of the tissue.

The processes we have considered are not without their influence on the circulation. The direct action of the bacteria, and the influence of the chemical changes they set up, tell at length on the vessel-walls within the affected region. The result is to disturb the circulation in various ways, chiefly in the way of inflammatory exudation and haemorrhage. In some instances the circulation is stopped altogether, and the preservation of the affected tissue is then impossible.

The inflammatory process set up by bacterial action (Fig. 76 e) may be of very different intensity and extent in different cases. It may be slight and transient, or it may be severe and issue in suppuration and necrosis. Not infrequently a more or less perfect granulation-tissue is formed as a result of the inflammation, as in tuberculosis. The extravasated cells often take up the bacteria into their substance.

199. The inflammation excited by the presence of bacteria often results in a great aggregation of living cells in the tissue affected. These may so act as to repel the continued advance of the fungi, which straightway perish, and the affection issues in healing and cicatrisation. The fixed tissue-cells of the region may likewise act so as to check the development of the bacteria, and may further suffice to make up any loss of tissue by their regenerative activity. If this does not happen the bacterial invasion continues to advance.

The bacteria spread first into the surrounding tissues, passing along the natural lines of division. Then they break into the lymphatics, and often into the blood-vessels also. If they can live in lymph or blood they go on multiplying; if not they perish. Many bacteria, like the micrococcus of erysipelas, flourish best in the lymphatics. Others, like the anthrax-bacillus, are more at home in the blood.

The extent to which the bacteria can spread within the lymphatic system is subject to no general rule. Many of them make a halt at the first gland they come to. Others pass beyond, and finally reach the blood-vessels by way of the thoracic duct. Their path is generally marked by degenerative and necrotic changes, and by the inflammatory reaction they excite. The degree and amount of these changes are determined partly by the nature of the bacteria, partly by their number.

They reach the blood either through the lymphatics or directly. In the latter case the walls of the veins in the invaded region are penetrated by the fungi, or they pass into the veins from the capillaries. Once in the current they are carried on by it to remote parts. Many of them perish in the blood, others again increase and multiply. Of the last some (anthrax-bacillus) thrive best in blood that is flowing; others (tubercle-bacillus, pyaemic micrococcus) prefer blood that is at rest, that is to say, they only

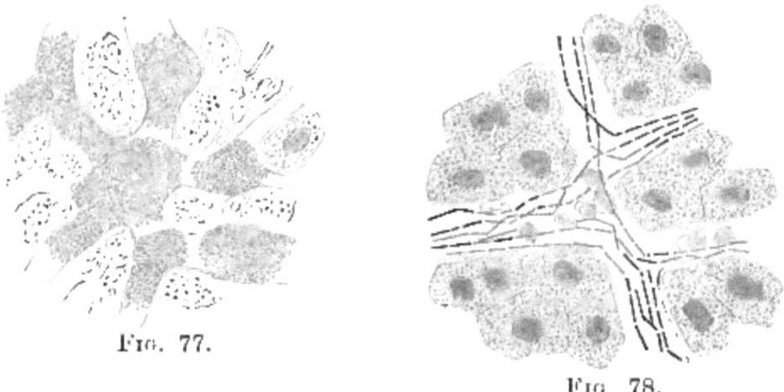

Fig. 77. Fig. 78.

Fig. 77. *Micrococcus septicus* in hepatic capillaries: Necrosis of the liver-cells. (× 350)

Fig. 78. *Bacillus anthracis*: liver-cells unaffected. (× 350)

grow when they have come to a standstill in some venule or capillary. It depends on the properties of the fungus, which of these events takes place; just as do the changes it calls forth in the course of its multiplication.

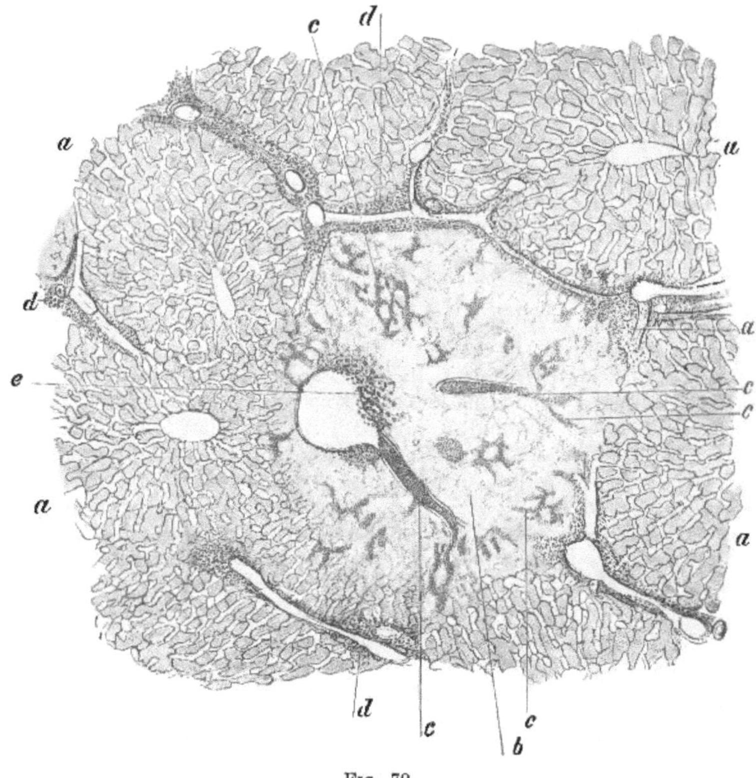

FIG. 79.

FIG. 79. HEPATIC ABSCESS: FIRST STAGE. (*Bismark-brown staining:* × 40)

a normal lobules
b necrosed lobules
c capillaries filled with micrococci
d small-celled infiltration of the interlobular tissue
e aggregation of small round-cells in a vein, into which opens an intralobular venule crammed with micrococci

The tissue-changes are the slightest in the case of bacteria which circulate and multiply in the blood (Fig. 78). Bacteria which settle in the smaller vessels give rise on the other hand to degenerations, necroses (Fig. 77 and Fig. 79 *e*), inflammations (Fig. 79 *d e*), and haemorrhages.

The spot where a lodgement takes place is mostly matter of chance; but it is to be noted that a bacterium may not be able to settle in every spot indifferently. One part of the vascular system may be more favourable to it than another. Many bacteria remain and multiply within the vessels. Others escape from them, and when the surrounding tissue is suitable they may multiply in it, and set up changes resembling those produced at the point of first invasion (as in tuberculosis).

References :—FRISCH, *Exp. Studien über d. Verbreitung der Fäulnissorganismen in d. Geweben* Erlangen 1874; KOCH, *Traumatic Infective Diseases* (Syd. Soc.) London 1880; PERLS, *Lehrb. d. allg. Path.* II.

We should mention with regard to the spread of bacterial infection within the system, that the mode of invasion and the number of the fungi present are points of importance. If mice or guinea-pigs be inoculated beneath the skin with a few oedema-bacilli, the resulting affection is merely local. If the bacilli be numerous the animals die of a general disorder. The bacilli of anthrax and those of 'rabbit-septicaemia' may be injected in small quantity into the ear of a rabbit without causing its death. In the quantity ordinarily used in inoculative experiments they are always fatal.

200. The facts just given (Arts. 198, 199) regarding the spread of bacterial infection within the system are derived from observations on pyaemia, erysipelas, anthrax, and tuberculosis. The greater number of the diseases now referred by many to the action of bacteria (such as typhoid, relapsing fever, diphtheria, the exanthemata, croupous pneumonia, acute atrophy of the liver, cholera, etc.) are as yet too little known to enable us to give the corresponding details for them. We do not exactly know how the poison finds entrance, where it is multiplied, and in what manner it spreads. We only know that in these affections we find at certain times in the blood or tissues definite bacterial forms; and we believe that they are the exciting cause of the disease. If this belief be correct, we must admit that many kinds of bacteria have the power to penetrate into the blood and other juices without leaving any traces at the point of entrance. This supposition is confirmed by the fact that in anthrax we are often unable to detect the point of entrance of the bacilli. In the case of these diseases we must likewise assume, as in the case of the others, that the bacteria find access through the mucous membranes or lungs, or through open wounds if any exist. Once the bacteria have entered the body they multiply in the blood or in some tissue, spread through the system, and call forth the special changes characterising the several diseases. It is worthy of remark that each poison has a corresponding special group of tissues, in which its mischievous effects are invariably and especially apparent. The anatomical changes produced in these diseases as in the others are of the nature partly of degeneration and necrosis, partly of inflammation or haemorrhage. Proliferous changes in the tissues may also ensue as secondary to the former.

201. We are not yet in a position to formulate a **theory of bacterial action** that will apply to all cases. The researches of

the last year or two have however enabled us to form some picture at least of the way in which bacteria affect the several tissues and the system in general.

The pathogenous bacteria are parasites which draw their nourishment from man's body. They withdraw this nourishment only from the tissues among which they are growing and multiplying. The effect of this withdrawal is in general not very grave. It can only become dangerous to life, when the bacteria multiply within the circulating blood and withdraw from it the indispensable oxygen it contains. The withdrawal of nutriment is not however the only result; it is seldom even the most important. Investigations show that the vital activity of the bacteria of necessity sets up extensive chemical change in their own nutrient materials. These changes are partly due to their direct action (Art. 191), partly to the action of the unorganised ferments which they form. Lastly, in the course of these changes matters are produced which act as poisons upon the system. This effect of the bacteria on their nutrient fluids, and the production of poisonous matters, have much more to do with the genesis of the symptoms in most of the microparasitic affections, than has the mere withdrawal of nutriment.

The influence of such factors is manifested in disturbances of the functional, formative, and nutritive activities of the organism. These activities are the expression of the cell-life of the tissues; hence the statement that bacteria disturb the vital actions of the tissue-cells. In Art. 81 we compared the life-history of the tissue-cells with that of the bacteria. We may not inopportunely refer to the comparison once more in this place. The nutritive activity of the tissue-cells is not confined to the replacement of used material by the absorption and assimilation of new material. Like the bacteria the tissue-cells act catalytically on their surroundings, partly by fermentive action (Art. 191), partly by the formation of unorganised ferments. Many cells have in addition the power of setting up synthetic processes.

When bacteria proceed to multiply within a tissue, a double influence is brought to bear on the common nutrient medium; the bacteria enter into conflict with the tissue-cells. We do not of course know in what exact way this conflict is carried on. But we may believe that the bacteria do not communicate to the organic compounds contained in the juices the same kinds of chemical motion as the tissue-cells. They will not therefore give rise to the same chemical changes as the latter. More or less serious disturbance of the normal metabolism of the tissues must ensue.

This is the first effect, but not the only one. Different kinds of fermentation cannot go on in presence of each other for any length of time. One is more and more repressed, and at length suppressed, as the other advances. This cannot of course happen without simultaneous injury to the corresponding ferment. Thus the prolonged presence of bacteria results in the suppression not alone of the nutritive activity, but also of the other functions of the tissue-cells; and at length their life itself is enfeebled or extinguished.

The products of the decomposition set up by the bacteria, the unorganised ferments and other poisons, also give rise to changes in the tissue-cells. It is possible that in many cases they only tend to modify the nutritive activity, *i.e.* the metabolism of the cells; but the other functions are doubtless often affected likewise. These modifications of the normal cell-life in their totality are manifested as disturbances of the functions of the organism, and we speak of them as symptoms of disease.

The mode in which the several symptoms are produced we cannot here stop to discuss. All we need say is that a disturbance of cellular activity is always at the bottom of a morbid symptom: mere alteration in an organic fluid is not enough to give rise to symptoms. Thus the origin of fever cannot be explained otherwise than by assuming the existence of some cellular disturbance. The chief factor in producing the elevation of temperature may be a change in the fermentive action of the cells, or it may be a disturbance of the functions of the central nervous system. That is a question which is open to discussion; but it does not touch the question of the ultimately cellular nature of the febrile process.

Inflammation itself is only to be explained by cellular change. In bacterial affections, inflammation appears as a specially beneficent process. By it a number of living cells are thrown out at the seat of danger, and they are the readiest instruments for checking the harmful influence of the fungi.

The issue of a bacterial affection is either the death of the patient, or the death and elimination of the bacteria. In the former case the bacteria interfere with the functions of cells so numerous or so essential to life, that life becomes impossible. In the latter case the tissue-cells gain the upper hand in the struggle for nourishment and existence, and the bacteria are at length deprived of the conditions essential to their continued life.

Observations on the infective diseases of man and on experimentally-produced bacterial diseases in animals have shown that a disease of the kind successfully withstood often leaves the tissues in a peculiarly unsusceptible condition. This condition may endure for months or years, and it ensures an immunity almost or quite complete against a fresh invasion of the same or kindred bacteria. We do not know whether this singular effect is due to a modification in the chemical constitution of the tissues, or to a change in the vital activity of the cells.

References:—VOIT, *Physiologie des Stoffwechsels* Leipzig 1881; NÄGELI, *Die niederen Pilze* Munich 1877, and 1882; BUCHNER, *Die Nägeli'sche Theorie der Infectionskrankheiten* Leipzig 1878; KLEBS, Article *Ansteckende Krankheiten*, *Realencyclopädie der gesammten Heilkunde von Eulenburg*, and *Cellular-Pathologie und Infectionskrankheiten, Tageblatt der Naturforscherversammlung in Kassel* 1878; VIRCHOW, *Krankheitswesen und Krankheitsursachen, Virch. Arch.* vol. 79; HILLER, *Die Lehre von der Fäulniss* Berlin 1879; WERNICH, *Die Entwickelung der organisirten Krankheitsgifte* Berlin 1880; KOCH, *Untersuchungen über Wundinfectionskrankheiten* Leipzig 1878, *Traumatic Infective Diseases* London 1880; WOLFF, *Zur Bacterienlehre bei accidentellen Wundkrankheiten, Virch. Arch.* vol. 81; TOUSSAINT, *Comptes Rendus* nos. 2 and 5, vol. 91; CHAUVEAU, *ibidem*, no. 16; DUCLAUX, *Ferments et Maladies* Paris 1882; BRIEGER, *Einige Beziehungen der Fäulnissproducte zu Krankheiten, Zeitsch. f. klin. Med.* III; BUCHNER, *Ueber d. Wirkung d. Spaltpilze im lebend. Körper, Zur Aetiol. d. Infectionskr.* Munich 1881; CHEYNE, *Antiseptic Surgery* London 1882; Discussion, *Trans. International Med. Congr.* vol. I, 1881; HORSLEY, *Rep. Med. Off. Loc. Gov. Board* 1881 (bibliography).

Of late years many experimenters have sought to furnish an experimental basis for the doctrine that individuals who have passed through an infective disorder are 'protected' against the same or a kindred disorder (as in the case of vaccinia and variola). They have attempted to make out that this holds for bacterial disease artificially communicated to animals.

PASTEUR was the first to make communications on this head (*Gaz. méd. de Paris* no. 18, 1880). TOUSSAINT refers the so-called fowl-cholera to the action of a certain micrococcus. Fowls die when inoculated with the bacteria cultivated in chicken-broth. If the poison be attenuated by letting it stay in the culture-liquid exposed to the air for eight or ten months, it is no longer fatal on inoculation: but the fowls become by one or more inoculations 'protected' against the unattenuated poison. PASTEUR further discovered that the activity of the anthrax-bacillus may be diminished by cultivation at a temperature of 42° to 43° C. Animals inoculated with the cultivated bacillus do not die, but are as it were 'vaccinated' against the unmitigated poison. After repeated inoculations sheep become at last quite unaffected by inoculation with the unaltered bacillus.

BOULEY communicated to the Paris Academy a research of TOUSSAINT'S, in which he found that the anthrax poison can be mitigated by warming infected blood to 55° C for ten minutes with the addition of 1 per cent. of carbolic acid. Young dogs, sheep, horses, and rabbits may be protected by inoculation with this blood. COLIN (Paris Academy, March 1, 1881) has disputed the force of these experiments, as it is known that some individual animals are specially 'refractory' with respect to the anthrax-poison, without any protective inoculation. The Royal Hungarian Ministry of Agriculture instituted at Buda-Pesth an extensive series of experiments superintended by one of PASTEUR'S assistants, and the results obtained confirmed on the whole what PASTEUR had announced (RÓSZAHEGYI, *Biolog. Centralb.* 5, 1882 and *Practitioner* Feb. and Mar. 1882). Similar successful experiments were made in Berlin in April 1882 (*Gaz. méd.* July 1882). OEMLER (*Arch. f. wiss. und pract. Thierheilk.* 1876—81) made similar inoculation-experiments without reaching any positive results. CHAUVEAU likewise experimented on sheep, but was not able to draw any certain inferences: he thinks however that an imperfect protection may be obtained by repeated inoculation. LÖFFLER (*Mitth. a. d. k. Gesundheitsamte* Berlin 1881) experimented on mice, rats, guinea-pigs, and rabbits, but was not able to verify PASTEUR'S and TOUSSAINT'S statements. He did not succeed either in attenuating the poison or in effectively 'vaccinating' the animals. He therefore disputes the force of their experiments, thinking that they must have lighted on sheep already immune against the poison. The experiments on fowl-cholera he thinks trustworthy. It was he who showed that when a mouse has lived through one attack of specific septicaemia it is protected against a further attack.

This specific septicaemia of the mouse is caused by a delicate bacillus, which can be 'purely' cultivated in nutritive gelatine, weakly alkalised with sodium phosphate and impregnated with 1 per cent. of peptone. The bacillus will infallibly kill a rabbit injected with it in from forty to seventy-two hours. If it be introduced into the tip of the ear it merely produces a plastic inflammation of the skin, and the animal does not die. Rabbits so inoculated are then protected for three or four weeks against any further inoculation with the same bacillus.

There are therefore some bacterial diseases in which one attack protects against a subsequent one, as in the case of small-pox, measles, and scarlatina. But this does not hold true of all bacterial diseases. KOCH and CARTER found that a monkey inoculated with the spirilla of relapsing fever gained no immunity against a second inoculation. SEMMER (*Centralb. f. med. Wiss.* 48, 1880 and *Virch. Arch.* vol. 83) asserts that rabbits may be protected against septicaemia by vaccination with bacteria heated to 55° C for fifteen minutes: LÖFFLER repeated the experiments and obtained opposite results. Experiments with the *Bacillus oedematis* (Art. 206) were likewise negative.

BERGMANN has recently (*Chirurgencongress* 1882) stated that in all infective disease, and in all intoxication with unorganised ferments, the white blood-cells become dissolved in the blood. This produces greater viscidity and coagulability of the plasma. He refers to this cause the local congestions in the capillaries of the lungs and intestine, and the echymoses of the serous membranes observed in the affections named.

202. The **infective diseases** form a group distinguished by their markedly specific character and their special mode of origin. The specific character is manifested in this—that the disease runs a similar course in each individual attacked, conditioned solely by the nature of the morbific virus. As to the genesis of the disease, it is always referable to the passage into the organism of a poison from without.

The infective diseases have been divided into miasmatic, contagious, and miasmo-contagious. In **miasmatic** disease the morbific virus is confined to certain localities, and developes outside the human body. When it passes into the body it sets up an affection which is not transmissible to other individuals. The malarial or intermittent fevers are classed as miasmatic.

In **contagious** disease the seat of the virus is in the affected organism. From this it is transmissible to others, either through the air directly, or by means of bodies acting as carriers (*fomites*), or by actual contact. Instances of contagious disease are scarlatina, small-pox, measles, vaccinia, typhus, diphtheria, glanders, syphilis, etc.

In **miasmo-contagious** disease the actual virus is derived from without, but the germs from which the virus developes must be furnished by a previous case of the disease. Of this kind are cholera, dysentery, yellow fever, and typhoid. In the case of the last it is probable, or at least possible, that the virus may be also derived from previously uninfected localities; in other words, that it may originate as a pure miasm.

203. Some of these diseases, especially the epidemic pestilences or plagues, have from ancient times been suspected to be due to organised poisons. The suspicion has now and again been re-expressed; but it is only within the last twenty years that, in a few instances at least, the fact has been demonstrated.

The strongest point of evidence in favour of the organic nature of the poisons that produce the infective diseases is their power of unlimited reproduction and multiplication. Thus, starting with the lymph from a single vaccine vesicle, we can vaccinate on indefinitely, continually generating new vaccine matter. Infection transmitted through the medium of the air (which certainly takes place), is scarcely to be explained if it be not that the air has had corpuscular particles suspended in it. Chemically active gases would very quickly become diffused through the atmosphere, and at short distances would become attenuated beyond the power of doing mischief.

The small quantity of infective matter required to set up the corresponding disease is another point in the evidence. The extraordinary potency of the matter can only be explained by the theory that the virus is reproduced and multiplied within the organism.

The researches of the last ten years have shown (as we have said in Arts. 198—201) that there are bacterial fungi which are able, by virtue of their specific properties, to affect the animal body and generate disease in it. On the other hand, we find such fungi in the blood and tissues of persons affected with infective disease. We must admit beforehand that the available observations on this head have not the extent or exactness which we could desire. Only in the case of a few diseases is the bacterial nature of the virus demonstrated by indefeasible histological and experimental investigation. In others the presence of bacteria has been demonstrated in single cases, but their causal relation to the disease has not been proved. In many others, neither the one point nor the other has hitherto been made out. As the question at present stands then, we can only say—that among the infective diseases there are certainly some which are due to the invasion of a microphyte, and that it is highly probable the others have a like origin.

If the microparasitic theory be correct, we must admit that some of the pathogenous bacteria are accustomed to develope and multiply without the body, while others only do so within it. The former kind we may describe as **ectogenous**, the latter as **endogenous**. The distinction must not however be over much insisted on. Sometimes the ectogenous bacteria proceed to multiply within the body, while the endogenous bacteria may meet with the necessary conditions for their growth (warmth and nutriment) outside it.

The fact that bacteria have not been found in most of the infective diseases, at least in number sufficient to account at all for the phenomena, is no proof that the affections are non-bacterial. It must not be forgotten that the demonstration of bacteria is often a very difficult matter, and the material obtained from the post-mortem table is by no means well-fitted for this purpose. The patients examined generally live on to a comparatively advanced stage of the disease. We know indeed in the case of many bacterial affections that, by the time the tissue-changes occasioned by the invasion are complete, all trace of bacteria has long disappeared.

204. The **micrococci** are among the most important of the pathogenous bacteria. They are the fungi most frequently found in connexion with infective disease. In the first place they occur in various wound-affections, such as pyaemia, and erysipelas simple or phlegmonous; and that not merely in the wound itself, but in its neighbourhood and even in distant organs. In this last case they are diffused through the lymphatics and blood-vessels. They also occur in internal suppurations like metritis, puerperal peritonitis, infective osteomyelitis and periostitis, and in strumous inflammations, meningitis, cerebral abscess, etc.

Among infective diseases of another kind we have to mention diphtheria, small-pox, measles, vaccinia, scarlatina, endocarditis, pyelitis, haemophilia neonatorum, acute atrophy of the liver, croupous pneumonia, gonorrhoea, etc. In all of these micrococci have been seen scattered through the tissues, partly as masses of zoogloea, partly as chains or chaplets. It would seem as if in some diseases zoogloea, in others chaplets or swarms, were chiefly formed. The spherules are of various sizes: but this character of size is not enough to enable us to distinguish between specific forms. We have as yet but few results of culture-experiments on these bodies, so that their life-history is little known. The micrococci are therefore distinguished merely by the disease to which they are related, and so we speak of *Micrococcus septicus, erysipelatis, variolae, diphtheriticus, etc.*

The part played by these micrococci (which are not found in every case) is by no means certainly determined. Of some we can only say that they are frequently or always found in connexion with the corresponding disease (small-pox, scarlatina, measles, haemophilia neonatorum). Of others (as in wound-infections) we know, by experimental investigations, that they are only able to attack the tissues when they find in the system poisonous products of tissue-necrosis, or of fermentive decomposition set up by bacteria like themselves. Of many (such as those found in simple and phlegmonous erysipelas) we have every ground for believing that they can develope in the system without any special auxiliary conditions (other than slight traumatic injury).

We shall here consider briefly the evidence for the bacterial nature of some of the infective diseases.

(1) *Purulent inflammations; cellulitis; purulent catarrh.*

There can be no doubt that micrococci are the exciting causes in many inflammatory processes associated with the formation of pus. This is true not only of purulent affections of the skin and mucous membranes, but also of suppurations in the deeper structures of the body. Many of these affections start in wounds, but in others it is impossible to make out any surface-injury, and we are constrained to admit that the micrococci have penetrated into the deeper tissues without entering through a wound. Purulent catarrh of the mucous membranes, when due to fungi at all, is generally excited by micrococci from without; but these may sometimes come from deeper organs already affected, as when the urinary tract is infected from the kidney. This also holds for phlegmonous or parenchymatous inflammations of the subcutaneous and submucous structures (cellulitis), associated with purulent, serous, or fibrinous exudations. In the case of deep-seated organs, the micrococci must be conveyed by the lymphatics or blood-vessels. If by the blood-vessels the affection should perhaps be described as pyaemic.

When the micrococci lie in the blood-vessels, they generally form colonies. In liquid exudations within the body-cavities they are found single or in chains; in solid structures they form swarms. In all places they occur both free and enclosed in cells.

It is a question whether in all the affections just cited the micrococcus met with is of the same species. Comparative examinations show that in the different cases the spherules vary in size. ZIEGLER found that the largest of all occurred in a case of spontaneous cellulitis of the face and neck, in which suppurating and haemorrhagic patches were found in the lungs.

References:—KLEBS, *Handb. d. path. Anat.* I (pyelitis), *Beiträge zur path. Anat. d. Schusswunden* Leipzig 1872, and *Arbeiten a. d. path. Inst.* Berne 1872 (pyaemia); VON RECKLINGHAUSEN, *Verh. d. Würzburger physic. Gesell.* 1871 (pyaemic foci); RINDFLEISCH, *Lehrb. d. path. Gewebelehre*, 1st Ed. (pyaemia); BIRCH-HIRSCHFELD, *Unters. üb. Pyämie* Leipzig 1873; KOCH, *Wundinfectionskrankheiten* Leipzig 1878, *Traumatic Inf. Diseases* (Sydenham Soc.) 1880; WOLFF, *Virch. Arch.* vol. 81; LÜCKE, *Deutsche Zeitsch. f. Chir.* IV; BRAIDWOOD and VACHER, *Brit. Med. Journ.* 1, 1882, with a very full summary of the contributions to this subject; KOCHER, *Arch. f. klin. Chir.* XXIII (osteomyelitis, infective periostitis, strumous inflammation); GREENFIELD ETC., *Trans. Path. Soc.* 1879; HAAB, *Corresp. f. Schweiz. Aerzte* 1881 (blennorrhoea gonorrhoica neonatorum, gonorrhoea); NEISSER, *Centralb. f. med. Wiss.* 28, 1879 (gonorrhoea); CHEYNE, *Brit. Med. Journ.* 1880 (gonorrhoea); PERLS, *Lehrb. d. allg. Path.* II; OGSTON, *Brit. Med. Journ.* 1, 1881; and under Art. 199.

(2) *Erysipelas.*

ZIEGLER has satisfied himself by his own researches that erysipelas is due to a micrococcus. It spreads chiefly by way of the lymphatics, which are sometimes seen to be crammed full of aggregated masses of spherules. Thence it penetrates into the tissues and forms chains or swarms. It excites inflammation and leads to tissue-necrosis. It can be transmitted to the rabbit, and spreads in it also by way of the lymphatics. The animal usually dies.

References:—NEPVEU, *Gaz. méd. de Paris* 1872; LUKKOMSKY, *Virch. Arch.* vol. 60; ORTH, *Arch. f. exp. Path.* I; KLEBS, *Arch. f. exp. Path.* IV; TILLMANNS, *Arch. f. klin. Chir.* XXIII; FEHLEISEN, *Deutsche Zeitsch. f. Chir.* XVI; KOCH, *Traum. Inf. Diseases* London 1880.

(3) *Septicaemia.*

This is a term which includes various rapid and fatal affections of the blood. Septicaemia in the human subject implies blood-poisoning with various chemical products of septic decomposition. It is a septic intoxication, but actual bacteria are not found in the blood. It is not progressive, and not infective in the strict sense of the word (BURDON SANDERSON, *Brit. Med. Journ.* 1, 1877). But the term is also applied by some to certain specific and infective affections of animals, in which bacteria grow and multiply in the blood itself.

Davaine's septicaemia is an infective disease of rabbits, produced by subcutaneous injection of septic matters (such as putrefying blood). It is characterised by a definite incubation-period, and a rapid course; it is transmissible to other animals of the same species. The blood is found to contain numerous oval bacteria.

Pasteur's septicaemia has been called by KOCH malignant oedema (*Acad.*

de méd. Feb. 1 and 8, 1881). It is produced in rabbits by inserting garden-mould under the skin of the abdomen. Death ensues in twenty-four to forty-eight hours. The blood itself seems to contain no organisms; but subcutaneous oedema results, and in the oedematous tissues a delicate motile bacillus is found. GAFFKY has cultivated the bacillus on slices of potato.

Mouse-septicaemia (KOCH) is a blood-affection generated in mice by inoculation with a certain delicate bacillus. The injection of human saliva produces in rabbits a form of septicaemia not, as it seems, identical with that of DAVAINE (RAYNAUD, PASTEUR). GAFFKY produced still another form of septicaemia in rabbits by injecting river-water (from the river Panke). The bacteria which developed and multiplied in the blood resembled *B. termo* (Art. 205).

References:—DAVAINE, *Acad. de méd.* Sep. 17, 1872; COZE and FELTZ, *Rech. exp. sur la présence des infusoires dans les maladies infect.* Strasburg 1866; SEMMER, *Virch. Arch.* vol. 83; KOCH, *Wundinfectionskr.* Leipzig 1878, *Traum. Inf. Dis.* (Sydenham Soc.) 1880; GAFFKY, *Mitth. a. d. k. Gesundheitsamte* Berlin 1881; RAYNAUD, *Acad. de méd.* Feb. 8, 1881; EWART, *Proc. Roy. Soc.* xxxii; TIZZONI, *Arch. per le scienze* 1880–81; STERNBERG, *Rep. of Nat. Board of Health* (*U. S.*) 1881; BRAIDWOOD and VACHER, *Brit. Med. Journ.* 1, 1882 (a full list of contributions to the subject of pyaemia and septicaemia is given).

(4) *Diphtheria.*

This is probably a specific infective disease. The anatomical changes are usually first discerned in the pharynx and in the neighbouring mucous membranes. They take the form of catarrhal, croupous, and diphtheritic inflammations (Arts. 423–426). They are probably caused by a micrococcus which settles in the tissues of the parts named (rarely elsewhere—as in the eye, or in wounds), and thence spreads through the system. This view is chiefly supported by the fact—that in and upon the affected mucous membranes we find micrococci scattered or aggregated as zoogloea, which do not occur under normal conditions. Occasionally it is possible to demonstrate the presence of micrococci in the swollen cervical glands or even in deeper organs. If these micrococci be experimentally introduced into animals, they produce a disease resembling diphtheria. The micrococci multiply mainly within the body, but they may also find a suitable soil for growth outside it.

The theory of the genesis of diphtheria is still defective in spite of the many investigations that have been made. Even what we have stated above regarding it is by no means beyond question.

References:—HÜTER and TOMMASI, *Centralb. f. med. Wiss.* 12 and 34, 1868; OERTEL, *Arch. f. klin. Med.* VIII, *Ziemssen's Cyclopaedia*, vol. II, *Die Aetiol. d. Diphtherie*, *Zur Aetiol. d. Infectionskr.* Munich 1881; TRENDELENBURG, *Arch. f. klin. Chir.* X; KLEBS, *Arch. f. exp. Path.* IV, Art. *Diphtheritis*, *Realencyclop. d. ges. Heilk.*; LETZERICH, *Virch. Arch.* vol. 68; NASSILOFF, *Virch. Arch.* vol. 50; EBERTH, *Zur Kenntniss d. bacter. Mycosen* 1872; WOOD and FORMAD, *Rep. of Nat. Board of Health* (*U. S.*) 1881–2.

BRIEGER (*Zeitsch. f. klin. Med.* III) has lately pointed out the fact that in pyaemia, erysipelas, diphtheria, and scarlatina, certain processes take place in the tissues nearly allied to those in bacterial putrefaction. He therefore calls the diseases in question putrefactive diseases.

(5) *Scarlatina* and *measles.*

We have no certain knowledge as to the causation of scarlatina. COZE and FELTZ (*Malad. infect.* 1872) and RIESS (*Reichert's Arch.* 1872) have seen micrococci in the blood, and by inoculation have generated a fever-like disease in rabbits. COZE and FELTZ also found micrococci in the blood of patients affected with measles; KEATING (*Philadelphia Med. Times*, Aug. 12, 1882) recently found them in an epidemic of malignant measles; RANSOME, and BRAIDWOOD and VACHER (*Brit. Med. Journ.* Jan 21, 1882) found them in the breath as well as in the tissues.

(6) *Endocarditis.*

In many forms of endocarditis the affected patches are covered with an abundant layer of micrococci. These are also found in metastatic patches if there be any. It is very probable that endocarditis may be set up by various causes, and as it would seem by various forms of micrococcus (Art. 282).

References :—R. MAIER, *Virch. Arch.* vol. 62; EBERTH, *Virch. Arch.* vol. 57; KLEBS, *Arch. f. exp. Path.* IV, IX; KÖSTER, *Virch. Arch.* vol. 72; KOCH, *Mitth. a. d. k. Gesundh.* Berlin 1882.

(7) *Variola* and *vaccinia.*

In both affections micrococci have been found in the vesicles. As to their real significance nothing certain is known.

References :—KEBER, *Virch. Arch.* vol. 42; ZÜLZER, *Berl. klin. Woch.* 51, 1872; WEIGERT, *Anat. Beitr. z. Lehre v. d. Pocken* 1874; KLEBS, *Arch. f. exp. Path.* X.

(8) *Haemophilia neonatorum.*

KLEBS (*Arch. f. exp. Path.* IV.) and EPPINGER (*Beiträge zur path. Anat. v. Klebs* 1878) have described a micrococcus in this disease, and have given it the name of *Monas haemorrhagicum.*

(9) *Acute yellow atrophy of the liver.*

KLEBS, WALDEYER, and EPPINGER (*Prag. Viertelj.* 1875) have published papers on the micrococcus found in this disease.

(10) *Croupous pneumonia.*

KLEBS (*Arch. f. exp. Path.* IV), KOCH (*Mitth. a. d. k. Gesundh.* Berlin 1881), and FRIEDLÄNDER (*Virch. Arch.* vol. 87) have seen micrococci in cases of this disease.

(11) *Acute catarrhal pneumonia.*

Micrococci are very often found in the alveoli and lung-tissue. They probably reach the lungs with other bacteria from the mouth-cavity (pneumonia by aspiration).

(12) *Sarcina.*

The fungus so called occurs chiefly in the stomach, lungs, pharynx, and urine. In the lungs it has been found by NAUWERCK in various pneumonic affections (*Corresp. f. schweiz. Aerzte* 1881). It is much smaller than the sarcina of the stomach. Nothing is known of its significance.

We may here refer to a disease of silkworms, which throws light on the development of bacteria within the body. It is called *pébrine, gattine*, or 'spotted disease'. It formerly produced enormous destruction among the silkworms in silk-producing districts. Investigations made in 1853–56 showed that it was associated with the presence of a micrococcus. NÄGELI called the fungus *Nosema bombycis.* PASTEUR proved experimentally that these organisms produced the disease, and also showed by what means it could be averted. The micrococcus is transmitted to the eggs: the moths are therefore isolated and after laying their eggs are microscopically examined. If the moths are found to be diseased the eggs are destroyed. Another disease of the silkworm, *maladie de morts-blancs*, which annually causes great losses to silk-growers, is very probably a bacterial affection.

TOUSSAINT and PASTEUR have shown (*Comptes Rendus* nos. 6, 17, 18, 1880) that fowl-cholera is caused by an invasion of micrococci. The organism can be cultivated in alkalised chicken-broth, which has previously been sterilised by being raised to a temperature of 110° to 115° C.

205. The two representatives of the class of *Microbacteria*, namely *Bacterium termo* and *Bacterium lineola*, can only develope in dead tissues and liquids. *B. termo* is frequently found in the

human body at places where necrosed tissue is accessible to the air. Putrefaction is in fact conditioned by the presence of this organism. It may become dangerous by setting free products of decomposition which excite inflammation or gangrene around the putrefactive focus, and when absorbed act poisonously on the system generally or on remote organs.

GAFFKY recently discovered a specific microbacterium (*Mitth. a. d. k. Gesundh.* Berlin 1881) which he was able to cultivate separately in sterilised gelatine impregnated with blood-serum, and in a cold infusion of boiled beef. He found the organism in river-water much polluted with sewage. The same bacterium is occasionally found in meat-washings and blood, as putrefaction sets in. It is a short rodlet which takes up aniline dyes at its poles only, the middle remaining clear. It is very like *B. termo.* Its spores have not been observed. Rabbits inoculated with it remain unaffected for ten or twelve hours, then high fever sets in, and death in twenty hours. The blood of the infected animals contains bacteria. Guinea-pigs, white rats, cats, and dogs are not susceptible, but sparrows, canaries, and chickens are. This bacterium does not set up putrefaction when 'purely' cultivated; it is therefore distinct from *B. termo.*

206. Of the *Desmobacteria* the typical example is the best known of all microparasites, the **Bacillus anthracis**. It is found in the blood of animals affected with anthrax or splenic fever, and it is certain that it is the sole cause of the affection. The organism can be cultivated outside the body (Art. 186), and anthrax can be produced by means of the cultivated specimens. All that is needful is to introduce the bacillus or its spores into the blood. No auxiliary conditions, such as the formation of septic products or the presence of chemical poisons, are necessary.

The spores are the commonest medium of infection, as they are hardier than the bacillus itself. Such spores develope in the blood of animals dead of anthrax even after burial (KOCH). If they are not deeply buried the spores may ultimately reach the surface of the ground. Cattle are then infected through wounds (such as scratches of the mouth caused by stubble or by insects), through the alimentary canal, or through the lungs. Death seems to result chiefly from abstraction of oxygen, and disturbance of the circulation.

In man the disease is only produced by transmission of the virus from infected animals living or dead. In England the infection is chiefly conveyed by means of the fleeces of diseased animals to persons engaged in handling them (woolsorters' disease). Anthrax in man usually continues as a local affection for a longer time than in the lower animals. Papules, vesicles, and pustules on a red and swollen base are developed in the skin. Numerous dark-red button-like nodules crammed full of bacilli then appear in the intestine. This haemorrhagic intestinal form also occurs in cattle. In human anthrax the blood usually contains much fewer bacilli than in the case of cattle.

ARMAUER HANSEN and NEISSER have lately succeeded in

demonstrating the presence of a bacillus (**B. leprae**) in the nodes and tubercles of leprosy. The constancy with which it occurs in leprous patches would indicate that it is the exciting cause of the disease (Art. 131).

KLEBS and TOMMASI-CRUDELI have likewise found a bacillus (**B. malariae**) in cases of malarial or intermittent fever, and have experimentally investigated its properties. They assert that it is to be met with in the soil and air of malarious districts, and can be demonstrated in the blood of affected patients. The significance of the bacillus has not however been fully made out.

In cases of typhoid fever KLEBS and EBERTH have discovered a bacillus lodging in recent infiltrations of the mesenteric and intestinal glands. KOCH and FRIEDLAENDER have verified the discovery, but the life-history of the bacillus is as yet unknown.

KOCH has recently made comprehensive researches into the aetiology of tuberculosis. He finds that bacilli (**B. tuberculosis**) are constantly present, not merely in tubercles, but in various diffuse inflammatory infiltrations and granulomatous growths, and in the sputa of phthisical patients (Fig. 80). He is also able to

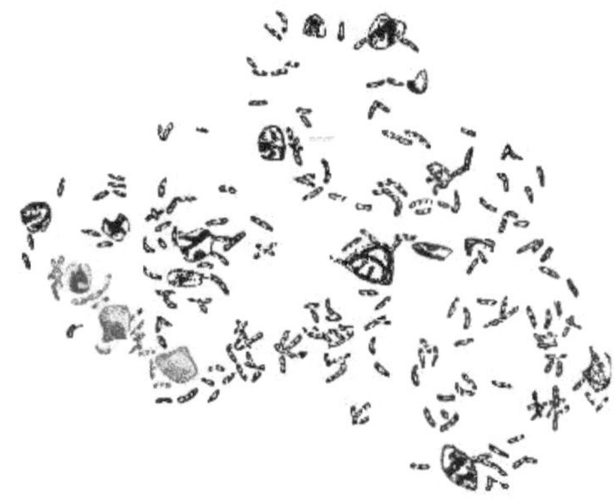

FIG. 80. *BACILLUS TUBERCULOSIS* IN PHTHISICAL SPUTUM.

(*Stained by* GIBBES'S *method with magenta and methylene-blue: the pus-cells appear blue, the bacilli crimson:* × 800 *circa*)

cultivate the bacilli in gelatine impregnated with blood-serum, and to produce tuberculosis with striking success by inoculation with the cultivated bacilli (Art. 127). It is probable that the bacillus is unable to develope outside the animal body; and that it forms spores within the body of its host (Art. 127).

(1) *Anthrax* (*splenic fever, malignant pustule, charbon*).

The *Bacillus anthracis* was first discovered by POLLENDER in 1849 (*Casper's Viertelj.* VIII, 1855) and BRAUELL (*Virch. Arch.* vol. 11, 1857). DAVAINE was the first to recognise it as the specific virus of splenic fever (*Comptes Rendus* vols. 57 (1863) and 77 (1873); *Archiv. gen.* Feb. 1868). Since then many investigators have examined the question of the significance of the bacillus (see BOLLINGER, *Splenic Fever, Ziemssen's Cyclopaedia* vol. III). KOCH has made the most careful researches on the subject (*Beiträge z. Biol. d. Pflanzen von Cohn* II, p. 277, and *Mitth. a. d. k. Gesundh.* Berlin 1881), and his experiments have thrown much light on the biology of the bacillus. TOUSSAINT also has lately published some elaborate researches (*Recherches expérimentales sur la maladie charbonneuse* Paris 1879). SPEAR and GREENFIELD have investigated anthrax in man as it occurs in the form of 'Woolsorters' disease' (*Med. Off. Report to Local Gov. Board* for 1880 and 1881).

The life-history of the anthrax-bacillus has already been given in Art. 186. It can only develope at a temperature over 18° C and in presence of a free supply of oxygen. Hence no spores are found in the bodies of animals buried more than a metre deep. Spores may however very readily be produced, if in burying the animal its blood or secretions (such as urine) be allowed to contaminate the superficial soil: in summer the temperature there may rise above 18° C (KOCH).

PASTEUR (*Bulletin de l'acad. de méd.* 28, 1880) thought that earthworms might carry spores from buried beasts to the surface, and eject them with their excreta. But KOCH regards this hypothesis as unlikely and unnecessary to explain the spread of the disease. The contamination of the surface-layers in the process of burial is enough. KOCH's experiments show that the transmission of the spores through the bodies of worms does not play the important part assigned it by PASTEUR, but they do not exclude it altogether. Other experiments prove that the bacillus may be cultivated on potatoes, in alkaline or neutral hay or pea-straw infusions, on crushed oats or barley, on turnip-juice, maize, beans, lentils, and many varieties of dead vegetable matter, if only sufficient water be provided. It is therefore probable that they may normally grow and develope outside the body of an animal. This takes place most readily in marshy spots and river-banks (KOCH). Spores are formed in summer, and persist through the winter. Inundations then carry the germs into the pasture-lands. If KOCH's views are correct, the invasion of the animal body by the bacillus is as it were an accidental incursion of an ectogenous organism. PASTEUR has shown that birds enjoy no immunity against anthrax.

(2) *'Symptomatic' anthrax (Rauschbrand).*

This disease is probably due to a bacillus found in the affected animals. It is shorter and thicker than the anthrax-bacillus, forms local aggregations in the tissues, and is accompanied by the development of gas. See KOCH (*loc. cit.*), and ARLOING, CORNEVIN, and THOMAS on *'Charbon symptomatique'* (*Paris Acad.* June 1881).

(3) *Malignant oedema.*

KOCH has occasionally found in putrefying matters a bacillus which produces in animals an affection resembling anthrax. He describes the affection as malignant oedema, and the bacillus as *B. oedematis.* It is fatal to mice and guinea-pigs. The site of inoculation becomes oedematous, and is beset with bacilli. These spread into the serous cavities, but except in mice the blood remains free of them. If mice be inoculated at the tip of the ear, they survive. The bacilli are somewhat narrower than anthrax-bacilli. It is possible that the bacilli found in certain affections due to poisonous meat (HUBER, *Arch. f. klin. Med.* XXV) are oedema-bacilli.

(4) *Intestinal mycosis.*

This is a term which includes several bacterial affections. Sometimes the affection is due to anthrax-bacilli, sometimes to oedema-bacilli. It is possible that other bacilli and micrococci (Art. 477) may give rise to similar disorders.

References:– E. WAGNER, *Arch. d. Heilk.* XV; LEUBE and MÜLLER, *Arch. f. klin. Med.* XII; BOLLINGER, *Beiträge zur vergl. Path. d. Hausthiere*

Munich 1872; BUHL, *Zeitsch. f. Biol.* VI; WALDEYER, *Virch. Arch.* vol. 52; FISCHEL, *Arch. f. exp. Path.* XVI.

Many instances of so-called 'meat-poisoning' are to be reckoned as cases of intestinal mycosis. They are very probably produced by various micro-organisms and their products. In some cases the poisoning is simply septic (Art. 204 (3)): in others it is apparently specific, and in some of these latter bacilli are certainly concerned. Exact investigations on the subject are still to be desired.

References:—ZANGGER, *Arch. f. Thierheilk.* XXIV (1871); ALBRECHT, *Wochensch. f. Thierheilk.* 1878; KUSSMAUL, *Arch. f. klin. Med.* IV; HUBER, *Arch. d. Heilk.* XIX; WALDER, *Berl. klin. Woch.* 1878; WYSS, *Corresp. f. Schweizer Aerzte* 1881; BOLLINGER, *Zur Aetiol. d. Infect.* Munich 1881; BALLARD and KLEIN, *Report of Med. Off. of Local Govt. Board* 1880.

(5) *Syphilis.*

KLEBS has a paper on a bacillus connected with syphilis in the *Arch. f. exp. Path.* X. He found microscopic rods and spherules in indurated chancres. From these he obtained bacilli by cultivation. Inoculating a monkey with these, he produced an inflammatory affection in some respects resembling syphilis, in other respects resembling tuberculosis. ZIEGLER made many similar experiments but was unable to corroborate KLEBS' statements. In 1878 he and VON RINECKER attempted to cultivate the substance removed with all care from indurated buboes, the attempt was repeated many times, but always with negative results. Various nutritive substances were used in the cultivation-experiments. See also AUFRECHT, *Cent. f. med. Wiss.* 13, 1881; BIRCH-HIRSCHFELD, *ibid.* 44, 1882.

(6) *Malaria.*

The *Bacillus malariae* was taken by KLEBS and TOMMASI-CRUDELI from the air over the Italian marshes by means of a special apparatus. Its properties were tested by culture and inoculation. They also found the fungus in samples of soil taken from the same districts. They conclude—that malarial disease can be reproduced in rabbits: that it is caused by an organism: that this is present in the soil of the malarious district before it produces fever in man: and that its passage into the air can be observed under favourable conditions. MARCHIAFAVA found the bacillus in the blood, marrow, and spleen of patients who had died of malarial fever.

The *Bacillus malariae* is an aërobious organism, which flourishes in soils of various kinds and may occur in places that are not marshy. It forms spores, and for its development requires a temperature of 20° C. LAVERAN found '*filaments mobiles*' in the blood of ague-patients.

References:—KLEBS and TOMMASI-CRUDELI, *Arch. f. exp. Path.* XI; CECI, *ibidem* XV; TOMMASI-CRUDELI, *La Malaria de Rome* Paris 1881, *Nuovi studj sulla natura della Malaria* Rome 1881, *Malaria and the Ancient Drainage of the Roman Hills, Practitioner* 2, 1881, *Istituzioni di anat. pat.* vol. I Turin 1882; MARCHIAFAVA and CUBONI, *Nuovi studj sulla natura della Malaria, Acad. dei Lincei*, Jan. 2, 1881; MARCHAND, *Virch. Arch.* vol. 88; LAVERAN, *Nature parasitaire des accidents d'impaludisme* Paris 1881; RICHARD, *Comptes Rendus* 1881; STERNBERG, *Rep. Nat. Board of Health* (*U. S.*) 1881.

(7) *Leprosy.*

Bacillus leprae was found in all the leprous nodules they examined by ARMAUER HANSEN (*Virch. Arch.* vol. 79 and *Q. Journ. Micro. Sci.* 1880) and NEISSER (*Breslauer ärzt. Zeitsch.* 1879 and *Virch. Arch.* vol. 84). The bacilli are rather longer than the semi-diameter of a red blood-cell: they lie partly within and partly without the cells of the leprous nodules. NEISSER cultivated them in blood-serum and extract of meat, and observed them develope into filaments. They form spherical spores which are seated at the ends of the rodlets, or form bright vacuoles in the middle of them. They spread through the system by way of the lymphatics, not of the blood-vessels. They are surrounded by a gelatinous envelope and at times seem to be motile. CORNIL and SUCHARD (*Annales de Dermat.* 1881) have confirmed the statements of the first observers.

(8) *Typhoid fever.*

KLEBS (*Arch. f. exp. Path.* XII, XIII) and EBERTH (*Virch. Arch.* vol. 81) have found bacilli in the diseased patches of the intestine, and in the mesenteric glands, in cases of typhoid fever. KOCH has confirmed the statement (*Mitth. a. d. k. Gesundh.* 1881). In the sloughs from the intestinal ulcers long and short bacilli have been seen, in the lymphatic glands only the short ones. The latter are found also in the vessels of various organs, especially the spleen, kidneys, and liver. They are probably the exciting cause of the disease. MARAGLIANO has found similar bacilli in the blood of living typhoid patients (*Cent. f. med. Wiss.* 41, 1882).

The above results seem at first sight to disagree with those of FISCHEL and EPPINGER (*Beiträge z. path. Anat.* II Prague 1880), LETZERICH (*Arch. f. exp. Path.* IX), and TIZZONI (*Studj di pat. sperim. sulla gen. d. tifo abdom.* Milan 1880). These observers detected micrococci. It is possible that micrococci may settle in the typhoid ulcers by way of a secondary invasion.

(9) *Tuberculosis.*

KOCH's *Bacillus tuberculosis*, mentioned already in Art. 127, grows in gelatine impregnated with blood-serum between the temperatures of 30° and 40° C, but not beyond these limits. It cannot therefore complete its development outside the body, at least in temperate climates. In most cases tuberculosis starts in the lungs, which become infected from the inspired air. The chief agent in contaminating the air is the sputum (Fig. 80) of phthisical patients which invariably contains the specific bacillus, either with or without spores. The infective power of the sputum is not destroyed by drying. It is highly probable that the spores are likewise unaffected thereby.

The tubercle-bacilli grow very slowly and therefore do not readily succeed in making a settlement on the surface of mucous membranes. Healthy tissues are besides at all times difficult to infect. The settlement is favoured by wounds, loss of epithelium, stagnating secretions, etc.

The tuberculosis of domestic animals and the 'pearly-disease' or 'grapes' of cattle are due to the same bacillus as the human disease (KOCH, *Berl. klin. Woch.* 15, 1882).

The bacilli grow well in sterilised ox-serum, but they develope and multiply very slowly. The colonies of fungi are only visible to the naked eye after ten days' growth: they then appear as dry whitish scales. These are made up of delicate rodlets. Each patch attains in three or four weeks the size of a poppy-seed, and then ceases to grow further until transplanted to a fresh substratum. This is owing to the fact that the bacilli have no power of locomotion, and so cannot spread over the nutrient gelatine.

207. Of *Spirobacteria* two forms are known to occur in man. The one, apparently quite innocuous, is the *Spirochaeta denticola:* it inhabits the mucous membrane of the mouth and nose. The other, the *Spirochaeta* (or *Spirillum*) *Obermeyeri* is found in the blood of patients suffering from relapsing fever, during the attacks. It is almost beyond doubt that the disease is caused by its invasion and multiplication within the blood. Quite lately the disease has been transmitted to monkeys by inoculation with the spirillum. Nothing certain is known of the habitat of the spirillum outside the body. It is easily detected by the microscope in the blood by

reason of its lively movements: these sometimes cause the red blood-cells to be driven and pushed about in the field of view.

The spirillum of relapsing fever was discovered by OBERMEYER in 1873 (*Centralb. f. med. Wiss.* 10, 1873 and *Berl. klin. Woch.* 33, 1873). Since then it has often been examined and described. See WEIGERT, *Deutsche med. Woch.* 1876; HEYDENREICH, *Der Parasit des Rückfallstyphus* Berlin 1877; MOCZUTKOWSKY, *Arch. f. klin. Med.* XXIV; GEDDES and EWART, *Proc. Roy. Soc.* xxvii. The successful inoculation of the monkey was performed by CARTER (*Deutsche med. Woch.* 16, 1879, *Lancet* I, 1880, and *Spirillum Fever* London 1882).

208. If we accept for a moment the hypothesis that all or most infective diseases (other than those due to animal parasites) are caused by the development of bacteria in some tissue or fluid of the body, we are met at once by the question whether in that case each specific form of disease has a corresponding specific bacterium. From a clinical standpoint this question must be answered in the affirmative. The most marked feature of the infective diseases is just this, that they run a typical and special course. Even though this may in individual cases be modified by various influences, it is in general so characteristic, so pathognomonic, that the disease can often be diagnosed by its course alone. We should therefore have no hesitation in inferring from the specific course of the disease that the virus which excites it is also specific.

Histological examination of the tissues of patients affected with bacterial disease has shown that in some cases (relapsing fever, anthrax, tuberculosis, leprosy) well-marked forms of fungi are always detected: and further that these forms of fungi, or at least forms belonging to one or other of their developmental stages, are the only ones constantly found.

In other cases such histological distinction has not yet been possible. The micrococci occurring in various infective diseases do not as yet afford us characters sufficiently well-marked to form a basis for distinguishing them into species. It must not however be assumed that these various micrococci are identical, and that it is merely the accidental association with them of this or that poison which makes them seem to have different properties.

If the micrococcus that is found be in fact the exciting cause of the disease, we must admit that it must be endowed *ab initio* with distinct properties. From the pathological point of view as well as from the clinical, we must regard it as belonging to a distinct species. As we pointed out in Art. 183, we are compelled to classify the bacteria into species on other grounds than those that apply to the higher plants. Our classification is based as yet on their morphological and physiological peculiarities. In the case of the micrococci we are confined almost entirely to the latter. We are compelled to set up physiological species. Thus as the chromatogenous micrococci are classified according to the colour they produce, so the infective micrococci are classified into species according to their pathogenous properties.

KOCH has shown that in the case of many bacterial affections it is possible to discover in the fungi well-marked morphological differences corresponding to the physiological differences (*Traumatic Infective Diseases* 1880). STRUCK's papers also contain many valuable contributions of this nature. See Arts. 204—207 for further references.

209. Each specific microparasitic disease presupposes a specific exciting cause, that is, a bacterium with special physiological properties.

In affirming this proposition we do not imply that the specific bacterium constitutes a distinct species in the biological sense. This is a question which cannot be answered by the physician: it belongs to the biologist. He will have to make out whether the properties attributed to the bacterium are constant, and whether these properties are the only ones possessed by the corresponding biological species.

On these points observers differ widely. KOCH from his culture-experiments has come to the conclusion that the pathogenous bacteria, like the non-pathogenous, do not alter in their properties. If bacteria be cultivated for several generations, the same developmental forms continually recur, and their physiological properties remain in every respect the same. Even when the nutrient medium is altered from time to time no recognisable differences are produced. KOCH does not dispute that mutability of species is possible among bacteria, but he holds that no adequate evidence has yet been brought to prove it.

This view has now many adherents, especially among clinical observers. Some go even further and assert that mutability of species is impossible.

The most important opponents of KOCH on this point are NAEGELI, DAVAINE, BUCHNER, and WERNICH. NAEGELI thinks that both the morphological and the physiological characters of the bacteria are mutable. A given bacillus does not invariably produce bacilli of the same structure, and does not always pass through the same developmental stages. A bacterium which under given conditions gives rise to a definite kind of fermentation may lose this property when cultivated under different conditions (Art. 192). Thus the same fungus can set up butyric acid fermentation or lactic acid fermentation according to circumstances. NAEGELI regards the various species of bacteria above described not as biological species, but as successive vegetative forms of a few as yet undetermined species.

References: NÄGELI, *Die niederen Pilze* Munich 1877 and 1882; BUCHNER, *Die Nägeli'sche Theorie* Leipzig 1878; BIRCH-HIRSCHFELD, *Schmidts Jahrbücher* 1875; WERNICH, *Die accommodative Züchtung der Infectionsstoffe*, *Kosmos* 4, 1880; *Die Entwickelung der organisirten Krankheitsgifte* Berlin 1880; *Desinfectionslehre* 1880; PASTEUR, *De l'atténuation des virus et de leur retour à la virulence*, *Comptes Rendus* vol. 92; KLEBS, *Arch. f. exp. Path.* XIII; BUCHNER, *Exp. Erzeug. d. Milzbrandbacillen aus Heubacillen* Munich 1880, *Münchener Acad. d. Wiss.* Jan. 12, 1882, and NÄGELI'S *Untersuch. üb. n. Pilze* Munich 1882; URLICHS, *Arch. f. klin. Chir.* XXIV; KOCH, *Traumatic Inf. Dis.* 1880, *Mitth. a. d. k. Gesundh.* Berlin 1881; GAFFKY, *ibidem*; FOKKER, *Virch. Arch.* vol. 88; WOLFF, *Virch. Arch.* vol. 81; SEMMER, *Virch. Arch.* vol. 83; DAVAINE, *Acad. de méd.* Paris 1872; GREENFIELD, *Proc. Roy. Soc. Edin.* 1880, *Journ. Roy. Agric. Soc.* 1880; KLEIN, *Rep. Med. Off. Loc. Gov. Board* 1881; MIQUEL, *Bull. Soc. Botan.* 1881.

WOLFF maintains that micrococci and short bacilli change into each other, and seeks to support this by showing that transitional forms exist. What he takes for transitional forms may very easily however be nothing more than germinating spores, or even rodlets viewed obliquely. His statement—that he obtained bacilli from a rabbit into whose peritoneal cavity he had injected micrococci—is explicable by supposing the injected matter to be impure. WERNICH also asserts that the various forms may be interchanged, and speaks of the circumstance as evidence of "unstable morphological equilibrium." He gives no other evidence in support of his idea. With regard to KLEBS and BILLROTH, and their views in this connexion, see Art. 185.

210. The defective state of our knowledge makes it for the present impossible to give a definite answer to the question of the **mutability of the bacteria**. It would however appear from the researches of NAEGELI and others that we are not absolutely justified in regarding all the various forms as representing distinct biological species. The idea of a species must be based on characters that are constant, not on those which may alter with the surroundings.

The researches of KOCH and his pupils do not prove that the properties of the bacteria examined by them are perfectly constant. They only show that the morphological and physiological qualities possessed by a bacterium at a given time are retained by it with some tenacity, even when a certain amount of variation takes place in its environment. On the other hand the researches of NAEGELI, BUCHNER, WERNICH, and others seem to afford evidence that this constancy is not shown under all conditions: that changes of the nutrient medium may have some effect on the form and size of the cells, on their mode of multiplication, and on their physiological or fermentive properties. Changes of this kind and extent do not however indicate that one species is transformed into another. We must rather conclude that one or other of the properties possessed by a biological species of bacterium may be brought into prominence by proper modifications of the external conditions.

The mutability manifested by a given bacterium will thus have definite limits. The bacterium cannot in any period of time within the extent of our observation acquire properties different from any of those possessed by the species to which it belongs. As to the extent of the cycle of varieties through which any one of the known bacteria may pass, we know indeed but little. It is possible that the properties of many of them admit of only the slightest variations from those with which we are acquainted. It is moreover probable that many of the varieties known to us constitute true biological species.

211. If we accept the hypothesis that different vital properties of the bacteria may be brought out by different external conditions, we have next to enquire whether the pathogenous bacteria may not be peculiar varieties of non-pathogenous forms. It is conceivable that in certain circumstances a bacterial virus might be developed from an innocuous bacterium, and might ultimately be transformed back to the innocuous form again. This view has been maintained by several authors (NAEGELI, BUCHNER, WERNICH) and has been supported by various experimental results. They have chiefly relied on the observation that many bacterial poisons appear to become more virulent by transmission from animal to animal (*e.g.* that of Davaine's septicaemia), in other words, that by continual inoculation the parasite learns to accommodate itself more and more completely to the conditions in which it is placed. The opponents of the theory of mutability diminish the force of this argument by showing that the increase of virulence corresponds with an increase in the 'purity' (or freedom from admixture with other bacteria) with which the fungus is cultivated. If a mass of mixed bacteria be injected into an animal, there will be at first several forms which develope simultaneously, and it is only after the virus has been transmitted through the living body twice or thrice that one form gets the upper hand, and developes to the exclusion of the others.

The theory of mutability, and especially that of the transformation of non-pathogenous into pathogenous forms, receives stronger support from an experiment of BUCHNER'S in which he seemed to show that anthrax-bacilli can be bred from hay-bacilli (*B. subtilis*) and conversely. KOCH, GAFFKY, and KLEIN dispute the validity of the experiment, but BUCHNER stands by it and claims to have confirmed it by fresh results of a like kind. The weight of evidence is for the present strongly against him.

At present we are unable to draw any certain conclusion regarding the relation of non-pathogenous to pathogenous bacteria. Clinical experience would indicate that the activity of the infective virus may vary within certain limits. And we must apparently admit that the infective bacteria have not always possessed their noxious qualities, but have acquired them somehow in the course of ages. But this is not enough to convince us that harmless bacteria can acquire infective properties rapidly, that is to say in the course of comparatively few generations. They appear rather to hold by their properties with a certain tenacity. We may therefore provisionally conclude that the transformation of innocuous into noxious bacteria can at most occur but rarely and under special conditions. In other words, the pathogenous bacteria, even if they do not represent biological species, are wont to maintain the pathogenous form for long periods of time.

DAVAINE, COZE, and FELTZ experimented on the septic poison obtained from putrefying blood. They at first asserted that its virulence increased with extraordinary rapidity, so that in the twenty-fifth generation one-trillionth of the amount of matter originally used in the inoculation was all that was necessary to produce the same infective results. DAVAINE became afterwards convinced that the virus attained its full power in the second or third generation. KOCH confirmed this, and explained it by showing that the original matter used in the inoculation was impure, *i.e.* contained other bacteria, and that the repeated inoculations gradually eliminated the admixture. GAFFKY's experiments brought out the same result. ROSENBERGER (*Centralb. f. med. Wiss.* 4, 1882) has lately found that the gradual increase of virulence is more protracted in the case of the *Bacillus oedematis.*

WERNICH finds that the potency of the *Micrococcus prodigiosus* (that is, its faculty of multiplying and producing red colouring-matter) can be increased by modifying the mode of cultivation. GAFFKY regards this fact as likewise due to the elimination of impurities.

BUCHNER first announced in 1880 that hay-bacilli could be transformed into anthrax-bacilli. If hay-bacilli are injected into the blood of animals they do not give rise to anthrax. If however they are bred for several generations in meat-extract and then in the arterial blood of a rabbit, they acquire noxious qualities and give rise to anthrax in mice after two to nine days' incubation. Conversely, if anthrax-bacilli are properly cultivated they can be transformed into bacilli whose properties are identical with those of hay-bacilli.

KOCH (*loc. cit.*) disputes the correctness of BUCHNER's observations, and suggests that he has been experimenting with the oedema-bacillus (Art. 206 (3)) instead of the *Bacillus anthracis*. According to KOCH the anthrax-bacillus and the hay-bacillus do not resemble each other. Hay-bacilli are rounded at the ends and possess cilia or flagella: anthrax-bacilli are as it were cut off square. BUCHNER's cultures were impure, they contained germs of other bacilli and these by degrees suppressed the original forms. While the hay-bacillus was supposed to be breeding in the blood the oedema-bacillus, or some other of similar action, was developed; in the converse process the so-called anthrax-bacilli were gradually suppressed by others.

In a later memoir (*Akad. d. Wiss.* Munich 1882) BUCHNER maintains his position and mentions fresh experiments bearing on it. In his view COHN's *Bacillus subtilis* includes several varieties; namely (1) hay-bacilli, (2) PASTEUR's butyric-acid ferment, (3) FITZ's bacterium (*Ber. deutsch. chem. Gesellsch.* IX, 1878) which converts glycerine into ethylic alcohol, (4) anthrax-bacilli. This fungus, which he regards as constituting a biological species, he calls *Bacterium subtile*. The properties of the variety which produces anthrax may be retained or withdrawn at pleasure by proper modes of cultivation. In the process of transformation transitional varieties appear representing intermediate stages between anthrax-bacilli and hay-bacilli. The middle forms only produce anthrax when injected in very large quantities. The process of transformation may be completed by cultivation in an alkaline solution of egg-yolk for twenty-four to forty-eight hours. The transformed bacillus (hay-bacillus) is distinguished by its energetic fermentive activity, and causes albumen to coagulate. It is inert when injected into the blood.

NÄGELI, in his recent book entitled *Untersuchungen über niedere Pilze* (Munich 1882), takes up the same position as BUCHNER with regard to the mutability of the bacteria. He believes that one and the same species may assume different forms according to the nutriment it is supplied with. These forms may exhibit different physiological and even morphological characters. The pathogenous bacteria are 'nutrimental' modifications of non-pathogenous species.

KLEIN in an important report (*Rep. Medical Officer to the Local Gov. Board* for 1881) communicates the results of a series of researches undertaken to test BUCHNER's hypothesis. He points out the probable sources of error in BUCHNER's work, and concludes that the anthrax-bacillus retains its full power to produce specific disease so long as it retains any power at all.

References:—see under Arts. 209 and 210.

CHAPTER XXXI.

HYPHOMYCETES AND BLASTOMYCETES (MOULDS AND YEASTS).

212. Mould-fungi and yeast-fungi, with their congeners, belong like the bacteria to the achlorophyllous Thallophytes. They appear to have no nearer affinity than this to the bacteria, and they have no phylogenetic relation to them. The mould-fungi and the yeast-fungi are however more nearly akin to each other, for it is probable that the yeast-fungi are the primitive forms from which the higher fungi have developed (BREFELD).

Moulds and yeasts, like bacteria, can only draw their nutriment from organic carbon-compounds. These they mostly find in dead organic matters, and they are therefore classed as Saprophytes. Some of them however are able to abstract nutriment from living tissues, and are therefore to be reckoned as Parasites. Both forms are met with in connexion with the human body.

The mould-fungi or Hyphomycetes are well known outside the body. They form the familiar flocculent covering or pellicle seen on decaying organic substances, and variously known as mould, mildew, mother, etc. They belong to several distinct genera and even to distinct sub-classes of the Thallophytes.

The yeast-fungi or Blastomycetes are also familiar organisms. They set up alcoholic fermentation, and form the yeasty scum which appears on the surface of brewed alcoholic liquors.

The systematic classification of the Thallophytes has in the last year or two undergone considerable modification.

The earlier classification, based on certain obvious characters of form and habit, was into *Algae*, *Lichenes*, and *Fungi*. This subdivision has been modified since the discovery of the reproductive organs, and in many cases of the entire life-history, of the various forms. No sharp line divides the algae from the fungi. Many families of so-called algae and fungi are really correlated, inasmuch as they agree in the characters of reproduction and 'alternation'. The lichens have been regarded as ascomycetous fungi which are parasitic on particular algae, the gonidia.

The absence of chlorophyll, and the variety of external forms (polymorphism) which occurs, are secondary characters; the latter especially being influenced by parasitism (SACHS, *Text-book of Botany* Oxford 1882; BREFELD, *Botanische Untersuchungen über Schimmelpilze* Leipzig 1874—77).

BREFELD's classification is—(1) *Phycomycetes*=algoid fungi; (2) *Mycomycetes*=true higher fungi; (3) *Myxomycetes*=gelatinous fungi; (4) *Blastomycetes*=yeast-fungi; (5) *Schizomycetes*=bacteria.

For pathological purposes it seems more convenient to retain, as we have done, the older and well-marked classes of bacteria, moulds, and yeasts.

The Hyphomycetes or Moulds.

213. **Morphology and physiology**. The mould-fungi are hyphomycetous, *i.e.* they are fungi characterised by the formation of a *mycelium.* As they occur in man they appear in the form (1) of simple or branched jointed or unjointed filaments of various thicknesses, and (2) of ovoid or spherical cells. These filaments are the *hyphae* (Fig. 81); the compact masses or tufts which they form are *mycelia;* the spherical, ovoid, or cylindrical cells, often strung into a kind of chaplet, are the *spores* or rather the *conidia.* Spores are more commonly found within the human body than any other of the vegetative forms: fructification is rarely observed. These fungi are classified according to the place in which they are found, and the affection which they produce. Their names are derived from the name of their discoverer, from the name of the disease they produce, or otherwise. Such a classification can only of course be a temporary expedient. The filaments and spores are not the plant, they represent merely a developmental stage of it, and by no means determine the species. To settle this the plant must be purely cultivated on a proper soil, and its various stages traced out.

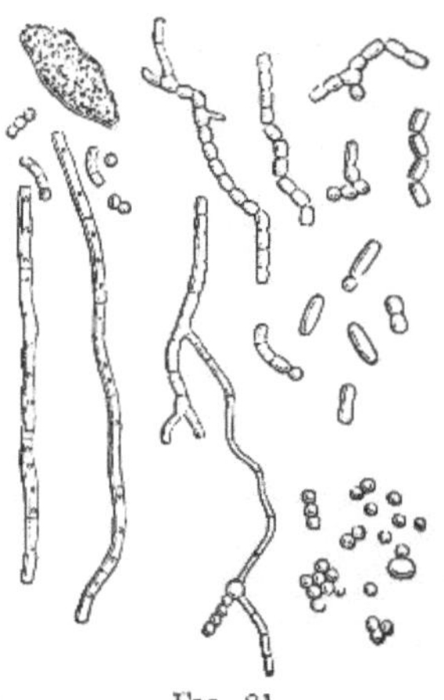

FIG. 81.
FUNGI FROM A FAVUS-PATCH. (*NEUMANN*)

In all cases the cell which we call the spore or conidium grows into a germinal tube or cylinder, and from it spring a greater or less number of ramifying unicellular or multicellular filaments or hyphae. These form a mass which, taken as a whole, is called the mycelium. This again may give rise asexually to reproductive cells, which develope into fresh mycelia. In other cases sexual organs are formed, and the product of the congress of the male and female elements is either a single spore (*zygospore*) or a fructification in which numerous spores (*ascospores*) are developed. From the zygospore, or from the ascospores, the new generation springs. The former is the case in *Mucor Mucedo;* the latter in *Aspergillus glaucus,* and *Penicillium glaucum*—the commonest of the ordinary moulds.

214. The genus *Oïdium* exhibits the processes of growth and multiplication in their simplest form. It forms a white downy covering on decaying organic substances, especially on animal excreta, fruit, grapes (*Oïdium Tuckeri*), and sour milk. According to GRAWITZ (*Virch. Arch.* vol. 70) *Oïdium lactis,* which grows upon the surface of milk, passes through the following stages of development. The conidia or spores, which are ovoid cells, lengthen out into one or more germinal tubes, which very soon become jointed and throw out lateral branches. These branches are at first cylindrical, but later on they become rounded off, and then appear as lengthened ovoids. Sooner or later they break up by transverse subdivision into chains or chaplets of conidia. The several conidia-cells then recommence the developmental cycle, which proceeds as before. No true *sporangia* or spore-capsules are formed, and no kind of sexual reproduction has been observed.

215. *Mucor Mucedo* is a mould-fungus which grows on all kinds of substances, but chiefly on excreta and on articles of food. It forms the familiar white mouldy covering. When the spores are numerous it takes on a brownish-yellow powdery look. If these spores be sown on the surface of a decoction of horse-manure, for instance, they proceed to germinate within a few hours. The long ovoid spores become larger and more spherical. Then they throw out their germinal tubes or hyphae in one or more directions. In twenty-four hours a dense interlacing weft of mycelium is already formed, made up of non-septate filaments (Fig. 82 *B m*), branching indefinitely into finer and finer expansions. The entire mycelium is thus one enormously branched cell.

When it reaches a certain point this vegetative growth ceases. The contents of the filaments become turbid, and draw towards the middle, from which springs a stouter branch than the rest, the *conidiophore* or *sporangiophore* (*g*). When this has grown somewhat, a button-like protuberance appears at its apex; this is the *sporangium.* It consists of an enclosing membrane and a protoplasmic core. The protoplasm becomes segmented and thus are formed a multitude of conidia (*A*). Septa then begin to develope in the filaments of the mycelium.

These sporangia are non-sexual structures. When ripe they consist of a membranous spherical envelope, containing a mass of spores agglutinated by a sticky intercellular substance. In water the membrane gives way, and the conidia are set free.

The mode of multiplication just described is the commonest: but there is also a sexual mode of propagation by means of what are called *zygospores.* The process is this:—the tips of two filaments rising from the mycelium are each marked off by a septum so that each ends in an apical cell (Fig. 82 *D aa*). These tips meet and the cells coalesce, and by absorption of the separating membranes the contents flow together. The single new cell thus produced is the zygospore. Its membrane becomes thickened and

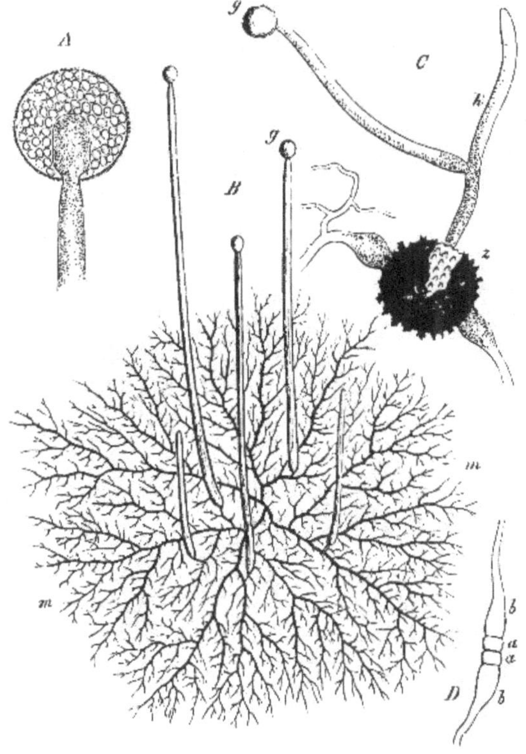

FIG. 82. DEVELOPMENT BY CONIDIA AND ZYGOSPORES.

A the conidiophore or conidia-bearing hypha of *Mucor Mucedo* in optical section
B mycelium of *Phycomyces nitens*; *g* conidiophore; *m* unicellular mycelium (*three days old: grown in plum-decoction and gelatine: the finest ramifications are left out in the drawing: from* SACHS)
C germinating zygospore (*z*) of *Mucor Mucedo*; the germinal tube or hypha (*k*) throws out a conidiophore (*g*)
D free conjugating branches (*bb*) whose tips (*aa*) have not yet coalesced, but are marked off by septa: the zygospore results from the coalescence of the cells (*aa*).

it grows to a considerable size. The thickened membrane is divisible into a blackish *exosporium* and a colourless *endosporium*. From this zygospore, which in the case of *Mucor* is also a resting-spore, there springs, after some weeks of cultivation, a germinal hypha (*C k*), which then developes a hypha bearing a sporangium (*g*).

We owe most of the details of our knowledge on this part of the subject to BREFELD (*Botan. Untersuch. über Schimmelpilze* Leipzig 1874—77): the foregoing account is taken from him. The mycelium of *Phycomyces* in the figure taken from SACHS agrees generally with that of *Mucor;* in the latter however only a single conidia-bearing hypha is developed.

216. The life-history of *Eurotium Aspergillus* (*Aspergillus glaucus*) and *Eurotium repens* is somewhat different. These two fungi are found on various substances, but chiefly upon cooked fruit. They form a finely filamentous jointed mycelium (Fig. 83 *A*), from which rise a great number of aërial hyphae or conidiophores (*c*). These end in a spherical knob, from the upper part of which sprout numerous densely-packed radial peg-shaped protuberances or *sterigmata* (*st*). Each sterigma gradually developes a long chain

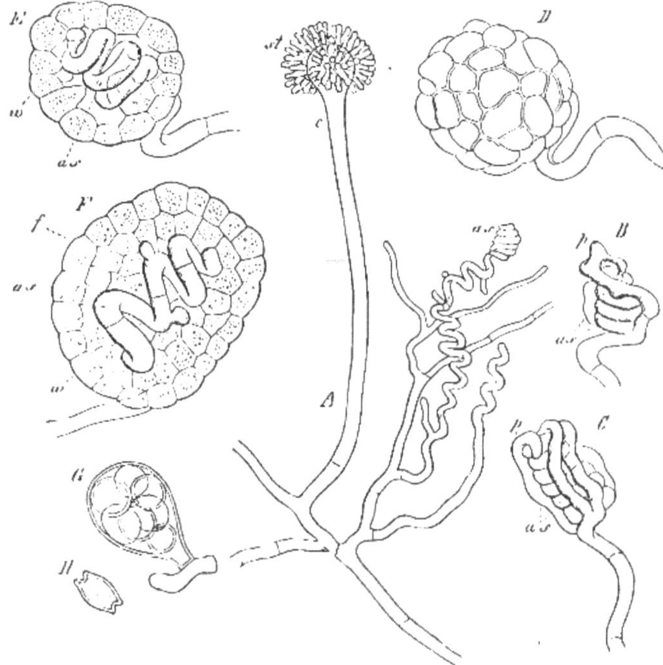

FIG. 83. DEVELOPMENT OF *EUROTIUM REPENS*, AND OF *ASPERGILLUS GLAUCUS*. (*After* DE BARY)

A small part of mycelium with a conidiophore (*c*) and young carpogonium (*as*)
B the spiral carpogonium (*as*) and pollinodium (*p*)
C the same with commencing growth of filaments to form the wall of the perithecium
D a mature perithecium
E and *F* young perithecia in optical section *w* wall-cells *f* 'packing-cells' or pseudo-parenchyma *as* ascogonium
G ascus *H* ascospore

of conidia so that the head of the conidiophore is at length covered with a sheaf of such chains.

While the conidia are developing, the sexual organs are being formed within the same mycelium. The end of a mycelial filament becomes twisted like a corkscrew (*A as*); and the spiral turns come closer and closer to each other, till at last they touch and form a hollow spiral tube. This is the female organ or *carpogonium* (*as*). From the lowermost turns of the carpogonium thin branches sprout out, which grow up over the outside of the spiral. One of these, growing more quickly than the rest, reaches the uppermost turn and applies its point closely to it (*B p*). This is the male part or *pollinodium*. Conjugation takes place between it and the carpogonium; the bounding membranes give way, and the contents coalesce. Thereupon from the lower part of the pollinodium and carpogonium spring new filaments, which increase rapidly in number and cling closely to the spiral (*C*) so as at length to cover it up completely. These tubular filaments subdivide transversely, and so an envelope of polygonal cells (*D*) is finally formed. This envelope is the *perithecium*, and it forms a hollow sphere (*E w*) containing the carpogonium. The cells multiply so as to fill up the cavity (*F*). Meanwhile numerous septa are formed in the carpogonium, and from the joints spring lateral branches (*ascogenous hyphae*) which ramify and subdivide (*F as*) between the surrounding cells. Their terminal twigs form the *asci* (*G*) (whence the fructifying carpogonium is named the *ascogonium*). The asci are tubular, and in each of them eight spheres (*ascospores*) are developed. As the ascogenous filaments develope the 'packing cells' or pseudo-parenchyma of the perithecium disappear. Ultimately the asci also vanish, and we are left with a hollow receptacle filled with spores. When ripe these last are lenticular or biconvex (*H*). On germinating they again form a mycelium, which produces both conidia and perithecia. There is no true alternation of generations between the sexual and asexual varieties.

217. The commonest of all mould-fungi, *Penicillium glaucum*, developes in a similar way. It grows on the most meagre soils. Until lately the mycelium with its conidia was the only form of it which had been recognised. BREFELD showed however that it is an ascomycetous fungus allied to the *Tuberaceae* or truffles.

The mycelium consists of jointed, much branched, uniform filaments. Some of these rise as conidiophores, which branch at the apex into sterigmata, and produce rows or chains of greenish-coloured conidia. *Penicillium* may pass through several generations all following this mode of propagation.

But there is also a sexual mode. As in *Eurotium* a spiral female carpogonium and a male pollinodium are developed. In the former the germs of the new plants are produced.

After fructification the carpogonium throws out thin sterile filaments which interlace to form an envelope for it; and also a thicker filament lying in the centre and constituting the germinal or sporiferous element, which takes the form of a branching tube. The densely-packed enveloping filaments subdivide freely, so as to produce a compact and coherent mass of cells. The cells increase greatly in size, and their walls become firm and hard; so that the structure appears at last as a firm ball or tuber, looking like a yellow grain of sand. This is called the *sclerotium*, and may be preserved in the dry state for many months together.

On germinating ascogenous filaments are developed within the carpogonium and grow out into threads, some of which are stout, while others are slender. The latter have to do with the absorption of nutriment from the enveloping capsular tissue, the former with the process of fructification. Clusters of asci are developed upon them, each containing eight spores. The whole of the enveloping tissue is ultimately absorbed, with the exception of the brownish outer layers. The asci and the filaments likewise vanish, and after some months we have left merely a hollow capsule filled with a multitude of bright yellow spores. From these spores or ascospores an ordinary mycelium is again reproduced.

218. The life-history of a few of the most common of the filamentous fungi, some of them occurring in the human body, exemplifies the fact that the various forms have various modes of development and reproduction. In some the process of reproduction is very simple. The mycelium gives rise by subdivision and abstriction to separate cells or conidia, which have the faculty of existing independently, and of developing a fresh mycelium. In others a second more complex but still asexual mode obtains: the mycelium shoots out specially constructed conidiophores or sporangiophores, and these bear sporangia, or sterigmata. In or upon these receptacles are developed reproductive cells, which we term conidia or spores.

But there is a third or sexual mode of propagation. In this two equivalent cells unite to form a new cell—the zygospore (as in *Mucor*) or true resting-spore: or a female organ developes—the carpogonium—which, fructified by the agency of a male organ or pollinodium, developes a germinal or ascogenous organ; and this again by a process of branching and subdivision produces asci or spore-tubes containing the true spores or ascospores. From these the cycle of development may begin once more.

This sexual reproduction may either go on simultaneously with the asexual modes, or an alternation of generations may take place. That is to say, from a conidium a mycelium is developed which possesses sexual organs, and from these is sexually generated an asexual plant. This bears ascospores, and they again form a mycelium which produces conidia. It is not to be forgotten, however, that strict alternation of this kind rarely occurs. Without prejudice to the plant the alternation may be pretermitted for many successive generations, as is the case with *Penicillium*. In any case, indeed, the number of asexual generations is much greater than the number of sexual ones.

Such an alternation of sexual with asexual generations is not peculiar to the fungi; it occurs in a much more definite manner among higher plants. No peculiar polymorphism is exhibited by the fungi. The idea of polymorphism has arisen from the fact that the asexual mode of reproduction is very common among fungi, while the sporangiophores or conidia-bearing organs assume very various forms. Moreover in all of the fungi there is more than one mode of asexual reproduction. The statement of various authors (like HALLIER)—to the effect that fungi possess a special and peculiar habit of polymorphism or 'pleomorphism'—rests mainly on error. They have either failed to cultivate 'purely' the plants studied, or they have been ignorant of the diverse modes in which they may be propagated.

The account just given by no means exhausts the various modes of sexual and asexual reproduction among the fungi. We have, for example, said nothing of the formation of *oospores*. Here a female cell or *oosphere* developes in an *oogonium*, and is fructified by a male cell or *spermatozoid* developed in an *antheridium*. From this is bred a plant like the parent plant, or else a multitude of germs which go to produce a new generation. For such details and others we must refer the student to SACH's *Text-book of Botany*, or to BREFELD's papers above cited. All we have here attempted is—to give such an account as would make clear the general modes of growth and reproduction of the mould-fungi, and enable the student to understand the allusions to them that are constantly occurring in articles on the fungous parasites of man.

219. The form and texture of the mycelium and the mode of multiplication depend greatly on the nature of the nutrient substratum. Thus the filaments of *Oïdium lactis* may be short or long, thin or thick, according to the proportion of sugar present and the reaction of the solution. If there is a dearth of nutriment, the formation of conidia is generally favoured. The free access of oxygen is also of import. According to BREFELD sexual reproduction can be induced in *Penicillium* if the access of air and light is prevented after the mycelium is formed.

If spores of *Mucor* be sown in a saccharine liquid with access of air, the mycelium developed on the surface is made up of branched non-septate hyphae, and the liquid absorbs oxygen (REESS, *Botan. Untersuch. über Alkoholgährungspilze* 1870; and FITZ, *Ber. d. deutsch. chem. Gesell.* Berlin 1873). If the mycelium be immersed, or oxygen withdrawn, the hyphae develope septa and break up into longer and shorter segments; these then multiply by budding like the yeast-plant, and form a kind of large-celled yeasty scum. This yeast has the power of decomposing sugar into alcohol and carbonic acid, but the fermentation ceases when a small proportion of alcohol is formed. The same is true of *Mucor racemosus*, but not of *Penicillium glaucum*.

If the composition of the nutrient substratum be gradually altered, the fungi may be got to grow on substances which they do not usually affect. Thus *Eurotium* and *Penicillium* may be transplanted from bread to solution of peptone, and can ultimately be made to grow on the surface of blood (GRAWITZ).

The limits of temperature, within which the mould-fungi can flourish, vary with the different forms. Some species of *Aspergillus* (*A. flavescens, fumigatus, nigrescens*) and some of *Mucor* grow very well at temperatures between 35° and 40° C; while *A. glaucus* and *Penicillium* only thrive below 34° C. The spores bear high degrees of heat: to kill them outright they must be kept at a temperature of 110° C to 115° C for an hour.

References:—GROHE, *Berl. klin. Woch.* 1, 1871; LÖFFLER, *Mitth. a. d. k. Gesundh.* Berlin 1881; GRAWITZ, *Virch. Arch.* vol. 81; LICHTHEIM, *Berl. klin. Woch.* 9, 1882; LEBER, *Gräfe's Arch.* XXV, and *Berl. klin. Woch.* 19, 1882; DUCLAUX, *Ferments et Maladies* Paris 1882; KOCH, *Berl. klin. Woch.* 52, 1881; KAUFMANN, *Lyon médical* 1882.

220. The **action** of the mould-fungi **on the nutrient soil** on which they grow is slow, and limited in extent. Thus the mouldy covering which forms on preserved fruit extends only to a slight depth below the surface. Mouldy articles of food acquire a peculiar unpleasant 'musty' taste. If the mycelium of a fungus gains access to an apple, for instance, the apple becomes rotten; *i.e.* a process of change and decay sets in, accompanied by purely chemical decompositions. Timber in which mould fungi develope becomes soft and brittle and breaks down into a dry 'mouldering' dust. Fungi which are specifically distinct may give rise to similar or identical decompositions in articles of food, timber, etc. The mycelium of *Merulius lacrimans* (dry-rot) destroys the wood-work of houses.

Moulds may likewise attack living plants, *i.e.* they may thrust their mycelia into living vegetable tissue. The changes they occasion are various. Sometimes they seem to exert no disturbing influence on the normal development of the tissue. In others they induce abnormal growths. The so-called 'witches' brooms' of the silver fir are produced by the settlement in the tree of the *Aecidium elatinum*. Often the cell-contents become altered: thus starch and cellulose may be converted into turpentine. HARTIG thinks the moulds may also act as organised ferments.

Not infrequently the fungi destroy altogether the plants they attack. Thus the *Oïdium Tuckeri* (vine-mildew) seizes on the green parts of the vine, and destroys it. If the spores of *Peronospora infestans* reach the tubers of the potato-plant, they drive their germinal hyphae into their substance, form a mycelium there, and so ruin the potato (DE BARY): this constitutes the 'potato-disease'. The 'leaf-rust' which destroys fruit-trees is likewise due to a fungus (*Roestelia cancellata*).

References:—SACHS, *Text-book of Botany* 1882; DE BARY, *Die gegenwärtig herrschende Kartoffelkrankheit* Leipzig 1861, *Journ. of Botany* 1876, *Botan. Zeitung* 1881; HARTIG, *Ueber die durch Pilze bedingten Pflanzenkrankheiten* Munich 1881.

221. **Pathological significance**. The mould-fungi do not act as producers of disease to anything like the same extent as the bacteria. The fact that they require abundance of oxygen and flourish best at temperatures below that of the body hinders their development within it. Moreover their growth and reproduction are much slower than in the case of the bacteria, and this also is a hindrance to the invasion of living tissues by them. Lastly, they do not usually find in living tissues their proper nutriment. At the same time the products of the decompositions set up by them are by no means so poisonous as those which result from the development of bacteria. For these reasons the effect of mould-fungi or their germs on the system is either *nil*, or very limited.

Multitudes of fungus-germs are received into the accessible cavities of the body with the air, water, and food. Most of these germs fail of development and perish, or are removed from the body. It is only now and then that they produce hyphae, and that only when they reach spots accessible to the air and containing necrotic tissues or other like matters. Such spots are the mouth, nostrils, and pharynx, and the external auditory meatus, the cornea, trachea, bronchi, and lungs. In the 'fur' of the tongue of patients whose mouths are not kept clean we often find not only bacteria but also the spores and hyphae of various filamentous fungi. In cases of bronchiectasis, vomicae, and pulmonary gangrene various forms of mycelial growths, such as *Mucor, Eurotium,* and *Aspergillus*, have been frequently described. They produce hyphae and conidia, and (rarely) the more complex conidiophores.

These fungi are not however to be regarded as the specific causes of the diseases in question. They are merely secondary growths developing on the dead tissues produced by antecedent morbid processes. They have merely sprung up on a soil which they found already prepared. They are not parasites, they are merely saprophytes. But their development in the necrotic matters, and the further decay they set up, may nevertheless tend to excite inflammatory action in the neighbouring tissues.

The fungi found occasionally in the stomach are in like manner to be regarded as secondary formations. They are not causally connected with the disease which they accompany. They are sometimes observed in cases where the gastric functions are gravely impaired, as in carcinoma and in dilatation of the stomach. The form of vegetative growth then met with is not the ordinary one: the fungi multiply by subdivision into short cells resembling those of the yeast-plant. This phenomenon we have already seen exemplified in the case of *Mucor* when grown under the surface of the nutrient liquid.

On mycoses (or fungus-affections) of the lungs see VIRCHOW, *Virch. Arch.* vol. 9; KÜCHENMEISTER, *Die in dem und an dem Körper des Menschen vorkommenden parasiten;* FRIEDREICH, *Virch. Arch.* vol. 10; PAGENSTECHER, *Virch. Arch.* vol. 11; COHNHEIM, *Virch. Arch.* vol. 33; FÜRBRINGER, *Virch. Arch.* vol. 66; LICHTHEIM, *Berl. klin. Woch.* 9, 1882; BOLLINGER, *Zur Aetiol. d. Infect.* Munich 1881; KITT, *Deutsche Zeitsch. f. Thiermed.* VII.

The *Aspergillus* which is found in the lungs is according to LICHTHEIM the *A. fumigatus.* It was formerly believed that *A. glaucus* occurred within the body. This cannot be the case however, for the body-temperature is too high. *A. glaucus* forms rounded conidia-spores 12—13 micromm. in diameter, with a thick warty yellowish envelope. Those of *A. fumigatus* are only 3—4 micromm. across, and are smooth. Invasions of the *Aspergillus* are very often observed in birds.

In the external meatus and middle ear the following are found—*Aspergillus fumigatus, nigricans, flavescens,* and *Trichothecium roseum.* They excite inflammation. The instillation of oil favours their development (BEZOLD, *Ueber Otomycosis, Zur Aetiol. d. Infect.* Munich 1881).

Aspergillus may grow on the injured surface of the cornea and lead to suppurative inflammation. LEBER (*Gräfe's Arch.* XXV) has cultivated it on the cornea and in the anterior chamber of rabbits. *Aspergillus* also occurs in the pelvis of the kidney.

222. Filamentous fungi are the exciting causes of certain skin-diseases. In Favus, Tinea tonsurans, Tinea versicolor, Tinea sycosis, and Onychomycosis deposits of hyphae and conidia are found in the epidermal layers of the skin.

In Favus, for example, the root and root-sheath of the affected hair (Fig. 84 *a b*) are beset with jointed filaments and spores. The other parts of the hair and skin are also interpenetrated with filaments and spores, and these tend to separate the constituent epidermal cells by loosening their cementing substance. Inflammation is set up and scales and crusts are formed on the surface. GRAWITZ asserts that the hyphae and conidia, which are met with in the above-named mycoses of the skin, all belong to the same species of fungus, which is identical with the *Oïdium lactis;* the differences observed in the various diseases being simply due to differences in the nutrient substratum. Most authors however maintain that they belong to different species. The fungus of Favus is called *Achorion Schönleinii,* that of Tinea tonsurans (or ringworm) is *Trichophyton tonsurans,* and that of Tinea or Pityriasis versicolor is *Microsporon furfur.*

Most of the parasitic filamentous fungi infesting man seldom penetrate beyond the superficial layers of the tissues affected. They can only do so under special and uncommon conditions, as in deep wounds. Some few, like *Aspergillus fumigatus* and *flavescens,* can germinate and throw out filaments into the blood, if they succeed in entering the vessels; but they do not multiply. As they grow they excite inflammation and necrotic changes. Only two fungi referred to this class are known to multiply in the substance of the tissues, and they cause wide-spread and highly destructive inflammations. One of these is the so-called *Actinomyces* or 'ray-fungus' which causes the disease known as Actinomycosis (Arts.

134—135). Its botanical position is not yet determined; if it is a mycelial fungus at all, it differs in many respects from its congeners.

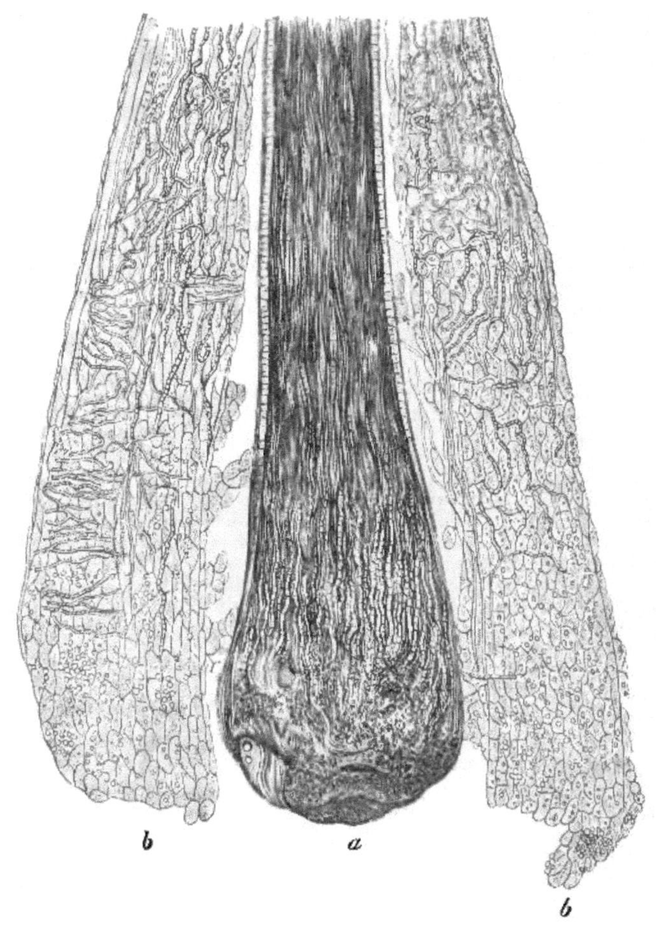

FIG. 84. HAIR AFFECTED WITH FAVUS (*after* KAPOSI).

a hair bulb and shaft
b root-sheath beset with hyphae and conidia

Some pathologists go so far as to question whether it is a vegetable. The other is the *Chionyphe Carteri*, which is found in tissues affected with the Indian disease known as 'madura-foot' or Mycetoma. Its mycelium penetrates the skin and subcutaneous tissue, and suppuration and ulceration are set up.

The earliest observation of filamentous fungi in the deeper organs was made by ZENKER (*Jahresb. d. Gesell. f. Natur- und Heilk.* Dresden 1861—2). He found them in cerebral abscesses.

GROHE (*Berl. klin. Woch.* 1, 1870) and BLOCK (*Ueber Pilzbildung in thier. Geweb.* In. Diss. Stettin 1871) made the first experimental researches on the behaviour of mould-spores introduced into the blood. They affirmed that the spores of *Aspergillus glaucus* and *Penicillium glaucum* germinate when injected into the blood, so that the tissues become penetrated with their filaments. Their experiments were again and again repeated, but their results were not confirmed until GRAWITZ took up the subject (*Virch. Arch.* vol. 81). He found that to obtain positive results the fungi must first be adapted to the conditions of the human body by cultivation in an incubator. KOCH, LÖFFLER, and LICHTHEIM (Art. 219), however, showed that this is not always necessary, for the conidia of various moulds, such as *Asp. fumigatus*, *A. flavescens*, and several of the *Mucorini*, have the power of developing within the body. Experiments made with a view to acclimatise other varieties to the conditions of the body were unsuccessful. GRAWITZ's results are vitiated by the fact that his cultures were probably 'impure'.

On Madura-foot see VANDYKE CARTER, *On Mycetoma* London 1874, and LEWIS and CUNNINGHAM, *The Fungus-Disease of India* Calcutta 1875, and *Quain's Dict. of Med.* 1882.

The affections induced by the mould-fungi have a totally different significance from those induced by the bacteria. No transmissible infective disease has yet been produced by the former class of organisms, for they do not multiply within the body. In all the experiments referred to what was obtained was at most the germination of conidia—never their fructification.

Among invertebrate animals diseases due to mycelial fungi are by no means rare. *Botrytis bassiana* sets up the so-called muscardine-disease in silkworms. *Cordyceps militaris* destroys the noxious pine-spider (*Gastropacha pini*). *Tarichium megaspermum*, a black fungus, is fatal to the noxious caterpillar *Agrotis segetum*. The genus *Empusa* is well-known: one of its species (*E. radicans*) attacks the caterpillar of the white cabbage-butterfly, another (*E. muscae*) the ordinary house-fly. These are often found completely beset and permeated with mycelial filaments.

The Blastomycetes or Yeasts.

223. The yeast-fungi consist of round or ovoid cells of various sizes (Fig. 85). The cell-protoplasm is granular, and often vacuolated. It is contained within a cell-wall.

Multiplication takes place by gemmation and abstriction. An outgrowth springs from some point of the surface of the parent-cell; this grows till it is about the size of the parent, and then it is abstricted. In some conditions (CIENKOWSKY, GRAWITZ) the cells grow out into filaments, but these do not become jointed or subdivided. If jointed threads seem to be formed, it is by a process of gemmation, like that which produces the rounder cells. Dilution of the nutrient liquid favours the development of filaments; abundance of sugar favours the development of spherical cells. REESS asserts that new cells may also be formed endogenously, by means of so-called brood-cells.

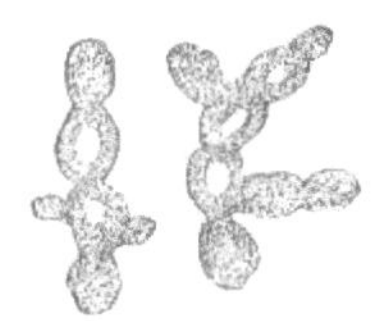

Fig. 85. *SACCHAROMYCES CEREVISIAE* (×400)

The organism which sets up alcoholic fermentation is a yeast-fungus (*Torula*). When it multiplies in a liquid containing sugar, alcohol and carbonic acid are generated. It has therefore been described as *Saccharomyces*. The scum which forms on the surface of alcoholic liquors and leads to their transformation into vinegar also contains a yeast-fungus: it is distinguished as *Mycoderma vini* or 'mother of vinegar.' NAEGELI maintains that *Torula* and *Mycoderma* are not distinct species.

SACHS classes the yeasts with the bacteria as *Protophyta*. BREFELD regards them as probably mere low forms of the moulds or filamentous fungi. CIENKOWSKY's paper on *Mycoderma* is in the *Mélanges biologiques...de l'acad. de St Pétersbourg* vol. VIII; GRAWITZ's in *Virch. Arch.* vol. 70. On *Saccharomyces* and alcoholic fermentation see REESS, *Bot. Untersuch. üb. d. Alkoholgährungspilze* Leipzig 1870; PASTEUR, *op. cit.* (Art. 191), *Studies on Fermentation* London 1879; MAYER, *Lehrbuch d. Gährungschemie* 1876; SCHÜTZENBERGER, *Fermentation* London 1876; BREFELD, *Phys. med. Gesellsch. zu Würzburg* V, 1873; HILLER, *Die Lehre von der Fäulniss* Berlin 1879. On the various theories of fermentation see Art. 191.

Yeast-cells not only set up fermentation directly, but they yield an unorganised ferment which changes cane-sugar into grape-sugar.

224. The yeast-fungi have but little pathological importance. They have no power of invading living tissue, and therefore they are only to be found in parts that are accessible from without. Even there it is only under specially favourable conditions that they are able to grow freely. There is usually no great supply of fermentable saccharine matter available for them. It is in the stomach that they are oftenest found, and there they may set up fermentation; the presence of the gastric acids does not check their development. If fermenting 'wort' or 'must' be drunk, the fermentation goes on in the stomach.

According to GRAWITZ the white patches known as 'thrush' (or sometimes aphthae) which form in the mouth, pharynx, and oesophagus of weakly children and debilitated patients are due to the presence of *Mycoderma vini*. The mycelial filaments and spores found in these patches have usually been regarded as belonging to an *Oïdium* distinguished as *O. albicans*. GRAWITZ has shown that on cultivation the filaments gemmate like *Torula* and *Mycoderma*. He has further proved experimentally that the latter can be grown in the epithelium of the mucous membrane. The subepithelial fibrous tissue is not usually invaded, and then only when by antecedent changes, constitutional or other, the resisting power of the tissues has been considerably diminished.

CHAPTER XXXII.

ANIMAL PARASITES.

Arthropoda.

225. **Arachnida**. The arachnoid parasites are mostly ectozoa: they inhabit the skin for a shorter or longer time. Only a single species *Pentastoma* is found (in the larval form) within the substance of the deeper tissues.

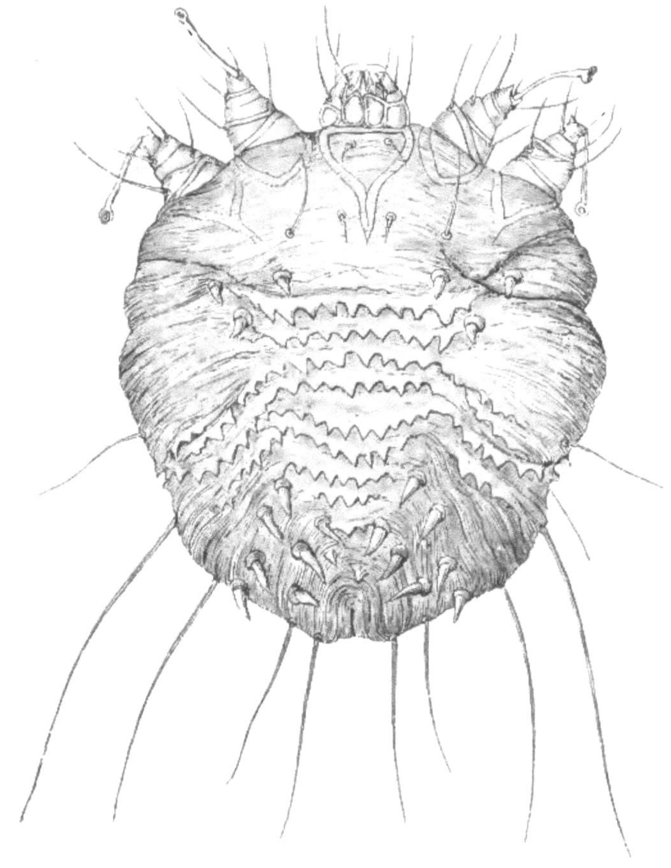

FIG. 86. FEMALE *ACARUS SCABIEI*, DORSAL SURFACE.
(*From* HEBRA'S *Atlas of Skin-Diseases*: × 200)

(1) *Acarus scabiei* (*Sarcoptes hominis*), or itch-insect. This mite is about the size of a small pin-head, and somewhat turtle-shaped. It has four pairs of legs springing from the ventral surface, each being furnished with bristly hairs (Fig. 86). The anterior pairs are prolonged into stalked suckers, as are also the posterior pairs in the male. The foremost of the two posterior pairs in the male and both posterior pairs in the female end in a long bristle. The border of the body behind is likewise furnished with bristles, and the dorsal surface is beset with tooth-like hooks and spines. The head is blunt and rounded, and beset with bristles. The female is about twice the size of the male.

The mite lodges in the epidermal layer of the skin, in which it excavates burrows or *cuniculi* that may run to 10 mm. in length. In these burrows the female lays her eggs. From the eggs the young acari are hatched *in loco*: they proceed to burrow further into the epidermis, and after changing their skin several times become sexually mature. The irritation caused by their presence produces inflammation of the skin. This again is greatly intensified by the scratching induced by the intolerable itching of the affected parts.

(2) *Leptus autumnalis*, or harvest-mite. This likewise infests the epidermis. It is red in colour, and thus is readily seen in spite of its smallness. It gives rise to the formation of papules and wheals. Two allied American species are the *Leptus Americanus* and *L. irritans*.

(3) *Acarus* (*Demodex*) *folliculorum* (Fig. 87). A third mite, which is found solitary or in small numbers in the sebaceous matter of the follicles in perfectly healthy skin. It is about 0·2 mm. long, and bears four pairs of short stumpy feet on the thorax. The head bears a proboscis and a pair of short antennae. It has no pathological significance.

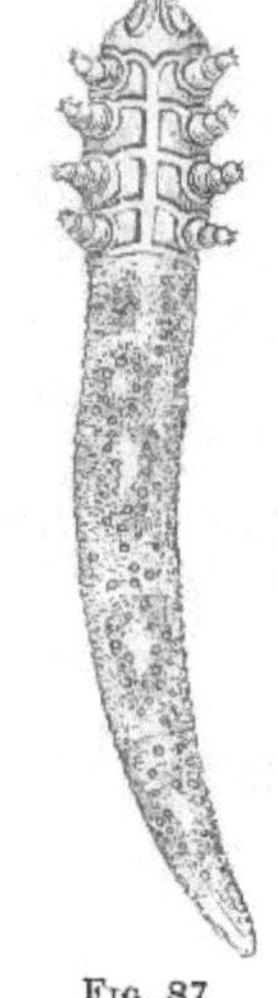

FIG. 87. ACARUS FOLLICULORUM. (*From* PERLS: × 300)

(4) *Ixodes ricinus* (*hominis*), or wood-tick, is also an occasional parasite of the skin. It buries its proboscis in the tissues and sucks its fill of blood. It belongs to the *Acarina*, as do also the American *I. unipunctata* and *I. bovis*.

(5) *Pentastoma denticulatum* (Fig. 88). This is an arachnoid, which in its larval state lodges in the internal organs. Its body is 4—5 mm. long, 1·5 mm. broad, squat and rounded, and possessing some ninety annular segments which are beset with spines at their margins.

The mouth is surrounded by four large hooks in chitinous sheaths. The larva chiefly inhabits the liver, more rarely the spleen, intestine, lung, or kidney. When looked for *post mortem* the animal has generally been dead for some time: it then appears as a nodule as big as a pea made up of a mortar-like chalky mass with a fibrous capsule. The mass often contains hooklets, but seldom the whole animal.

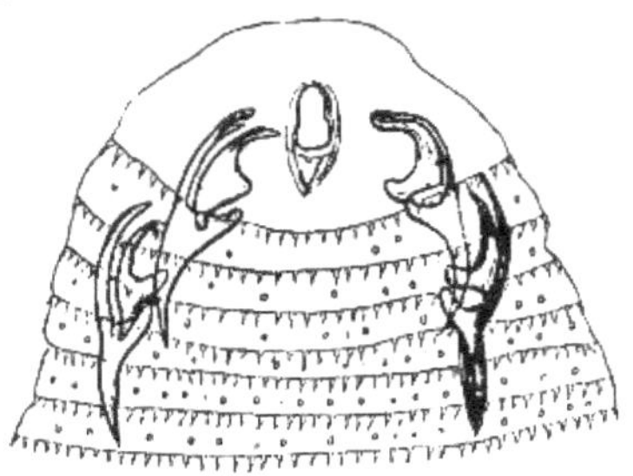

FIG. 88. HEAD-END OF *PENTASTOMA DENTICULATUM*.
(*From* PERLS: ×40)

According to LEUCKART, *Pentastoma denticulatum* is the larva of *Pentastoma taenioides*, a lanceolate arachnoid inhabiting the frontal sinuses of various animals, chiefly the dog. The female is 60—85 mm. long, the male 16—18 mm.; the breadth of each is about 3 mm. The mature animal resembles the larva, but it has no hooklets.

Pentastoma constrictum has also been met with as a larva in the liver and in the lungs (VON SIEBOLD; AITKEN, *Science and Pract. of Medicine* 1882).

226. **Insecta.** The parasites belonging to this class are nearly all epizoa. Some settle on the skin for a brief time only, in order to extract nutriment from it: others are stationary and make use of the epidermal structures for the deposit of their eggs. Of the many insects which afflict man we need name only the following.

(1) *Pediculus capitis*, or head-louse. This inhabits the hairy scalp, and extracts from it by means of its proboscis the blood on which it feeds. It fastens its eggs to the hairs by means of a chitinous covering. The 'nits' are easily seen as small greyish oval bodies, tightly affixed to the hair. The young louse emerges in about eight days, or less. The irritation induces scratching, which may set up somewhat severe inflammation or eczema.

(2) *Pediculus pubis*, or crab-louse, inhabits the hairy parts of the body and extremities, more especially about the genitals. Its mode of life is much like that of the head-louse, but it is smaller, and often more difficult to detect.

(3) *Pediculus vestimentorum*, or body-louse, infests the under-clothing, and lays its eggs there. It passes to the surface of the body merely in order to feed. It is somewhat larger than *P. capitis*.

(4) *Cimex lectuarius*, or bed-bug, infests bedding, bedsteads, old floors and walls, cupboards, etc. and betakes itself to its human victim at night in order to suck blood from him. It produces wheals on the skin.

(5) *Pulex irritans*, or common flea, also draws blood from the skin. At the point attacked is found a small punctiform haemorrhage surrounded by a reddened areola. More marked swellings or wheals are sometimes formed. The eggs are laid in the crevices and cracks of flooring-boards, in saw-dust, etc.

(6) *Pulex penetrans*, or sand-flea, (chigoe or chigger) is found in the sands of South Africa. The female buries itself and lays its eggs beneath the skin, and so produces intense inflammation.

(7) *Culicida* and *Tipulida* (midges and mosquitoes), *Tabanida* (gad-flies), and *Stomoxys calcitrans* also take blood from the skin and excite transient exudative inflammations. Some flies (*Oestrida*) lay their eggs occasionally in accessible body-cavities or in wounds. This occurs oftener among the lower animals than among men. *Oestrus hominis* (a doubtful species) lays its eggs beneath the human skin, and the larvae (maggots or bots) set up violent inflammation. *Haematopota pluvialis* is the Scotch 'clegg': it attacks men and beasts indifferently.

The above account has been chiefly taken from LEUCKART, *Die menschlichen Parasiten* Leipzig 1863—76 and 2nd Ed. vol. I, 1879—81; HELLER, *Ziemssen's Cyclopaedia* vols. III, VII; KLEBS, *H. d. path. Anat.*; PERLS, *Lehrb. d. allg. Path.* II Stuttgart 1879. Other comprehensive works are—KÜCHENMEISTER and ZÜRN, *Die Parasiten d. Menschen* Leipzig 1882; DAVAINE, *Traité des Entozoaires* Paris 1877; MÜLLER, *Statistik d. menschlichen Parasiten* Erlangen 1874; STEIN, *Die parasitären Krankheiten d. Menschen* vol. I Lahr 1882; PERRONCITO, *Parasiti d. uomo e d. animali utili* Milan 1882; COBBOLD, *Parasites* London 1879.

Scolecida, or Worms.

227. **Nematoda.** The parasitic round-worms and thread-worms are all nematoids. They have slender cylindrical elongated (sometimes filiform) bodies, without segments or appendages. The cuticle is thick and elastic. The mouth is placed at the anterior extremity, and is provided with soft or horny lips according to the species. The intestine is straight and, with the pharyngeal and gastric portions, extends from end to end of the body-cavity, terminating on the ventral surface just in front of the acuminate tail. The genital organs and their orifices are on the ventral side. The female genital orifice is usually placed at about the middle-point of the length; more rarely it is anterior or posterior to this. The male orifice coincides with that of the anus: it is provided with a chitinous investment, which serves also as a prehensile organ during copulation. The males are usually smaller than the females. Development is direct, and the metamorphic variations slight. The nematoids parasitic on man are some of them harmless inhabitants of the intestine, while others are highly dangerous when they invade the deeper organs.

228. *Ascaris lumbricoides*, the common round-worm or maw-worm (Fig. 89, p. 325), is a cylindrical worm with pointed ends: it is light brown or red in colour. The female (*A*) is 25—40 cm. long; the male (*B*) is considerably smaller, and its tail-end is bent into a hook provided with two *spicula* (*c*) or chitinous spines. The mouth is surrounded by three muscular lips bearing very delicate teeth. The female genital orifice (*a*) is anterior to the middle of the length. The eggs, which the female bears in enormous numbers, have when mature a double shell (Fig. 90) surrounded by an albuminous coating. It is about 50—60 micromm. in diameter. The worm is found in all parts of the alimentary canal, but chiefly in the small intestine. When the females are mature great numbers of eggs are shed and are found in the faeces. They are very tenacious of life, and are not killed by drying or freezing. The life-history of the worm is not fully known. It is possible that the eggs after ejection from the intestine require to pass through the body of an intermediate host before they can take up their abode in another human body. Their presence in the intestine does not usually give rise to any serious trouble. Only when they are very numerous do they cause intestinal catarrh, vomiting, and nervous irritation, chiefly in children. At times they pass through normal or morbid openings in the intestinal wall, and give rise to more serious disturbances. Thus an ascaris in the common bile-duct may obstruct the outflow of bile and so induce jaundice. Or if it pass through an ulcerated opening into a hernial sac, or into the peritoneal cavity, it may excite inflammation in the corresponding tissues. According to LEUCKART it may even penetrate the wall of the intestine where there is no pre-existing wound. It is often voided *per anum*, and occasionally *per os* during vomiting.

Ascaris mystax, or round-worm of the cat, is a very rare inhabitant of the human intestine. It is considerably smaller than the common round-worm (COBBOLD, *Entozoa*, 1864—69).

229. *Oxyuris vermicularis*, the thread-worm, seat-worm, or maggot-worm (Fig. 91), is a small round-worm. The female (*A*) is 10 mm. long, and acuminate at the tail: the male (*B*) is 4 mm. long and blunt at the tail, which is furnished with a single spiculum at the anus.

The eggs (*C*), often seen in great multitudes within the body of the female, are 50 micromm. long and 24 micromm. broad. One side is flat and the other rounded. The shell is covered

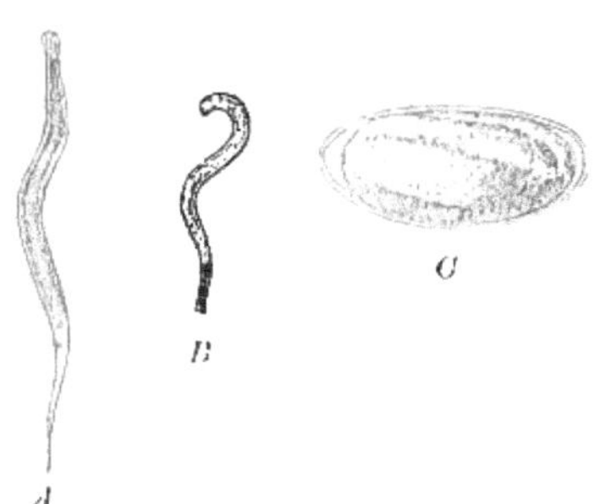

FIG. 91. OXYURIS VERMICULARIS. (*From* LEUCKART)
A female and *B* male, magnified fivefold
C egg magnified 350-fold

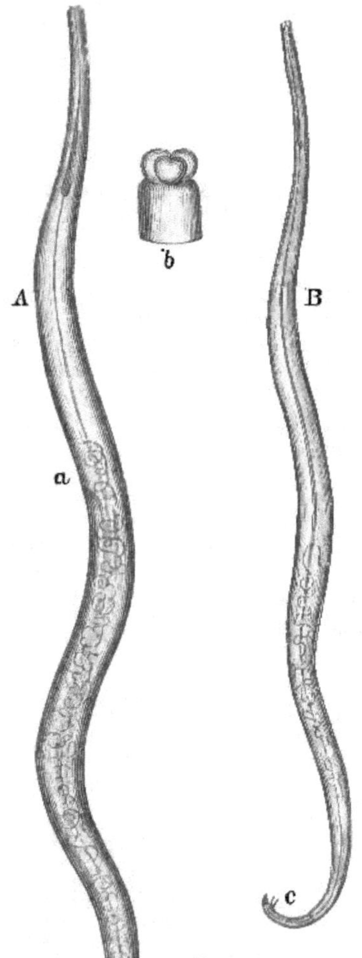

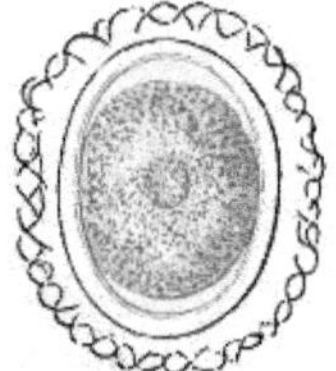

FIG. 90.

EGG OF *ASCARIS LUMBRICOIDES* WITH ITS SHELL AND ALBUMINOUS COATING.

(*From* LEUCKART: ×300)

FIG. 89. *ASCARIS LUMBRICOIDES.*

(*From* PERLS*: natural size*)

A female *B* male

a female genital orifice
b head end with the three lips, magnified
c male orifice with spicula

with a thin albuminous coating. The thread-worm inhabits the upper part of the colon and lower part of the ileum. According to ZENKER and HELLER the mature egg-bearing females affect the colon and caecum, the younger ones and the males affect the ileum. They are of very common occurrence and are often found in vast numbers. They are apt to migrate from the rectum into neighbouring parts, and may so enter the vagina. The irritation they cause induces violent scratching, and this again brings about inflammation of the skin and other disagreeable consequences.

When the eggs have been ejected from the body with the faeces, they must be taken up into the stomach of an animal before they can develope. It is not improbable that the individual host may re-infect himself; for eggs may stick under his finger-nails after he has been scratching himself, and may thus be inadvertently carried to the mouth.

The eggs are not destroyed by being dried, and in this condition they may be carried from place to place.

230. *Trichocephalus dispar*, or whip-worm (Fig. 92), is a common but innocuous parasite inhabiting the caecum and neighbouring parts of the intestine. DAVAINE says that half the inhabitants of Paris are infested with it. Both male and female are 4—5 cm. long. The anterior part of the body is very fine and thread-like. The posterior part, which contains the genital organs,

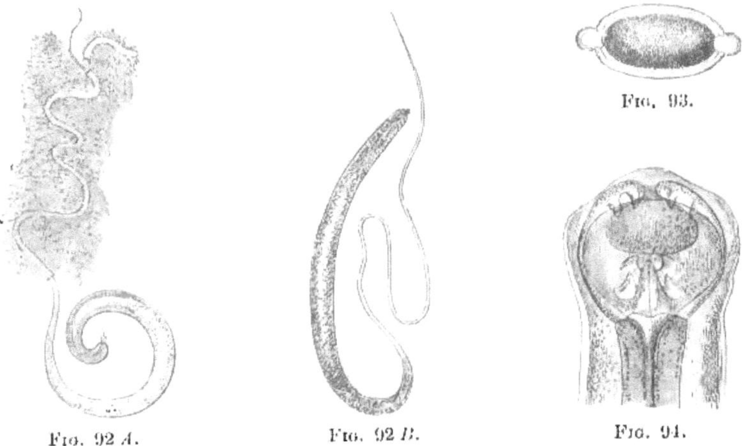

Fig. 93.

Fig. 92 *A*. Fig. 92 *B*. Fig. 94.

Fig. 92. *TRICHOCEPHALUS DISPAR*. *A* male *B* female

(*From LEUCKART: somewhat magnified: the male is anchored in the mucous membrane by means of his whip-like anterior part*)

Fig. 93. Egg of *TRICHOCEPHALUS DISPAR*. (*From HELLER*: ×350)

Fig. 94. Head-end of *DOCHMIUS DUODENALIS*. (*From LEUCKART: magnified*)

is much thicker; in the female (*B*) it is straight and cylindrical, in the male (*A*) it is rolled into a flat spiral and furnished with a spiculum.

The eggs (Fig. 93) are prolate spheroids, 50 micromm. in length. They have a thick brown shell, with a peg-shaped glassy-looking projection at each pole.

The first stage of development is passed in water or moist earth. It is very protracted, lasting even in the warm season for four or five months; and in cold weather for a longer time still. The eggs resist cold and drying extremely well.

231. *Anchylostoma* or *Sclerostoma duodenale* (*Dochmius* or *Strongylus duodenalis*) is a small worm infesting the upper part of the small intestine. The female is cylindrical and 6—18 mm. long, the male 6—10 mm.

The head-end (Fig. 94) is bent towards the dorsal surface and is furnished with a bulging oral capsule. This is cleft almost throughout on the dorsal surface, the cleft being covered by two chitinous lamellae. On the ventral lip are four curved teeth, on the dorsal lip are two straight ones. These are all held together by chitinous clasp-like structures. Beneath the dorsal cleft a conical projection rises from the interior of the capsule.

The male at its posterior end has a three-lobed bursa, and two thin spicula looking like slender fish-bones. The posterior part of the female becomes gradually thinner and ends in an awl-shaped spine. The vulva lies behind the middle point. The oval eggs are 44—67 micromm. long and 23—40 broad. They pass through their first developmental stages in the human intestine; in the next stages they inhabit dirty or muddy waters; thence they again obtain access to the alimentary tract, and there grow to maturity. Their presence in the small intestine is not free from danger. The worm gnaws into the mucous membrane with its teeth until it reaches the submucous coat, and thence it sucks its fill of blood. The point attacked is recognisable as a small ecchymosis, in the middle of which is a white spot with a central punctate aperture. This aperture has contained the head. Occasionally small blood-filled cavities are found in the mucous membrane, each containing a coiled-up worm. When present in number these parasites give rise to serious haemorrhages, which produce intense anaemia in the patient (the Egyptian chlorosis). The parasite is common in the tropics. According to GRIESINGER and BILHARZ a great proportion (something like 25 per cent.) of the natives of Egypt suffer from it. WUCHERER says it is also common in Brazil. McCONNELL has met with it in India (*Lancet* 1, 1882). Within the last few years it has been very frequently observed among the workmen engaged in the St. Gothard tunnel.

References to *Anchylostoma*:—GRIESINGER, *Arch. f. phys. Heilk.* 1854; WUCHERER, *Arch. f. klin. Med.* XII, 1872; BILHARZ, *Zeitsch. f. wiss. Zool.* IV;

LEUCKART, *op. cit.*; GRASSI and PARONA, *Annali univ. di med.* 1878; BOZZOLO and PAGLIANI, *Giorn. d. Soc. ital. d' igiene* II Milan 1880; SONDEREGGER, *Corresp. f. Schweiz. Aerzte* 1880; BUGNION, *Anchylostome duodénal et anémie du St.-Gothard, Rev. méd. de la Suisse rom.* I, 1881; PERRONCITO, *Arch. p. l. scien. med.* V, Turin 1881; LONG, *Trans. Int. Med. Congress* I, 1881; MÉGNIN, *Soc. de Biologie* March 1882; COBBOLD, *Human Parasites* 1882, Art. *Sclerostoma, Quain's Dict. of Med.* 1882.

Among the rarer nematoid parasites are the following. *Eustrongylus gigas* or palisade-worm; the female attains a length of 1 metre, the male of 35 cm.; the colour is blood-red. It has been found a few times in the pelvis of the human kidney; but it is commoner in the seal, marten, wolf, and dog. The immature worms dwell chiefly in fresh-water fishes. *Strongylus longevaginatus (bronchialis)*, a thread-like worm 26 mm. long. It has once been found in the lung of a boy. *Anguillula (Rhabditis) stercoralis*, a minute round-worm 1 mm. long, indigenous in Cochin-China. It infests the entire alimentary tract, bile-ducts, and pancreatic duct, and gives rise to chronic diarrhoea. PERRONCITO (*loc. cit.* and *Micr. Soc. Journ.* 1882) found it in the tunnel-workmen at St. Gothard. See PERLS, *Allg. Path.* II; DAVAINE, *Traité des Entozoaires* 1877; LIEBERMANN, *Dysenterie chronique de Cochin-chine, Gaz. des Hôp.* 1877; NORMAND, *Arch. de Méd. Navale*, 1877.

232. *Trichina spiralis*, or flesh-worm of pork, appears in two forms according as it inhabits the intestine or the muscles. The intestinal form (Fig. 95) is the sexually mature worm. It is a minute filiform creature, scarcely visible with the naked eye, and white in colour. The female (*A*) is 3 mm. long; the male is considerably smaller.

In both sexes the hinder part of the body is straight: the male (*B*) has on the dorsal side of its tail two mammillary protuberances which are turned toward the ventral aspect and include between them four wart-like nodules. There is no spiculum: in copulation the muscular cloaca is everted and protruded.

The alimentary canal begins with a muscular pharynx which widens as it passes into the oesophagus. This latter is surrounded throughout its length with a series of large cellular masses. The stomach passes without notable change of structure into the intestine. In the male this terminates,

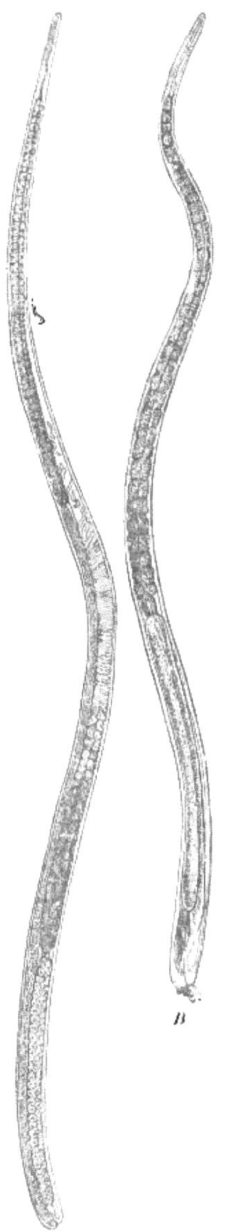

FIG. 95.
MATURE *TRICHINAE*.
(*From LEUCKART: magnified*)
A female *B* male

with the seminal ducts, in the cloaca. The testis consists of a tube which commences caecally at the tail-end, extends forward to the cellular bodies round the oesophagus, and then bends back to be joined by the seminal ducts. The genital organs of the female (*A*) consist of a simple ovary, uterus, and vagina: the latter opens at a quarter of the whole length from the head-end. The ovary, like the testis, is a tube commencing posteriorly and passing forwards to join the tubular uterus.

The eggs develope into embryos in the uterus, and these are born in the free state.

The trichina of muscle (Fig. 96) is a small worm 0·7 to 1·0 mm. in length: it inhabits the fleshy muscles. It is usually coiled up into a spiral, and lies in a fibrous capsule or cyst, which sometimes also contains calcareous matter. A finely granular substance surrounds the coils of the worm. One capsule may enclose two to five trichinae.

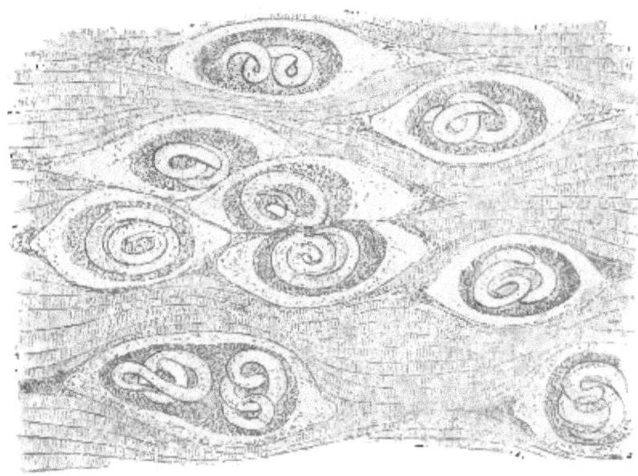

FIG. 96. TRICHINAE ENCYSTED IN MUSCLE, SHOWING THE CAPSULE AND ITS CONTENTS. (*From* LEUCKART: *magnified*)

233. The following is the life-history of the trichina. When a piece of muscle containing live encysted trichinae reaches the stomach of a host, human or other, the capsule is dissolved and the trichinae set free. They come to maturity in the intestine in about 2½ days; when they proceed to pair. The birth of embryos begins on the 7th day and continues for some time, it may be for weeks. A single worm may bring forth 1000 to 1300 young. These then migrate from the intestine in search of striated muscle. They do so in various ways. Most of them seem to pass directly through the wall of the intestine, the peritoneal cavity, and the subperitoneal connective tissues. Others gain access to the lymph and blood, and are thus conveyed to remote organs. Once in the muscle they penetrate the primitive bundles, reduce the contents to mere detritus, and in 14 days or so become mature

muscle-trichinae. At first they are only enclosed by the evacuated sarcolemma. Afterwards a cyst is formed, consisting partly of a chitinous secretion of the animal, partly of hyperplastic fibrous tissue.

The intestinal trichinae live but a short time (5 to 8 weeks). The muscle-trichinae on the other hand may live for a very long time, perhaps indeed for a time limited only by the death of their host. After a while calcareous salts are generally deposited within the cyst; this gives the cyst a lustrous white appearance by reflected light, and a dark or turbid appearance by transmitted light. If for any reason the trichina dies, the contents of the capsule become calcified.

Trichinae are met with in man, in the pig, cat, rat, mouse, hamster, pole-cat, fox, marten, badger, hedgehog, and racoon. By feeding on trichinous flesh, muscle-trichinae may be acquired by rabbits, guinea-pigs, sheep, dogs, etc. Human beings are infected by eating uncooked pork. Trichinosis in man is attended with very various symptoms. Intestinal catarrh follows upon the introduction of the trichinous flesh into the alimentary tract. The invasion of the muscles is marked by swelling, oedema, partial paralyses, and not uncommonly fever. The symptoms are at their height in the fourth or fifth week. Death not infrequently ensues. The violence and gravity of the symptoms depend generally on the number of trichinae which have entered the muscles.

The trichinae are found most abundantly in the diaphragm, intercostal, cervical, and laryngeal muscles; they are least abundant in the muscles of the limbs. They are usually crowded together at the points of attachment of the muscle to its tendon.

The worm was first discovered by PAGET at St Bartholomew's Hospital in 1834; see *Lancet* 1, 1866. OWEN named and described it shortly afterwards.

The literature of trichinosis is very abundant: we can only refer to a few of the chief works on the subject.

OWEN, *Zool. Soc. Trans.* 1835; ZENKER, *Virch. Arch.* vol. 18, *Arch. f. klin. Med.* VIII; VIRCHOW, *Die Lehre von den Trichinen* Berlin 1866; LEUCKART, *Die Parasiten des Menschen*; HELLER, *Ziemssen's Cyclopaedia* vol. III; COBBOLD, *Entozoa* 1869; GLAZIER, *Report on Trich.* Washington 1881; WENDT, *Chronic Affect. following Trich.*, *New York Med. Rec.* 1879. For further references see COBBOLD, *Human Parasites* 1882.

234. *Filaria (Dracunculus) medinensis*, (Fig. 97) or Guinea-worm, is a fine thread-like worm from 60 to 100 cm. in length. Only the female is known. The anterior end is rounded; the posterior terminates in a pointed tail curved over ventrally. The outer covering consists of a firm cuticle thickened at the head-end into a kind of shield. The intestine is narrow, and there is no anus. The gravid uterus occupies nearly the whole of the body-cavity. The embryos have no envelope; they have a stout cuticle and an acuminate tail. They use as intermediate hosts certain small crustaceans (*Cyclops*) that inhabit drinking-water, and so

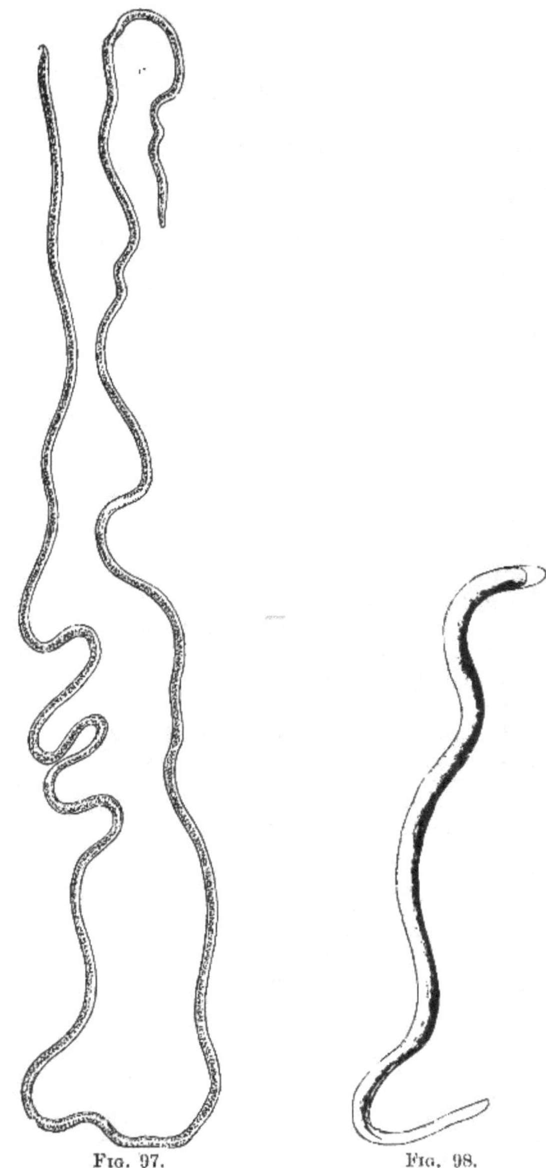

FIG. 97. FIG. 98.

FIG. 97. *FILARIA (DRACUNCULUS) MEDINENSIS.*
(*From* LEUCKART: *natural size*)

FIG. 98. EMBRYO OF *FILARIA SANGUINIS HOMINIS.* (*From* LEWIS: ×400)

they ultimately reach the human stomach. In Africa and Asia they are very common. They develope to maturity under the skin, giving rise to cutaneous abscesses. They are most commonly found in the legs and feet, especially in the neighbourhood of the heel.

See LEUCKART, *op. cit.*; DAVAINE, *Entozoaires* etc.; COBBOLD, *Entozoa* 1864. The guinea-worm disease has been identified with the *dracontiasis* of PLUTARCH, and with the endemic disorder attributed to 'fiery serpents' in the book of Numbers.

235. *Filaria sanguinis hominis* (LEWIS) or *sanguinolenta* in its sexually mature form is a filiform worm 8 to 10 cm. long. According to MANSON it inhabits the lymphatics, especially those of the scrotum and lower limbs. It gives rise to obstructions of the lymph-current and to peculiar inflammations, which end in elephantiasis of the tissues with oedema and lymphangiectasis. Suppurative inflammations, lymphatic abscesses, buboes, chylous hydrocele, and chylous ascites have all been observed as consequences of its presence.

The embryos, which are about 0·35 mm. long (Fig. 98), pass from the lymphatics into the blood and induce haematuria and chyluria. Both conditions result from the lodgement of the embryos in number within the kidneys. The embryos may be ejected with the urine. MANSON finds that they are spread by the agency of mosquitoes, who take up the filariae with the blood they suck. The filariae pass through an intermediate developmental stage in the body of the mosquito; thence they pass into water, and thence again into the human body. It is thus probable that they reach the vessels and tissues from the intestine.

The *Filaria sanguinis* appears to be indigenous only within the tropics (Brazil, Egypt, India, Guadaloupe, etc.).

See LEWIS, *On a haematozoon inhabiting human blood: its relation to chyluria and other diseases* Calcutta 1872, *Lancet* 2, 1877, *Quart. Journ. Mic. Sci.* 1879, Art. *Chyluria*, *Quain's Dict. of Med.* 1882; BANCROFT, *Trans. Path. Soc.* 1878; MANSON, *Lancet* 1, 1878 and *Trans. Path. Soc.* 1881; COBBOLD, *Parasites* 1879 and *Human Parasites* 1882; *Journ. Quekett Micros. Club* 1880; BARTH, *Annales de Derm. et Syph.* 1881.

Several other rare species of *Filaria* are known. References to them will be found in the standard works of LEUCKART, DAVAINE, and COBBOLD, already cited.

236. **Trematoda.** The flukes, or suctorial worms, are flattened or tongue-shaped worms. They possess suctorial pores by which they can adhere to surfaces, and in some cases they have also hook-like processes. The intestine is usually bifurcated, and terminates caecally. The development is direct or by alternate generations. In the latter case an intermediate host is necessary. This is usually a mollusc; while the mature worms almost all find lodgement in vertebrate animals. The intermediate larval stage is usually preceded by a period of active locomotion. The trematode larvae are furnished with a propelling tail, and swim about freely as *cercaria*.

237. *Distoma hepaticum*, the liver-fluke (Fig. 99), is a leaf-shaped trematode 28 mm. long and 12 mm. broad. The head-end projects like a beak, and bears a small suctorial disc in which the

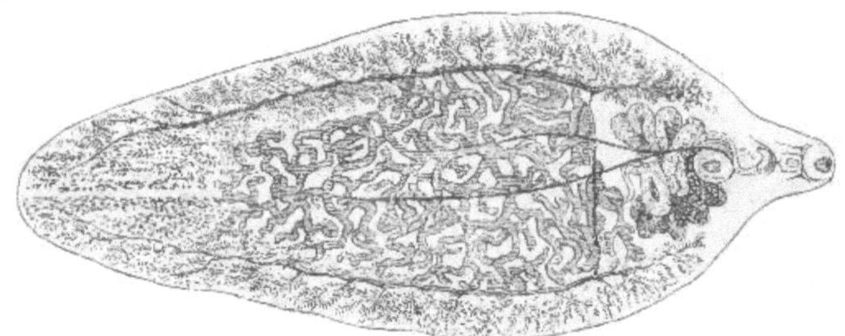

FIG. 99. *DISTOMA HEPATICUM* WITH MALE AND FEMALE GENITAL ORGANS. (*From LEUCKART*: ×2½)

orifice of the mouth is visible. Immediately behind this on the ventral surface is another suctorial disc. The genital orifice lies between the two discs.

The uterus is a convoluted tube lying behind the posterior disc. The ovaries lie on each side of the hinder part of the body, and between them lie the deeply bifurcated testes. The intestinal canal is also bifurcated and much branched.

The eggs (Fig. 100) are oval, 0·13 mm. long and 0·08 mm. broad. When placed in water a globular embryo is developed,

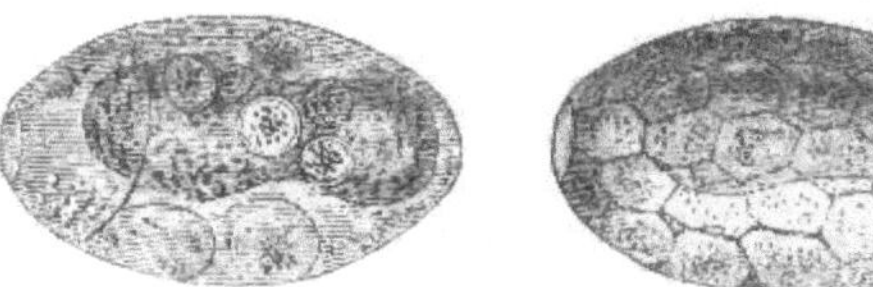

FIG. 100. EGG OF *DISTOMA HEPATICUM*. (*From LEUCKART*: ×200)

which swims freely by means of its ciliated envelope. The details of its life-history are not certainly known. The adult animal infests the biliary ducts: more rarely it is found in the intestine or in the vena cava. It is rare in man, but very common among the ruminants: it causes the 'rot' in sheep. The consequences of its invasion, especially in great numbers, are obstruction of the biliary ducts, accumulation of bile, dilatation and incrustation of the ducts with biliary matters, inflammation around them and hyperplasia of the hepatic connective tissues, with associated atrophy of the liver-cells.

238. *Distoma lanceolatum* is only 8 or 9 mm. long and 2 to 2·5 mm. broad. It is lancet-shaped, and the head-end does not markedly project. The integument is naked. The two lobulated

testes lie close behind the posterior disc and in front of the ovary and uterus: the coils of the latter are seen through the transparent

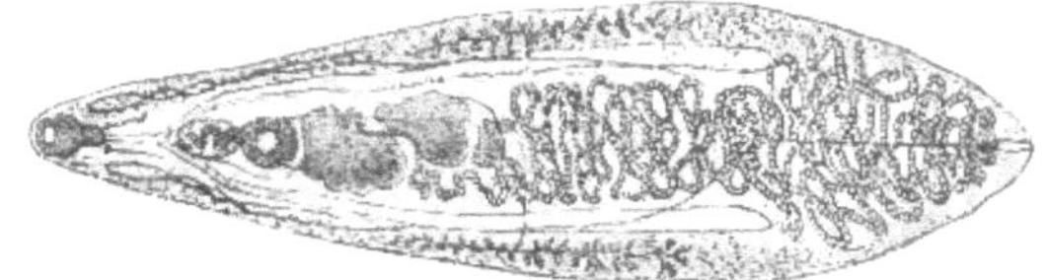

FIG. 101. *DISTOMA LANCEOLATUM* WITH ITS INTERNAL ORGANS. (*From* LEUCKART: ×100)

body-walls. The more anterior coils which are filled with eggs look black, the remaining coils are russet-coloured. The yellowish-white ovaries lie about the middle of the lateral margin.

The eggs (Fig. 102) are 0·04 mm. long. The embryo is visible in them before they have left the uterus, but it only escapes some

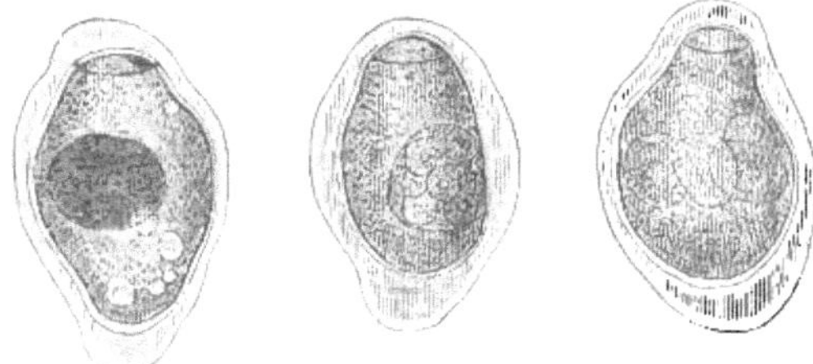

FIG. 102. EGGS OF *DISTOMA LANCEOLATUM* SHORTLY AFTER THE SHELL IS FORMED. (*From* LEUCKART: ×400)

weeks after they are deposited. Its metamorphoses are unknown. This fluke like the other infests the biliary ducts, but it is rarely found in man. It is commonest in sheep and cattle, but as it is usually present in small numbers, it rarely gives rise to any grave disturbances of health.

239. *Distoma haematobium* or *Bilharzia haematobia* (Fig. 103) is a species of fluke in which the sexes are distinct. The oral and ventral discs are close to each other, and the fore-end of the body is slender. The sexual orifice in each sex lies just behind the ventral disc. The male is 12—14 mm. long. The body is flattened, but its posterior part is rolled laterally into a kind of tube or gynaecophoric canal (Fig. 103) into which the female is received. The female is 16—19 mm. long and almost cylindrical in form. The eggs are prolate (Fig. 104) and 0·12 mm. long. They are furnished with a spine which may be either terminal or lateral.

These worms are found in the inferior vena cava, in the portal vein, in the splenic vein, in the mesenteric veins, and in the vessels of the rectum and bladder. They feed on the blood, and infest man and the monkey. They are very common in Egypt and

Abyssinia, the Cape, and Natal, where they give rise to the disease known as 'endemic haematuria.' The cercaria abound

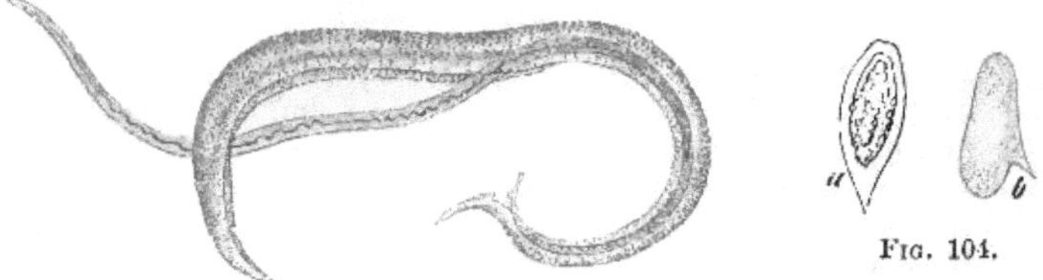

FIG. 103. FIG. 104.

FIG. 103. *DISTOMA HAEMATOBIUM* MALE AND FEMALE, THE LATTER WITHIN THE GYNAECOPHORIC CANAL OF THE FORMER. (*From* LEUCKART: ×10)

FIG. 104. EGGS OF *DISTOMA HAEMATOBIUM*. (*From* LEUCKART: ×150)
a with terminal spine *b* with lateral spine

in canals and rivers, and gain access to the body in drinking-water. The embryos mature quickly and permeate the mucous and submucous coats of the ureters, bladder, and bowel, and occasionally the kidney and liver. They set up inflammation of the bladder and ureters, associated with ulcerations, incrustations, and concretions. Haematuria is always produced. Cylindrical ciliated embryos may develope within the urinary tract.

References :—GRIESINGER, *Arch. f. phys. Heilk.* XIII, 1854; BILHARZ, *Wien. med. Woch.* 4 and 5, 1856, and *Brit. For. Med. Chir. Rev.* 1856—58; SONSINO, *Arch. gén. de méd.* 1876; COBBOLD, *Parasites* 1879; GUILLEMARD, *Endemic Haematuria* London 1882; ZANCAROL, *Trans. Path. Soc.* XXXIII (1882).

240. **Cestoda.** The cestoids, or tape-worms, are flat compound 'worms,' destitute of a mouth or alimentary canal. They multiply by gemmation from a pyriform 'head' or 'nurse.' The budded individuals or segments remain for a long time connected with the head, forming a jointed chain. The several members (*proglottides*) of this colony are hermaphrodite. The older segments increase in size as they are gradually pushed away from the place at which they were formed by the constant development of new segments. In other respects they resemble each other exactly; while the head is distinguished by possessing two or four suckers or *oscula*, and generally a circlet of claw-like hooks. By means of these the tape-worm fastens itself to the intestinal wall of its host, which is probably always a vertebrate. The head developes from a rounded embryo having four to six hooklets. These embryos (*proscolices, hydatids*) are found in the various parenchymatous organs of the intermediate host; and thence by what we may call passive migration they reach the intestine of their final host.

The cestoids parasitic on man belong to the families of *Taeniada* and *Bothriocephalida*. The former infest man both as hydatids and as tape-worms; the latter only as tape-worms.

The development of the Cestoda is exhaustively treated in the handsome work of HEIN, *Die parasitären Krankheiten des Menschen* 1882; see also DAVAINE, *Les Cestoïdes*, *Dict. ency. sciences méd.* 1874; COBBOLD, *Tapeworms* 1874.

241. *Taenia solium* when fully developed is 2 to 3 metres long. The head (Fig. 105 *A*) is the size of a small pin-head; it is globular and the suckers project somewhat. The vertex is not uncommonly pigmented and is surrounded with a pretty large *rostellum* or circlet of some 26 hooks (Fig. 105 *B*). The hooks are

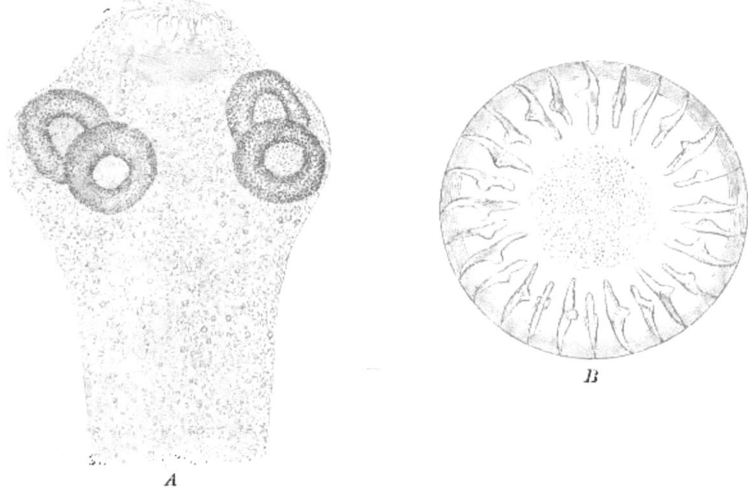

FIG. 105. *A* HEAD OF *TAENIA SOLIUM* WITH ROSTELLUM PROTRUDED. (*Carmine staining; mounted in Canada Balsam*: × 50)
B CIRCLET OF HOOKS MAGNIFIED (*LEUCKART*).

short, broad, and appressed, with a small projection at the root. The head is followed by a filiform neck an inch or so in length. At a certain distance from the head the joints begin to be traceable. The first joints are very short, the more advanced ones are longer (Fig. 106): they then become square, and finally the length is greater than the breadth. About 130 cm. beyond the head the mature segments begin, though the sexual organs have been fully developed in earlier segments. The ripe segments (Fig. 107) are 9—10 mm. long and 6—7 mm. broad: their corners are rounded off. The genital opening lies at the side, somewhat behind the middle. The ovary has seven to ten lateral branches separated by considerable intervals; each branch breaks up into a series of dendritic ramifications. The ovary is filled with eggs. The parenchyma of the body both in ripe and unripe segments is divisible into a peripheral and a central layer. The central layer contains the generative organs and the water-vascular system.

The latter is an excretory apparatus; it takes the form of two lateral canals running along the margins of the entire chain of segments and connected by cross-canals at both ends of each segment. Fine ramifications pass from these into the parenchyma.

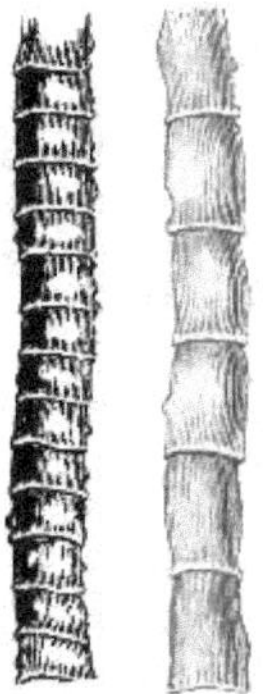

FIG. 106.

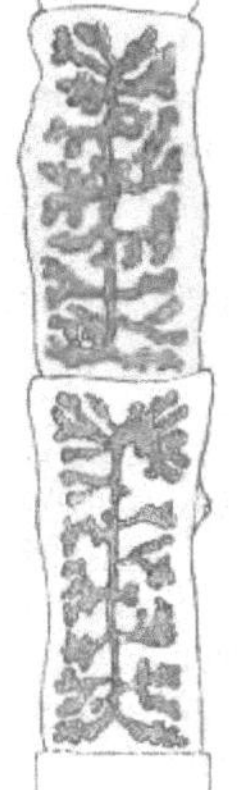

FIG. 107.

FIG. 106. IMMATURE AND MATURE PROGLOTTIDES.
(*From* LEUCKART: *natural size*)
FIG. 107. TWO PROGLOTTIDES SHOWING THE UTERUS.
(*From* LEUCKART: × 2)

The male and female sexual organs lie close to each other. The testis is a clear or whitish convoluted tube with vesicles, lying in the fore-part of the segment. It passes into the vas deferens, and this into a *cirrus* or retractile extremity, which is rolled up within a muscular pouch or cloaca at the middle of the lateral margin. The cirrus can be everted and protruded through the genital orifice. The opening of the female organ lies close behind the male opening in the same genital cloaca. From this the vagina passes backwards towards the hinder border of the segment. Before reaching the border it communicates with a copulative sac or *receptaculum seminis*, and receives the duct of the germ-bearing organ or true ovary. Then turning forwards it passes into an oviduct, into which opens the duct of the so-called vitelligenous organs. The entire ovigenous organ (which must be studied in unripe segments) is thus made up of an unpaired germ-bearing portion or true ovary and a pair of yolk-bearing or vitelligenous glands, all lying in the hinder part of the segment. The oviduct having received the ducts of these glands passes then into the dilated matrix or uterus, which in sexually mature segments forms a simple straight tube. The egg-germs leaving the true ovary become impregnated by spermatozoa from the seminal receptacle, and passing onwards are invested with yolk-substance from the vitelligenous glands. Being then complete ova they pass into the uterus, which as it gradually fills throws out the numerous lateral caeca characteristic of the ripe segment. As this happens the other generative organs gradually disappear.

The peripheral layer is essentially muscular, but it contains a greater or less number of calcareous granules. These indeed are not entirely absent in the central layer. The muscular tissue is made up of non-striated fibres; in the neighbourhood of the sucking-discs of the head they form peculiar bunches or groups. The surface of the tape-worm is covered with a transparent cuticle, from which the hooklets of the head are developed.

242. The egg-germs as they leave the ovary are pale thin-walled spherical cells. In the oviduct they are transformed into yellowish globules, which become covered over with a somewhat opaque envelope or shell thickly beset with minute spicula (Fig. 108 *a*). It is frequently found to be invested by a second covering (*b*) made up of an albuminous layer with granules, and enclosed in a fine membrane (primitive vitelline membrane). Without this envelope the egg is 0·03 mm. in diameter. With the second envelope the egg already contains the partly developed embryo, whose six hooklets can be distinguished. Thus the embryonic development begins within the uterus; the ripe segments are in fact viviparous animals.

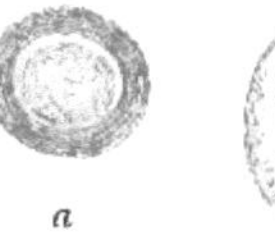

FIG. 108.
EGGS OF *TAENIA SOLIUM*.
(*From* LEUCKART: × 300)
a without the primitive vitelline membrane
b with it

The further development of these embryos, which are now enclosed in a brownish envelope, does not take place within the body of the original host: they must pass into a new one. When they reach the stomach of a pig, the envelope is dissolved, and the liberated embryo bores its way into the wall of stomach or intestine. Thence it migrates, either by way of the vessels or directly, into one or other of the organs. When at last it settles, it passes through various metamorphoses, and at the end of two or three months is transformed into a vesicle filled with serum (Fig. 109), from the inner surface of the wall of which springs a new head or scolex, enveloped in a second membrane or *receptaculum scolicis*.

This cyst or vesicle containing the head of the tape-worm is called a 'measle' or *cysticercus cellulosae*. The scolices have already their circlet of hooks, sucking-discs, water-vascular system, and calcareous granules. If the scolex reaches the stomach of a man, the cyst-membrane is dissolved, and from the scolex is developed a chain of proglottides, forming a new tape-worm.

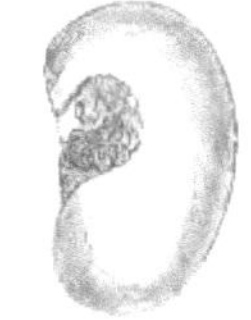

FIG. 109. *CYSTICERCUS CELLULOSAE* WITH THE HEAD AND ITS MEMBRANE. (*From* LEUCKART: *natural size*)

243. *Taenia solium* inhabits the small intestine of man, and is acquired by eating ill-cooked pork. The corresponding measle is found in man and in the pig exclusively, or nearly so. In the intestine the worm is generally solitary, but cases in which two or more have coexisted are not very rare. In some instances from thirty to forty have been found in one person. The tape-worm gives rise to irritation of the mucous membrane, colic, and reflex nervous disturbances.

The measle or cysticercus also occurs in man, as we have already indicated. It is found in the most various tissues, in the muscles, brain, eye, skin, etc. Its pathological significance depends on its seat; but it is usually slight. Even in the brain it does not always give rise to serious consequences. It excites a local inflammation, which induces a fibrous thickening of the tissues round the cyst. It maintains its vitality for years. After the death of the scolex the cyst shrinks, and chalky masses are deposited within its cavity. The hooklets may be found long afterwards. Cystic infection depends necessarily on the introduction of eggs or proglottides into the stomach.

Cysticercus racemosus is a measle of the brain. It is distinguished by the fact that it remains sterile and forms grape-like bunches of vesicles (HELLER, *Ziemssen's Cyclopaedia* vol. III; ZENKER, *Henle's Beiträge* Bonn 1882).

Abnormalities of development are very often observed in individual tapeworms.

244. *Taenia mediocanellata* or *saginata* exceeds *T. solium* not only in length (it may reach 4 metres) but in width and thickness, as well as in the size of the separate proglottides (Fig. 110 p. 340).

The head (Fig. 111) has neither hooklets nor rostellum. Its vertex is smooth and furnished with four large sucking-discs, usually surrounded with a dark pigmented border.

The eggs are like those of *T. solium*. The uterus (Fig. 112) has a large number of lateral diverticula, running close to each other and branching dichotomously, not like *T. solium* in dendritic ramifications. The genital opening lies below the middle of the lateral margin. The segments which break loose are generally empty of eggs.

The corresponding cysticerci infest the muscles and organs of cattle. The development follows the same course as in the case of *T. solium*. Malformations of the worm are very frequently observed.

Man acquires this tape-worm by eating uncooked beef. It is more widely diffused than *T. solium*.

Taenia cucumerina or *elliptica* is 15 to 20 cm. long: its head has a circlet of hooks and a rostellum. It is often found in cats and dogs, rarely in man. Its cysticercus infests the dog-louse.

Taenia nana is a small tape-worm 15 mm. in length: its head has four sucking-discs and a circlet of hooks. It has been found in Egypt.

The frequent malformations to which *Taenia* is subject have led to the multiplication of species, or rather of specific names. Many of these refer to what are at best mere varieties.

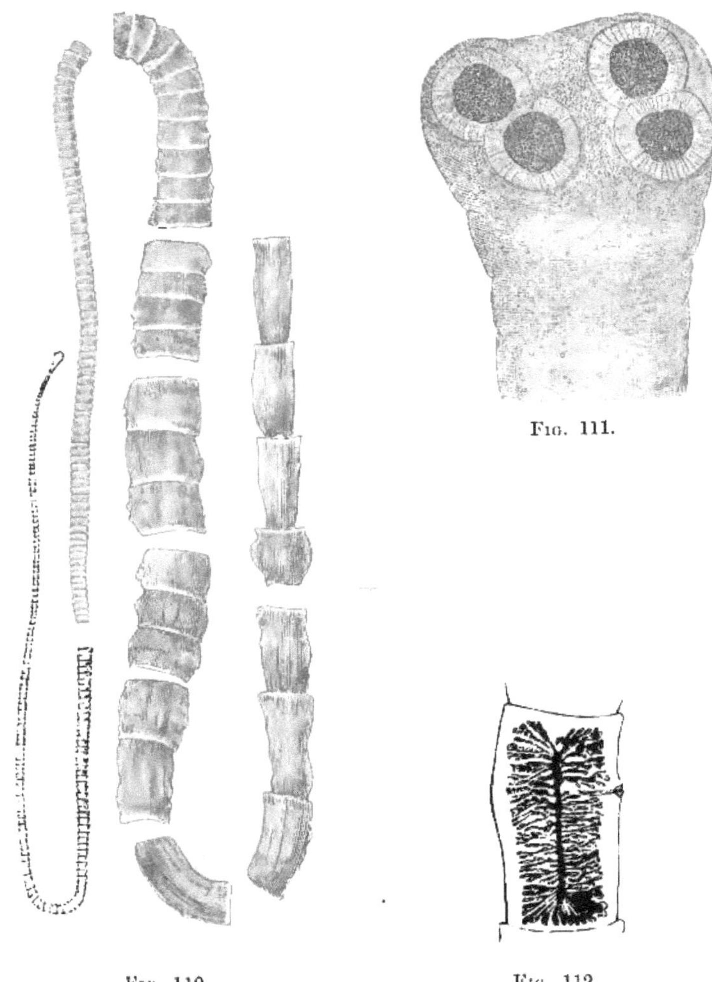

Fig. 111.

Fig. 110.

Fig. 112.

Fig. 110. Fragments of a *Taenia saginata.*
(*From Leuckart: natural size*)

Fig. 111. Head of *Taenia saginata* retracted; with dark pigment in and between the sucking-discs. (*Unstained glycerine preparation:* × 30)

Fig. 112. Segment of *Taenia saginata.* (*From Leuckart:* × $1\frac{1}{2}$)

245. *Taenia echinococcus* inhabits the intestine of the dog. It is 4 mm. long, and possesses only four segments, of which the last is larger than all the rest of the body (Fig. 113).

The hooklets have a blunt process at the base, and are seated on a somewhat prominent rostellum. There are some thirty or forty of them.

Only the cystic form or hydatid is known to occur in man; he acquires it by the introduction of the eggs into the alimentary canal.

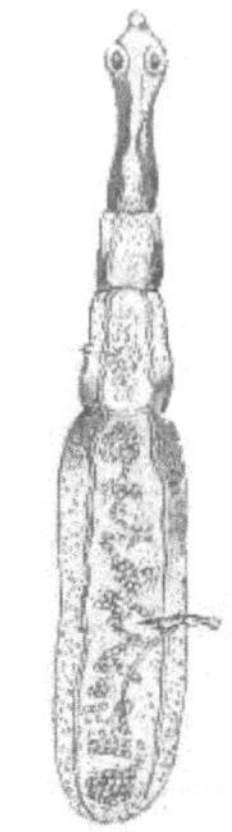

Fig. 113. Full-grown *Taenia echinococcus.* (*From Leuckart*: × 12)

When the embryo migrates from the intestine to some other organ, it is transformed into a cyst incapable of active motion. The **hydatid cyst** consists of an external lamellar highly-elastic cuticle, and an internal lining of body-parenchyma consisting of granular matter, cells, muscle-fibres, and a vascular system. When the cyst reaches the size of a walnut (or in some cases sooner) it begins to develope from the parenchymatous layer a series of smaller vesicles (brood-capsules). The wall of these is likewise two-fold; but the cuticular layer is within and the parenchymatous layer without. On these brood-capsules develope numbers of heads or scolices (Fig. 114). According to Leuckart they are formed out of sacculated outgrowths from the external wall of the capsules (see the left side of Fig. 114).

When the rudimentary head has become fully developed into a scolex (sometimes even sooner), it is retracted within the cyst which it thereby invaginates (Fig. 114). What was before the

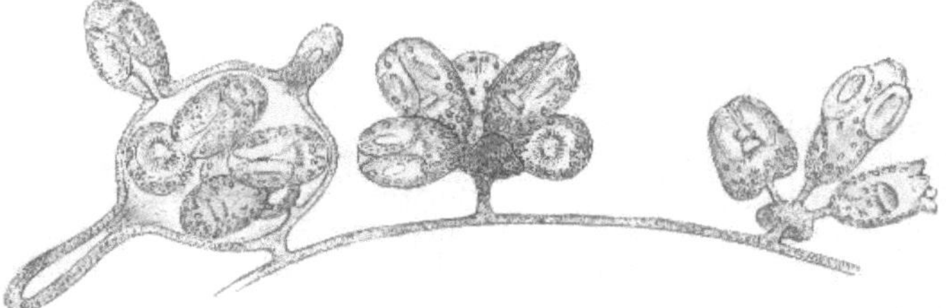

Fig. 114. Brood-capsules of *Echinococcus* in connexion with the parenchymatous layer of the cyst.

(*From Leuckart: some of the capsules are closed, some have been burst open in making the preparation*: ×50 *circa*)

internal or cuticular surface of the head now becomes the outer surface. The original outer surfaces, which are parenchymatous, come now into contact and adhere to each other. The head is then about 0·3 mm. long, and has a rostellum with tiny blunt hooklets, four sucking-discs, a water-vascular system, and numerous calcareous granules in its parenchyma. The fore-part of the body is often invaginated within the hind-part.

In many cases these echinococcus-cysts remain single. The only change they undergo is that they grow larger as fresh capsules and scolices are formed, so that they at length reach the size of a big orange, or of the closed fist. The surrounding tissues form, by condensation and thickening, a pseudo-cyst round the cuticular membrane. The cavity of the cyst is filled with clear liquid which is not coagulable by heat or acid. The brood-capsules are always seated on the inner surface, unless they are shaken loose mechanically. They appear as small white points lying in the transparent parenchyma. Occasionally the cyst may remain altogether sterile.

246. In many cases 'daughter-cysts' are formed. They develope in the thickness of the cuticle independently of the proper parenchymatous layer. Between two lamellae of the cuticle is formed an aggregation of granules which becomes surrounded with a secondary cuticle. This forms the starting-point of a new series of layers. As the layers multiply the inner cavity increases in size and its contents at length become clear and liquid. As the daughter-cyst grows it forces out the wall of the parent cyst like a hernial sac, until it at length gives way and sets the daughter-cyst free. Escaping thus into the tissues round the parent cyst it receives from them an external fibrous envelope, and proceeds to develope brood-capsules in the same way as the primary cyst derived from the six-hooked embryo.

An echinococcus which is thus reproduced exogenously is called *Echinococcus granulosus* or *scolecipariens* (KÜCHENMEISTER). It is also described as *E. veterinorum*, as it often occurs in domestic animals.

A second compound echinococcus is the *E. hydatidosus*. It is characterised by the formation of internal daughter-cysts. NAUNYN (*Dorpat. med. Zeitsch.* 1870) asserts, and LEUCKART agrees with him, that the scolices and brood-capsules may undergo a cystic transformation, and so become daughter-cysts. NAUNYN goes on to say that these endogenous daughter-cysts may migrate from the parent cyst and so produce the *E. granulosus*; but this LEUCKART disputes. The internal daughter-cysts sometimes develope daughters of their own or 'granddaughter-cysts.' Each of the cystic forms of which mention has been made may reach to a very considerable size.

247. The third form, or *Echinococcus multilocularis*, only forms small cysts, from the size of a millet-seed to that of a pea. They are always present in very large numbers.

The *E. multilocularis* appears as a hard tumour seated in the liver. It is built up of a multitude of alveoli separated by dense scar-like fibrous tissue. The contents are transparent and jelly-like or semi-fluid. The alveoli are spherical or irregular in form. Here and there the tissues may have softened and broken down, and thus ulcerated cavities are formed. In other places the vesicles are shrunken and calcified, or the tissues are bile-stained. The distinct alveolar texture of the growth led to its being regarded as a tumour, and it was described as **alveolar colloid** of the liver. VIRCHOW (*Verh. d. phys. med. Ges. zu Würzburg* VI, 1855) was the first to make out its real nature, and he showed that the colloid masses were made up of echinococcus-cysts. The smallest vesicles merely contain granular matter, the larger contain liquid. The granular pseudo-parenchymatous covering of the cuticle seldom contains scolices, most of the cysts being sterile.

E. multilocularis is possibly an abnormal variety or 'sport' from the exogenous form.

References :—VIRCHOW, *Virch. Arch.* vol. 6; LEUCKART, *Parasiten* vol. I; KLEBS, *Handb. d. path. Anat.*; BOLLINGER, *Deutsche Zeitsch. f. Thiermed.* II, 1875; PROUJEANSKY, *Die multiloculäre Echinococcusgeschwulst* In. Diss. Zurich 1873; MORIN, *Deux cas de tumeurs à échinocoques* In. Diss. Berne 1875; HUBER, *Arch. f. klin. Med.* I, IV, V, XXIX. WALDSTEIN (*Virch. Arch.* vol. 83, with beautiful illustrations) brings forward evidence to show that the dissemination of the echinococcus may be effected through the lymphatics of the liver. He gives full reference to previous memoirs.

248. The occurrence of hydatids in man implies that the eggs of the corresponding canine tape-worm have somehow gained access to his body. The liver is the commonest seat, but hydatids are found in all organs. Apart from the local inflammation and fibrous hyperplasia they induce, they often cause no trouble to the patient. When a hydatid reaches a certain size, it sometimes dies and the cyst shrivels up. Its contents are changed to a fatty or cheesy mass, often becoming mortar-like as it calcifies. The hooks remain for a long time unchanged.

In other cases the hydatid becomes larger, especially when it forms exogenous or endogenous daughter-cysts. It may then become dangerous by its mere size. Sometimes if the cyst is wounded or bursts, its contents pass into one or other of the body-cavities and set up severe inflammation. It may even break into a blood-vessel. In the most favourable case it breaks into the intestine or upon the exterior of the body.

The *Echinococci* are widely diffused, but not very frequent: they are commonest in Iceland, where the inhabitants are in constant contact with their dogs. It is somewhat surprising that the multilocular variety is chiefly observed in Switzerland and Southern Germany.

NEISSER gives a summary of the various cases of hydatids that have been published (*Die Echinococcus-krankheit* Berlin 1877). See also PERLS, *Handb. d. allg. Path.* II.

249. *Bothriocephalus latus* is the largest of human tape-worms. It measures 5 to 8 metres in length, and consists of three to four thousand short wide segments (Fig. 115). The largest segment is about 3·5 mm. long and 10 to 12 mm. broad. Towards the 'tail' the breadth diminishes and the length increases. The body is thin and flattened like a ribbon. The central part of each segment projects somewhat; it is here that the uterus lies, in the form of a simple tube coiled into numerous convolutions. When this is full of eggs the coils lie in contiguous loops, forming a kind of rosette. The genital openings are in the mesial line of the ventral surface, somewhat anteriorly; the female opening being close behind the male.

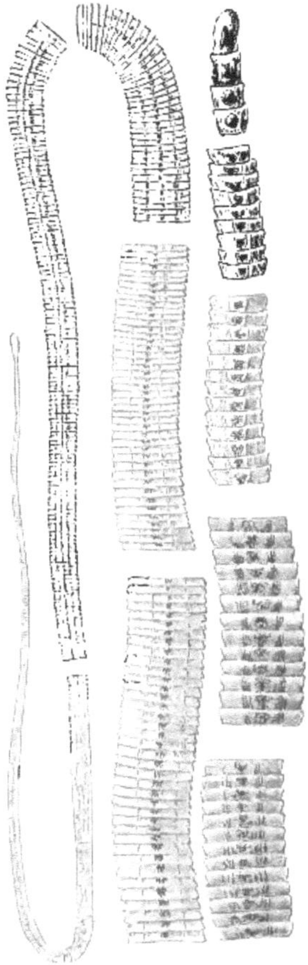

The testis consists of a series of sacculations lying along the lateral margins of the central layer of the body. The general structure of the body resembles that of the Taeniada.

Anteriorly the worm becomes gradually more and more slender and at length thread-like. The head, which is 2·5 mm. long and 1 mm. broad, is club-shaped or oval in outline, and somewhat flattened. Along each lateral margin is a chink-like suctorial groove.

FIG. 115. FRAGMENTS OF A *BOTHRIOCEPHALUS LATUS.* (*From LEUCKART: natural size*)

The eggs (Fig. 116) are oval; they measure 0·07 mm. by 0·045 mm. They have a thin brown shell furnished at the anterior pole with a lid or cap, which is in general easily seen.

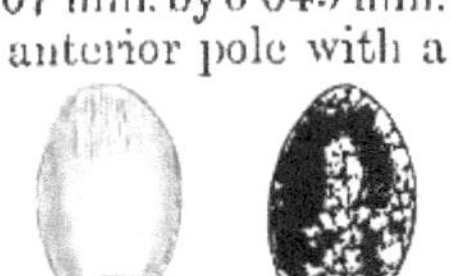

B. latus occurs chiefly in Switzerland and in the north-east of Europe: it is occasionally met with in Ireland. It lives like the Taeniada in the small intestine. The first development of the eggs takes place in water. After some months an embryo is hatched, which is provided with six booklets and a ciliated cuticle.

FIG. 116. EGGS OF BOTHRIOCEPHALUS LATUS. (*LEUCKART*) One is emptied of its contents and shows the lid.

This enters the body of the pike, the trout, or the eel-pout (*Lota vulgaris*) (BRAUN, *Virch. Arch.* vol. 88), and developes in the muscles or viscera into an asexual tape-worm. If it thence reach the alimentary canal of man, it proceeds to develope further and becomes sexually mature.

It has been maintained that *B. latus* represents the mature form of the cestoid of the trout, known as *Ligula nodosa.* See DUCHAMP, *Les Ligules* Paris 1876; KIESSLING, *Troschel's Arch.* 1882.

In Greenland another form, *B. cordatus,* occurs. It is only 1 metre long and has a heart-shaped head.

B. cristatus, 2 to 3 metres long, with a crest-like rostellum, has been found in France.

Protozoa.

250. **Protozoa** are not rarely found in the cavities of the body accessible from without, such as the mouth, lungs, intestine, vagina, etc.: they are most common in patients suffering from chronic disease. The forms observed belong to the *Rhizopoda, Infusoria,* and *Psorospermia* or *Sporozoa,* respectively.

Of parasitic *Amoebae* one species only has been described, the *Amoeba coli.* It occurs in the intestine, and is simply a motile cell with a granular protoplasm containing a nucleus and several vacuoles.

LÖSCH and SONSINO found the *Amoeba coli* in the dejections of a patient suffering from dysentery.

Among *Infusoria* the *Ciliata* and the *Flagellata* are represented. *Paramoecium* (or *Balantidium*) *coli* is a large ciliated organism occasionally met with in the large intestine and in the faeces. *Cercomonas intestinalis* (DAVAINE) is a pyriform infusorian, with a spine-like process at its smaller end and a *flagellum* at its larger end. It is found in the intestine in cases of catarrh, of typhoid, and of cholera. KANNENBERG discovered *Cercomonas* in the sputa from a patient affected with gangrene of the lungs. In the same sputa he also found *Monas lens,* a spherical flagellate infusorian. *Trichomonas* is another flagellate infusorian; it is oval in shape and provided with a comb-like row of cilia. One species (*T. vaginalis*) is found in the vagina, another (*T. intestinalis*) in the intestine.

These protozoa are not to be regarded as the exciting cause of the affections with which they are associated. They may possibly however maintain or intensify the morbid processes, when present in considerable numbers.

Of parasitic *Psorospermia* we have here to mention the *Coccidia.* According to LEUCKART, they are when young simple non-capsulated inhabitants of the epithelial cells. When they reach maturity they become invested with a kind of membranous capsule. In this condition they leave their first lodging, and generally their host at the same time. Their contents are then transformed into 'spores' containing granular masses and peculiar rod-like embryonic forms. The spores are round or ovoid. *Coccidium oviforme* (Fig. 117) is a parasite of the intestine and bile-ducts, especially those of the rabbit. In a few cases it has been found in the human subject. It leads in the liver of the rabbit to the formation of whitish nodules, which may be as large as a hazel-nut. The nodules consist of a puriform or cheesy mass, containing multitudes of coccidia. The granular contents of the coccidium are uniformly spread throughout its body, or rolled into a ball in the middle of it. The changes produced in the human liver by the presence of the parasite in the few cases observed have been similar to those met with in the rabbit.

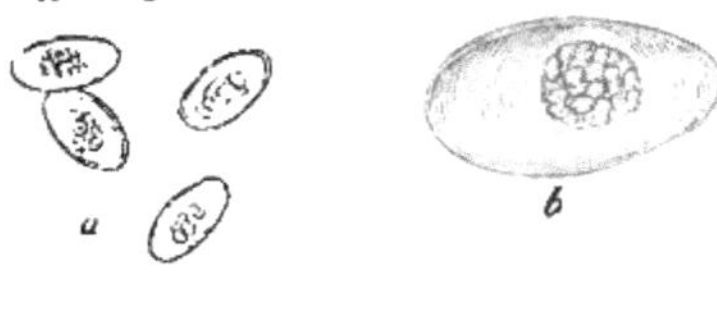

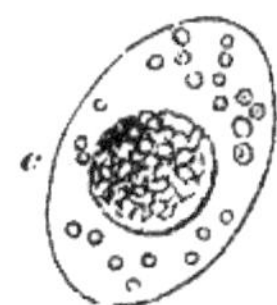

FIG. 117. *COCCIDIA* FROM THE HUMAN LIVER. (*From LEUCKART*)
a is magnified 300-fold,
b and *c* 1000-fold

Our knowledge of the organisms known as 'Miescher's cylinders' or 'Rainey's corpuscles' is still very defective. They are cylindrical or tube-like bodies found not infrequently in the muscles of the pig, ox, sheep, and mouse. They contain an innumerable multitude of small oval or reniform corpuscles. Nothing is known of their effect on the human system.

References to memoirs on *Coccidia* and *Psorospermia* generally :— LEUCKART, *Die Parasiten des Menschen*, 2nd Ed.; LIEBERKÜHN, *Arch. f. Anat. u. Phys.* 1854; EIMER, *Ueber die ei- oder kugelförmigen Psorospermien der Wirbelthiere* Würzburg 1870; KLEBS, *Virch. Arch.* vol. 32; STIEDA, *Ueb. die Psorospermien d. Kaninchenleber*, *Virch. Arch.* vol. 32; WALDENBURG, *ibidem* vol. 40; RIVOLTA, *Dei parasiti vegetali* Turin 1873.

According to our present information the parasitic protozoa take no important share in the production of human disease. It is however not impossible that further research may considerably alter our views in this regard. This is perhaps suggested by the fact that animal parasites are every now and then detected in the blood of vertebrate animals. Thus RÄTTIG (In. Diss. Berlin 1875) describes a ciliated infusorian in frog's blood. KLEBS (*Eulenburg's Realencyclop.* Art. *Flagellata*) has found in the blood of scurvy-patients very minute organisms, which he refers to the *Infusoria* and names *Cercomonas globulus* and *C. navicula.* LIEBERKÜHN (*Ueb. Bewegung. d. Zellen* Marburg 1870) found an amoeba (*A. rotatoria*) in frog's blood. LEWIS (*Quart. Journ. micros. Science* XIX, 1879) found in rat's blood, and WITTICH (*Centralb. f. med. Wiss.* 4, 1881) in hamster's blood, a mobile organism resembling the spermatozoon of the frog. KOCH (*Mitth. a. d. k. Gesundh.* Berlin 1881) describes a fusiform granular-looking structure with one or two flagella found in hamster's blood. He regards it as a flagellate infusorian.

INDEX OF AUTHORS CITED

(The numbers refer to the articles)

(*The numbers refer to the articles*)

(*The numbers refer to the articles*)

(*The numbers refer to the articles*)

(*The numbers refer to the articles*)

INDEX OF SUBJECTS

(The numbers refer to the articles)

(*The numbers refer to the articles*)

(*The numbers refer to the articles*)

(*The numbers refer to the articles*)

(The numbers refer to the articles)

(*The numbers refer to the articles*)

(*The numbers refer to the articles*)

(*The numbers refer to the articles*)

(*The numbers refer to the articles*)

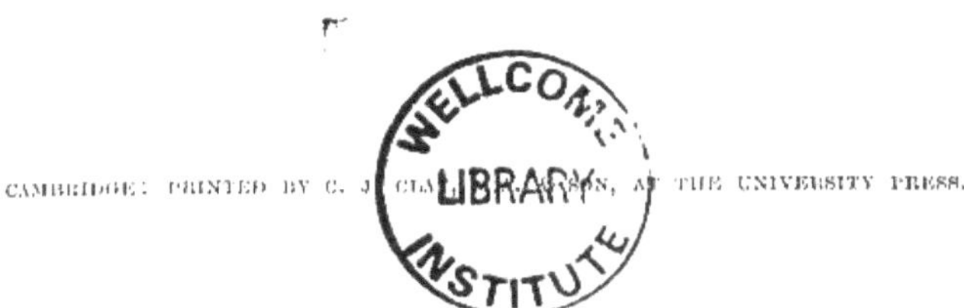

CAMBRIDGE: PRINTED BY C. J. CLAY, M.A. & SON, AT THE UNIVERSITY PRESS.

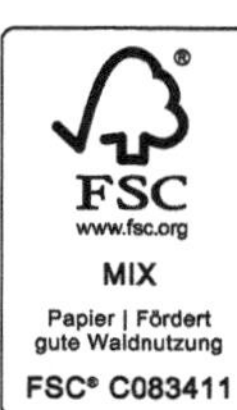

Zeitfracht Medien GmbH
Ferdinand-Jühlke-Straße 7
99095 Erfurt, Deutschland
produktsicherheit@kolibri360.de